Core Topics in Thoracic Surgery

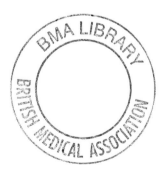

Core Topics in Thoracic Surgery

Edited by

Marco Scarci
Papworth Hospital, Cambridge, UK

Aman S. Coonar
Papworth Hospital, Cambridge, UK

Tom Routledge
Guy's Hospital, London, UK

Francis Wells
Papworth Hospital, Cambridge, UK

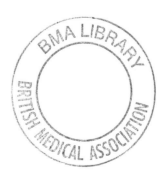

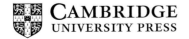

CAMBRIDGE
UNIVERSITY PRESS

University Printing House, Cambridge CB2 8BS, United Kingdom

Cambridge University Press is part of the University of Cambridge.

It furthers the University's mission by disseminating knowledge
in the pursuit of education, learning and research at the highest
international levels of excellence.

www.cambridge.org
Information on this title: www.cambridge.org/9781107036109

First published 2016

Printed in the United Kingdom by Clays, St Ives plc

A catalogue record for this publication is available from the British Library

Library of Congress Cataloging-in-Publication Data
Names: Scarci, Marco, editor. | Coonar, Aman, editor. | Routledge, Tom,
editor. | Wells, F. C., editor.
Title: Core topics in thoracic surgery / edited by Marco Scarci, Aman
Coonar, Tom Routledge, Francis Wells.
Description: Cambridge, United Kingdom ; New York : Cambridge
University Press, 2016. | Includes bibliographical references and index.
Identifiers: LCCN 2016011202 | ISBN 9781107036109 (Hardback)
Subjects: | MESH: Thoracic Surgical Procedures
Classification: LCC RD536 | NLM WF 980 | DDC 617.5/4–dc23 LC record
available at http://lccn.loc.gov/2016011202

ISBN 978-1-107-03610-9 Hardback

....

Contents

List of contributors   vii

Section I Diagnostic work-up of the thoracic surgery patient

1 **Lung function assessment**   1
John E. Pilling

2 **Endobronchial and endoscopic ultrasound for mediastinal staging**   11
Robert C. Rintoul and Nicholas R. Carroll

3 **Staging of lung cancer: mediastinoscopy and VATS**   17
Gaetano Rocco and Giuseppe De Luca

4 **Access to the chest cavity: safeguards and pitfalls**   25
Laura Socci and Antonio E. Martin-Ucar

Section II Upper airway

5 **Therapeutic bronchoscopy**   39
Keyvan Moghissi

6 **Tracheal stenosis, masses and tracheoesophageal fistula**   48
Timothy M. Millington and Douglas J. Mathisen

Section III Benign conditions of the lung

7 **Congenital and developmental lung malformations**   57
Naziha Khen-Dunlop, Guillaume Lezmi, Christophe Delacourt and Yann Revillon

8 **Lung volume reduction surgery for the treatment of advanced emphysema**   69
Nathaniel Marchetti and Gerard J. Criner

9 **Surgical aspects of infectious conditions of the lung**   86
Elaine Teh and Elizabeth Belcher

10 **Treatment of haemoptysis**   105
Odiri Eneje and Katharine Hurt

Section IV Malignant conditions of the lung

11 **Evaluation of solitary pulmonary nodule**   115
Dustin M. Walters and David R. Jones

12 **Lung cancer staging**   121
Bilal H. Kirmani and Aman S. Coonar

13 **Pathological considerations in lung malignancy**   127
Doris M. Rassl

14 **Medical treatment of lung cancer (neo and adjuvant chemoradiotherapy)**   140
Athanasios G. Pallis and Mary E. R. O'Brien

15 **Superior vena cava obstruction: etiology, clinical presentation and principles of treatment**   150
Federico Venuta, Marco Anile, Miriam Patella and Erino A. Rendina

16 **Robotics in thoracic surgery**   158
Marlies Keijzers, Peyman Sardari Nia and Jos G. Maessen

17 **Pulmonary metastasectomy**   167
Michel Gonzalez, Jean Yannis Perentes and Thorsten Krueger

Section V Diseases of the pleura

18 **Tube thoracostomy: evidence-based management of chest drains following pulmonary surgery**   179
Alessandro Brunelli

v

19 **Primary spontaneous pneumothorax** 188
Giuseppe Cardillo, Gerard Ngome Enang,
Francesco Carleo, Bernardo Ciamberlano,
Pasquale Ialongo, Aldo Morrone and
Massimo Martelli

20 **Bronchopleural fistula management** 193
Steven M. Woolley and Susannah M. Love

Section VI Diseases of the chest wall and diaphragm

21 **Surgery for pectus and other congenital chest wall disorders** 199
Jakub Kadlec, Jean-Marie Wihlm and
Aman S. Coonar

22 **Eventration, central bilateral diaphragmatic paralysis and congenital hernia in adults** 209
Françoise Le Pimpec-Barthes, Pierre Mordant,
Alex Arame, Alain Badia, Ciprian Pricopi,
Anne Hernigou and Marc Riquet

Section VII Disorders of the esophagus

23 **Benign esophageal disease** 221
Donn H. Spight and Mithran S. Sukumar

24 **Esophageal cancer** 234
Gail Darling

25 **Esophageal perforation** 240
Michael J. Shackcloth and George John

Section VIII Other topics

26 **Thoracic trauma** 253
Gregor J. Kocher and Ralph A. Schmid

27 **Thoracic sympathectomy in the treatment of hyperhidrosis** 267
John Agzarian and Yaron Shargall

Index 275

Contributors

John Agzarian MD MPH
Department of Surgery, McMaster University,
Hamilton, Ontario, Canada

Marco Anile MD
Università di Roma Sapienza, Policlinico Umberto I,
Fondazione Eleonora Lorillard Spencer Cenci,
Cattedra di Chirurgia Toracica, Rome, Italy

Alex Arame MD
Department of Thoracic Surgery, Georges
Pompidou European Hospital, Descartes University,
Paris, France

Alain Badia MD
Department of Thoracic Surgery, Georges
Pompidou European Hospital, Descartes University,
Paris, France

Elizabeth Belcher PhD MRCP FRCS(CTh)
Department of Thoracic Surgery, Oxford University
Hospitals NTS Trust, Oxford, UK

Alessandro Brunelli MD
Department of Thoracic Surgery, St. James's
University Hospital, Leeds, UK

Giuseppe Cardillo FRCS FETCS
Unit of Thoracic Surgery, Carlo Forlanini Hospital,
Azienda Ospedaliera San Camillo Forlanini,
Rome, Italy

Francesco Carleo MD
Unit of Thoracic Surgery, Carlo Forlanini Hospital,
Azienda Ospedaliera San Camillo Forlanini,
Rome, Italy

Nicholas R. Carroll MA FRCP FRCR
Department of Radiology, Addenbrooke's Hospital,
Cambridge, UK

Bernardo Ciamberlano MD
Unit of Thoracic Surgery, Carlo Forlanini Hospital,
Azienda Ospedaliera San Camillo Forlanini,
Rome, Italy

Aman S. Coonar MD MRCP FRCS
Division of Thoracic Surgery, Papworth Hospital,
Cambridge, UK

Gerard J. Criner MD FACP FACCP
Department of Thoracic Medicine & Surgery,
Temple University School of Medicine,
Philadelphia, PA, USA

Gail Darling MD FRCSC FACS
Division of Thoracic Surgery, University of
Toronto, Toronto General Hospital, Toronto,
Ontario, Canada

Christophe Delacourt MD PhD
Department of Paediatric Pulmonology,
Necker-Enfants Malades Hospital, Paris, France

Giuseppe De Luca MD
Division of Thoracic Surgery – Department of
Thoracic Surgery and Oncology, National Cancer
Institute, Pascale Foundation, Naples, Italy

Gerard Ngome Enang MD
Unit of Thoracic Surgery, Carlo Forlanini Hospital,
Azienda Ospedaliera San Camillo Forlanini,
Rome, Italy

Odiri Eneje MRCP
Department of Respiratory Medicine, Brighton &
Sussex University Hospitals NHS Trust, Brighton, UK

Michel Gonzalez MD
Division of Thoracic Surgery, Centre Hospitalier
Universitaire Vaudois, Lausanne, Switzerland

Anne Hernigou MD
Department of Radiology, Georges Pompidou
European Hospital, Descartes University, Paris,
France

Katharine Hurt MRCP
Department of Respiratory Medicine, Brighton &
Sussex University Hospitals NHS Trust, Brighton, UK

Pasquale Ialongo MD
Department of Radiology, Carlo Forlanini Hospital,
Azienda Ospedaliera San Camillo Forlanini,
Rome, Italy

George John MS FICS
Division of Thoracic Surgery, Hospital Kuala
Lumpur, Kuala Lumpur, Malaysia

David R. Jones MD
Division of Thoracic Surgery, Memorial Sloan
Kettering Cancer Center, New York, NY, USA

Jakub Kadlec FRCS(CTh)
Department of Surgery, University of Toronto,
St Joseph Hospital, Toronto, Ontario, Canada

Marlies Keijzers MD PhD
Department of Cardiothoracic Surgery,
Maastricht University Medical Center, Maastricht,
Netherlands

Naziha Khen-Dunlop MD
Department of Paediatric Surgery, Necker-Enfants
Malades Hospital, Paris, France

Bilal H. Kirmani BSc MBChB MRCS
Division of Thoracic Surgery, Papworth Hospital,
Cambridge, UK

Gregor J. Kocher MD
Division of General Thoracic Surgery, University
Hospital Berne, Berne, Switzerland

Thorsten Krueger MD
Division of Thoracic Surgery, Centre
Hospitalier Universitaire Vaudois, Lausanne,
Switzerland

Françoise Le Pimpec-Barthes MD
Department of Thoracic Surgery, Georges Pompidou
European Hospital, Descartes University, Paris,
France

Guillaume Lezmi MD
Department of Paediatric Pulmonology,
Necker-Enfants Malades Hospital, Paris, France

Susannah M. Love
Liverpool Heart and Chest Hospital, Liverpool, UK

Jos G. Maessen MD PhD
Department of Cardiothoracic Surgery,
Maastricht University Medical Center, Maastricht,
Netherlands

Nathaniel Marchetti DO
Department of Thoracic Medicine & Surgery,
Temple University School of Medicine, Philadelphia,
PA, USA

Massimo Martelli MD
Unit of Thoracic Surgery, Carlo Forlanini Hospital,
Azienda Ospedaliera San Camillo Forlanini,
Rome, Italy

Antonio E. Martin-Ucar MD FRCS(CTh)
Department of Thoracic Surgery, Nottingham City
Hospital, Nottingham, UK

Douglas J. Mathisen MD
Division of Thoracic Surgery, Massachusetts General
Hospital, Boston, MA, USA

Timothy M. Millington MD
Division of Thoracic Surgery, Dartmouth Geisel
School of Medicine, Lebanon, NH, USA

**Keyvan Moghissi BSc MD MS(Ch) FRCS FRCSEd
FETCS Membre (Etranger) Academie de
Chirurgie (Paris)**
The Yorkshire Laser Centre, Goole & District
Hospital, Goole, UK

Pierre Mordant MD PhD
Department of Thoracic Surgery, Georges Pompidou
European Hospital, Descartes University, Paris,
France

Aldo Morrone MD
Unit of Thoracic Surgery, Carlo Forlanini Hospital,
Azienda Ospedaliera San Camillo Forlanini,
Rome, Italy

Mary E. R. O'Brien MD FRCP
The Lung Unit, Royal Marsden Hospital, Sutton, UK

Athanasios G. Pallis MD MSc PhD
European Organization for Research and Treatment of Cancer Lung Cancer Group, Brussels, Belgium

Miriam Patella MD
Università di Roma Sapienza, Policlinico Umberto I, Fondazione Eleonora Lorillard Spencer Cenci, Cattedra di Chirurgia Toracica, Rome, Italy

Jean Yannis Perentes MD PhD
Division of Thoracic Surgery, Centre Hospitalier Universitaire Vaudois, Lausanne, Switzerland

John E. Pilling BMedSci FRCS(CTh)
Department of Thoracic Surgery, Guy's Hospital, London, UK

Ciprian Pricopi MD
Department of Thoracic Surgery, Georges Pompidou European Hospital, Descartes University, Paris, France

Doris M. Rassl FRCPath
Department of Pathology, Papworth Hospital, Cambridge, UK

Erino A. Rendina MD
Università di Roma Sapienza, Policlinico Umberto I, Fondazione Eleonora Lorillard Spencer Cenci, Cattedra di Chirurgia Toracica, Rome, Italy

Yann Revillon MD
Departments of Paediatric Surgery, Necker-Enfants Malades Hospital, Paris, France

Robert C. Rintoul PhD FRCP
Department of Thoracic Oncology, Papworth Hospital, Cambridge, UK

Marc Riquet MD
Department of Thoracic Surgery, Georges Pompidou European Hospital, Descartes University, Paris, France

Gaetano Rocco MD FRCSEd
Division of Thoracic Surgery – Department of Thoracic Surgery and Oncology, National Cancer Institute, Pascale Foundation, Naples, Italy

Peyman Sardari Nia MD PhD
Department of Cardiothoracic Surgery, Maastricht University Medical Center, Maastricht, Netherlands

Ralph A. Schmid MD
Division of General Thoracic Surgery, University Hospital Berne, Berne, Switzerland

Michael J. Shackcloth FRCS
Liverpool Heart and Chest Hospital, Liverpool, UK

Yaron Shargall MD BSc FRCSC FCCP
Department of Surgery, McMaster University; Division of Thoracic Surgery, St Joseph's Healthcare, Hamilton, Ontario, Canada

Laura Socci MD
Cardiothoracic Surgery Unit, Northern General Hospital, Sheffield, UK

Donn H. Spight MD
Department of Surgery, Oregon Health Sciences University, Portland, OR, USA

Mithran S. Sukumar MD
Division of General Thoracic Surgery, Oregon Health Sciences University, Portland, OR, USA

Elaine Teh MRCS MD
Department of Cardiothoracic Surgery, Plymouth Hospitals NHS Trust, Plymouth, UK

Federico Venuta MD
Università di Roma Sapienza, Policlinico Umberto I, Fondazione Eleonora Lorillard Spencer Cenci, Cattedra di Chirurgia Toracica, Rome, Italy

Dustin M. Walters MD
Division of Thoracic Surgery, University of Washington, Seattle, WA, USA

Jean-Marie Wihlm MD
Division of Thoracic Surgery, Cochin University Hospital, Paris, France

Steven M. Woolley FRCS(CTh) MD
Liverpool Heart and Chest Hospital, Liverpool, UK

Lung function assessment

John E. Pilling

History and examination

All patient assessment, including that of lung function, begins with a history and clinical examination.

Cough, sputum production, haemoptysis, wheeze and chest pain should be discussed. As well as a detailed history of breathlessness, chronicity, variability and severity are important. For a chest surgeon, an objective measure of breathlessness is useful, such as the Medical Research Council Dyspnoea Scale (Table 1.1) or exercise tolerance. While exercise tolerance can be limited by mechanical factors such as knee pain, if these are absent, the number of flights of stairs a patient can climb without stopping is useful as a comparable and reproducible value. It is also worth enquiring what stops the patient stair climbing: dyspnoea, angina, claudication or general fatigue.

Eliciting any history of cardiovascular disease is also vital as this may be the cause of breathlessness and is often the cause of post-operative complications in the thoracic surgical patient. Significant weight loss will result in muscle wasting, including the respiratory muscles.

It is imperative to discuss smoking history; a patient's number of pack-years allows an expression of both the quantity and duration of smoking. Many diseases that cause post-operative complications are caused by smoking. Pulmonary complications after thoracic surgery fall dramatically if the patient has abstained from smoking for 6 weeks prior to surgery. All smokers being considered for surgery should be made aware of the benefits of stopping, encouraged to do so and given every assistance, both psychological and pharmacological.

Examination of the patient begins with watching him or her walk from the waiting room into the consultation room. It should include looking for breathlessness on exertion, chest wall deformity and signs of respiratory disease. It may include observing the patient exercise or climb stairs.

Lung volumes

Upon maximal inspiration, the volume of gas contained in the lungs is the total lung capacity (TLC). Upon forcible exhalation, not all the air in the lungs

Table 1.1 Medical Research Council Dyspnoea Scale

Category 0	No dyspnoea
Category 1	Slight degree of dyspnoea (troubled by shortness of breath when hurrying on level or walking up a slight hill)
Category 2	Moderate degree of dyspnoea (walks slower than people of the same age on level because of breathlessness)
Category 3	Moderately severe degree of dyspnoea (has to stop because of breathlessness when walking at own pace on level)
Category 4	Severe degree of dyspnoea (stops for breath after walking 100m yards or after a few minutes on level)
Category 5	Very severe degree of dyspnoea (too breathless to leave the house or breathless dressing or undressing)

Core Topics in Thoracic Surgery, ed. Marco Scarci, Aman Coonar, Tom Routledge and Francis Wells. Published by Cambridge University Press. © Cambridge University Press 2016

can be exhaled; after expelling the forced vital capacity (FVC), the residual volume (RV) remains. During normal, quiet breathing, the volume inhaled and then exhaled is the tidal volume (TV), the volume left in the lungs at this point is the functional residual capacity (FRC), which is made up of the residual volume and expiratory reserve volume (ERV).

Investigations

Spirometry

Spirometry comprises a relatively simple set of tests. The results can be used for diagnosis, following the course of a disease, assessing response to treatment and, most commonly by thoracic surgeons, to predict risk of death, complications and breathlessness after pulmonary resection.

Rationale for spirometry

The thoracic surgical patient must tolerate trauma to his or her chest wall and possible pulmonary resection and is at high risk of developing pulmonary complications; the development of atelectasis is dependent on the closing volume (CV). CV is the volume of lung inflated when the small airways in the dependent parts of the lung begin to collapse during expiration. The dependent parts are affected as the intrapleural pressure is more negative at the apex and less negative at the base. In active expiration, the small airways at the base, which lack cartilaginous support, collapse prior to RV being reached. Usually, the CV is about 30% and FRC about 50% of TLC. As patients age and their lungs lose elasticity, the closing volume rises such that airway closure occurs at the end of tidal volume in the mid-40s while supine and in the mid-60s while erect. As well as increasing age, tobacco smoking, fluid overload, bronchospasm and airway secretions all increase the closing volume. A reduction in FRC or a rise in CV leads to closure of small airways during expiration, atelectasis and increased work of breathing. A thoracotomy reduces the FRC by 35%; hence thoracic surgical patients are at high risk of developing atelectasis, hypoxia and its sequelae, infection. An understanding of the patient's spirometry allows assessment of the likelihood of the development of complications and his or her ability to tolerate them.

Common measurements

The two values commonly measured are forced expiratory volume in 1 second (FEV1) and forced vital capacity (FVC). In the pre-operative thoracic surgical patient, these should be tested either standing or sitting upright after an inhaled beta agonist (if it is safe for the patient to do so). The spirometer should have been subjected to calibration, for example, syringe calibration for volume. The patient is asked to inspire to TLC and then exhale as hard as he or she can to RV. Flow rate at the mouth, volume exhaled and time are recorded. Two or three reproducible test manoeuvres should be obtained; graphical results should be superimposable and numerical results (FEV1, FVC) should be within 0.15 L of each other (0.1 L if FEV1 or FVC < 1 L). Exhalation to RV should be completed within 6 seconds.

Expiratory airflow can be expressed either by a volume over time curve or a flow-volume curve. The ratio of FEV1 over FVC can then be calculated. The flow-volume loop is generated by having the patient inhale deeply to TLC, forcefully exhale until the lungs are emptied to RV and rapidly inhale to TLC; flow is plotted on the y-axis and volume on the x-axis. Flow climbs rapidly to peak expiratory flow; once reached, the flow rate falls in an almost linear fashion, independent of patient effort, as any increased effort by the patient causes dynamic compression of small, unsupported airways (more so as lung volume falls), and so the flow cannot be increased by increased effort.

In patients with reduced FEV1 two patterns are recognized: reduced FEV1 with normal or increased FVC and a FEV1/FVC ratio less than 0.7, which is an obstruction, as in COPD (Figure 1.1). Where both the FEV1 and FVC are reduced, the ratio remains above 0.7, and the pattern is described as restrictive (Figure 1.2), as seen in pulmonary fibrosis or pleural thickening. In reality, many patients present with a mixed restrictive and obstructive picture, so they cannot simply be classified by their spirometric data. The flow-volume loop is also used to diagnose and assess fixed upper airway obstruction (Figure 1.3) as seen in post-intubation tracheal strictures, tracheal tumours and goitres.

When spirometry was being investigated as a predictor of morbidity and mortality post lung resection, the studies were performed on a population of patients undergoing surgery for lung cancer who were predominantly male[1]. It was said that a patient should be left with 800 ml of FEV1 after pulmonary resection. The normal values of FEV1 and FVC for men and women of different heights

(a)

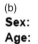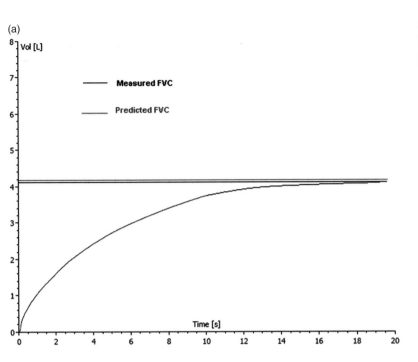

Figure 1.1 A Volume-time curve of a patient with obstructive lung disease: the FEV1 is reduced while the FVC is normal but takes longer than 6 seconds to reach.

(b)

Sex:	**male**	**Height:**	**166 cm**
Age:	**50 years**	**Diagnosis:**	**Emphysema**

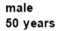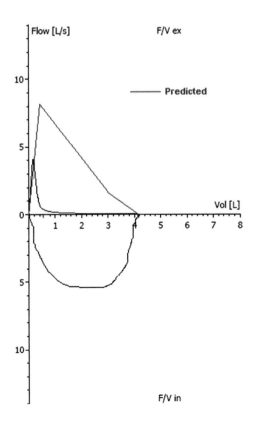

Figure 1.1 B Flow-volume loop of a patient with obstructive lung disease: the peak flow rate is reduced and the flow rate is very low in relation to lung volume, giving the curve a concave appearance.

(a)

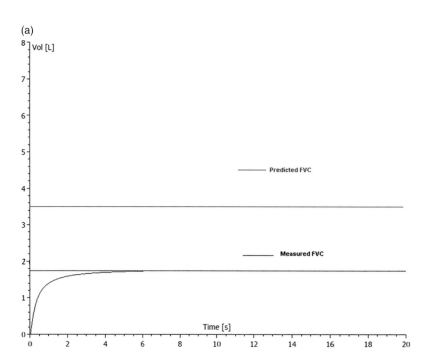

Figure 1.2 A Volume-time curve of a patient with restrictive lung disease: the FEV1 and FVC are reduced; the duration of expiration is normal.

and ages are known, so FEV1 and FVC can be expressed as a percentage of the normal value for that patient. By using percentage predicted values rather than absolute values of volume, discrimination against female and small patients is avoided. A 5-foot-tall, 80-year-old woman with an FEV1 of 1.5 L has normal lung function (96% predicted); a 6-foot-tall, 40-year-old man with the same FEV1 has severe COPD (39% predicted).

Transfer factor

Gas exchange between the capillaries and alveoli occurs by simple diffusion from high to low partial pressure across the capillary membrane. This is governed by Fick's law, which states the volume of gas diffusing across a membrane per unit time is proportional to the area of the membrane; the diffusion constant (also known as permeability coefficient) of the gas and the difference in partial pressure of the gas either side of the membrane are inversely proportional to the thickness of the membrane.

To measure the transfer factor across the alveolar capillary membrane, a gas is needed which does not build up on the capillary side and so is only limited by diffusion – carbon monoxide (CO) binds avidly to haemoglobin, and hence there is little rise in its partial pressure in the capillary.

The transfer factor is the volume of gas transferred per minute from alveoli to capillary divided by the difference of the partial pressures of gas in the alveoli and the capillary. It is dependent on the area, thickness and diffusion properties of the blood gas barrier and is measured using a single-breath-holding technique. The patient takes one breath of dilute CO, which is held for 10 seconds and then exhaled, allowing the rate of disappearance and alveolar partial pressure to be measured; the capillary partial pressure is assumed to be zero.

The transfer factor is given in ml/min/mmHg and is the value for the whole ventilated lung volume. Thoracic surgeons rarely use the absolute value but more commonly use the percentage of predicted for the patient's gender, age, height and weight. The kCO is the transfer factor per unit lung volume and is most commonly used by physicians following patients with interstitial lung disease and its treatment.

Lung volumes

Lung volumes can be measured in two ways: gas dilution and body plethysmography.

Gas dilution

The patient is connected to a spirometer of known volume containing a known concentration of helium,

(b)

Sex: male   **Height:** 169 cm
Age: 74 years   **Diagnosis:** Pleural disease

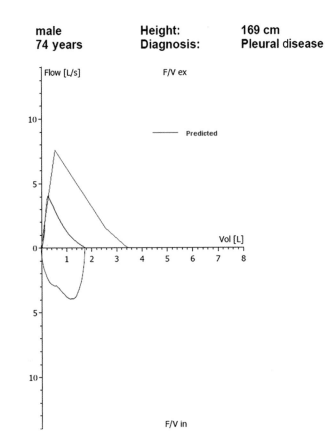

Figure 1.2 B Flow-volume loop of a patient with restrictive lung disease: the peak flow rate and total volume exhaled are reduced.

(a)

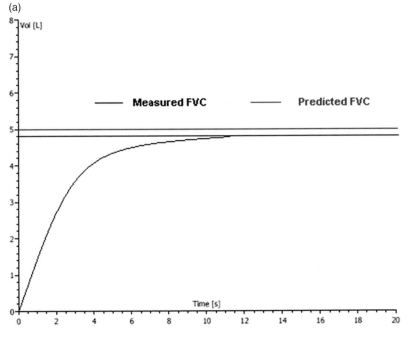

Figure 1.3 A Volume-time curve of a patient with a fixed upper airway obstruction: consider this diagnosis if the peak flow is close to the FEV1.

5

(b)

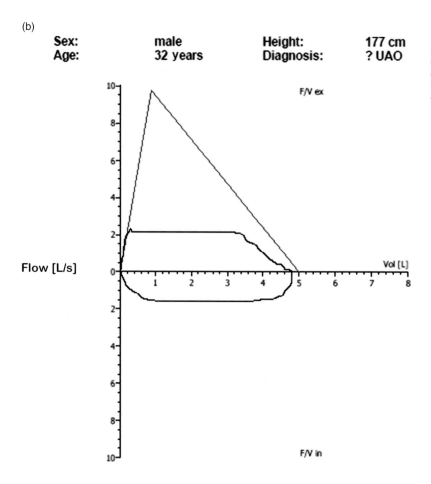

| Sex: | male | Height: | 177 cm |
| Age: | 32 years | Diagnosis: | ? UAO |

Flow [L/s]

Figure 1.3 B Flow-volume loop of patient with a fixed upper airway obstruction: the lack of change of calibre of the obstruction in both inhalation and exhalation causes similar flattening of both inspiratory and expiratory portions of the loop.

chosen because it is insoluble in the blood. After a number of breaths, the concentrations in the spirometer and the patient's lungs equalize and can be measured. The product of the initial concentration and volume of the spirometer is equal to the product of the new concentration and the sum of the volumes of the spirometer and the patient's lungs. This only measures the volume of ventilated parts of the lung.

Body plethysmography

Also known as the body box, the body plethysmograph is a large airtight box in which the patient sits with his or her mouth connected to a tube which exits the box. At the end of normal expiration, a shutter closes on the mouthpiece and the patient inhales, expanding the gas in his or her lungs and changing the volume and pressure in the box. Boyle's law (pressure multiplied by volume is constant, at constant temperature) is applied to both the patient's lungs and the box. The volume in the box is known; the

pressures in the box before and after inspiratory effort are measured, so applying Boyle's law to the box allows the change in volume with inspiratory effort to be calculated. The mouthpiece pressure before and after inspiration is measured so Boyle's law can be applied to the patient's lungs. The initial pressure multiplied by the lung volume is equal to the new pressure multiplied by the sum of the change in volume in the box and the lung volume; the change in volume in the box has been calculated by applying Boyle's law to the box. This method of calculating lung volume includes non-ventilated segments of lung.

Predicted post-operative (ppo) lung function

Chest surgeons are interested in their patient's lung function after resection, which is dependent on the extent of resection and the pre-operative function.

Ppo lung function can be estimated in two ways: segment counting and quantative VQ scan.

Segment counting

Segment counting is the simplest method of determining post-operative lung function once the extent of pulmonary resection required has been determined. The pre-operative FEV1 or transfer factor is multiplied by the number of remaining ventilated segments after surgery divided by the number of ventilated segments prior to surgery. Atelectatic segments on CT or obstructed segments at bronchoscopy are excluded as they did not contribute to the pre-operative lung function and if not resected will not contribute to the post-operative lung function.

Quantitative VQ scan

Quantitative VQ scan is especially useful in patients who may undergo pneumonectomy. It can be more accurate than segment counting or estimating using a 55% right, 45% left lung split; central tumours or tumours with hilar nodal disease (for which pneumonectomy may be required) often cause pressure on the pulmonary artery (a high-flow but low-pressure system) to the lung and significantly reduce the proportion of the flow to the affected lung. Following quantative VQ scan, the pre-operative FEV1 and transfer factor are multiplied by the proportion of perfusion to unaffected lung to give ppo values.

Upper, middle and lower zone perfusion can be calculated for patients undergoing lobectomy, but this is unhelpful as the fissures are oblique; oblique views can be used to illustrate the perfusion and ventilation to various lobes but not for calculating lobe-specific perfusion values or ppo values.

PpoFEV1 predicting operative risk

A number of small case series have shown a ppoFEV1 of less than 40% to place patients at a substantial risk of post-operative death and complications compared with those whose ppoFEV1 was greater than 40%. The relationship of low ppoFEV1 to increased pulmonary complications was confirmed in a large series of 331 patients by Kearney et al. (1994)[2]. There have been studies showing that patients with ppoFEV1 < 40% can successfully undergo anatomical pulmonary resection without excess risk, and so ppoFEV1 alone cannot be used to deny patients access to curative surgery.

Ppo transfer factor predicting post-operative risk

Initially shown by Ferguson et al. (1988), a ppo transfer factor of less than 40% is a strong predictor of post-operative mortality[3]. Transfer factor is often low in patients with a low FEV1 but is not always preserved in patients with normal spirometry. Brunelli et al. (2006) showed that a ppo transfer factor < 40% in patients with normal spirometry was a reliable predictor of post-operative complications[4]. Hence transfer factor should be measured as routine when assessing candidates for lung resection, not just in those with a poor FEV1.

Confounding factors

The ppo value of FEV1 overestimates the patient's lung function in the initial recovery after surgery as this value is affected by chest wall trauma and pain. It also underestimates the value in the long term, especially after lobectomy where the remodelling of the chest and expansion of the remaining lung mean values higher than the predicted values by a year. Ppo values seem to be most accurate between 3 and 6 months after pulmonary resection.

Another confounding variable in considering ppo lung function is the possibility of having a 'lung volume reduction effect' as a side effect of lobar resection for lung cancer. Most patients with lung cancer have an element of pulmonary emphysema, and if a carcinoma contained in a severely emphysematous upper lobe is resected, the same beneficial effect of reducing intra-thoracic hyper-expansion and removing non-functioning lung tissue may be seen, as is seen with a pure lung volume reduction operation. This allows patients with severely reduced pre-operative lung function to be considered for surgery and makes ppo values of FEV1 and TLCO (transfer factor for the lung for carbon monoxide) inaccurate. There is growing evidence that this effect is evident early after surgery, having been shown on the first post-operative day and at discharge.

Exercise testing

Exercise testing is theoretically attractive to the thoracic surgeon wishing to effectively counsel his patients about their ability to withstand post-operative complications, which are commonly respiratory and cardiovascular in nature. Testing the patient's physiological ability to deliver oxygen to respiring tissues, utilize it and expel carbon dioxide seems to closely mimic the post-operative situation. There are a number of tests involving exercise of varying complexity.

Simple

Stair climbing

While this test is not sophisticated, if performed by the surgeon, it allows for assessment of the patient's motivation and 'fighting spirit', which are difficult to quantify but play a significant role in coping with recovery after pulmonary resection. Patients are stood at the bottom of a set of stairs and their saturation and pulse are measured. They are then asked to climb the stairs at the pace of the surgeon, using the hand-rail only for balance and aiming to climb two floors. If they manage to climb two floors without stopping, having angina or desaturating by more than 4%, then they are fit for thoracic surgery. Investigators have tried to standardize this simple test by reporting altitude climbed in metres; it seems that those climbing less than 12 m have a 50% risk of complications[5].

Intermediate

Shuttle Walk Test (SWT)

The patient walks between two cones placed 9 m apart in time to a set of beeps played on a CD. With turning distance, one shuttle is 10 m. The walking speed required to keep up with the beeps increases incrementally. The number of completed shuttles is recorded, and the test ends when patients are too breathless to continue or they are more than 0.5 m from the cone at a beep for two shuttles. Completing 25 shuttles (250 m) is considered to imply average risk for pulmonary resection, as by regression this is thought to imply a VO2max of 10 ml/kg/min. This has not been consistently shown in practice, and while passing an SWT is a good sign that a patient has an acceptable risk for pulmonary resection alone, it should not be used to exclude patients.

Six-minute walk test (SMWT)

Over a flat track of at least 25 m in length, patients are asked to walk as far and as fast as they can in the 6 minutes. The result is the distance covered. Encouragement is given, and if patients have to stop, for a non-sinister reason, then they are asked to continue when able. As there is an element of learning in performing the test, it should be done twice and the best result used. The predictive normal values for SMWT are based on sex, age, height and weight. It has not been evaluated fully enough to use in pre-operative evaluation for pulmonary resection for lung cancer.

Complex

The cardio-pulmonary exercise test (CPET) allows measurement of the maximal oxygen uptake (VO2max). It requires a means of exercising the patient – usually a cycle-ergometer (a cycle on which the work rate of the patient can be determined and varied by the examiner), continuous electrocardiogram and oxygen saturation measurement, the ability to continuously measure exhaled carbon dioxide and oxygen, and non-invasive blood pressure testing. The patient's expected maximal heart rate is determined, and then he or she is incrementally exercised until this is reached, the patient gives up or a medical complication intervenes. The maximum oxygen uptake during the test is reported in ml/kg/min; it can also be given as a percentage predicted.

This test is complex and demands a lot of time, expensive equipment and highly trained technical staff. It also requires a patient who can pedal a stationary cycle or walk on a treadmill. It is an indirect test of the patient's motivation. Most pre-operative assessment algorithms submit patients whose ppo spirometry is borderline to this test. Unfortunately, these patients are likely to have a borderline result on this test also. A result of > 15 ml/kg/min (or 60% predicted) means the patient's risk of death and complications after surgery is average; those whose VO2max is < 10ml/kg/min (or 40% predicted) have a prohibitively high risk. The difficulty lies in dealing with a result between 10 and 15 ml/kg/min, which is where the majority of patients with borderline spirometry will fall.

Using lung function tests in pre-operative assessment

A number of learned societies have published guidance for surgeons on selection of patients for surgical treatment of lung cancer (see Box). While these can only be used as guidance and the surgeon must discuss the individual risks and benefits of a proposed procedure with the patient, these documents are helpful in informing our approach.

In patients with borderline ppo lung function tests, the surgeon is more likely to recommend surgery to a patient in whom he feels that surgery stands a good chance of curing the disease.

Guidelines for assessing fitness for radical surgery for lung cancer

European Respiratory Society (ERS), European Society of Thoracic Surgery (ESTS):
Brunelli A, Charloux A, Bolliger CT. ERS/ESTS clinical guidelines on fitness for radical therapy in lung cancer patients (surgery and chemoradiotherapy) *Eur Respir J* 2009; 34:17–41.

British Thoracic Society (BTS) and the Society for Cardiothoracic Surgery (SCTS) in Great Britain and Ireland:
Lim E, Baldwin D, Beckles M, et al. Guidelines on the radical management of patients with lung cancer. *Thorax* 2010; 65 (Suppl. 3).

American College of Chest Physicians (ACCP):
Brunelli A, Kim, AW, Berger DJ, et al. Physiologic evaluation of the patient with lung cancer being considered for resectional surgery: Diagnosis and Management of Lung Cancer, 3rd edition: American College of Chest Physicians evidence-based clinical practice guidelines. *Chest* 2013; 143 (Suppl. 5):e166S–e190S.

ACCP

FEV1 and TLCO should be measured in all patients and the ppo values calculated; if both are > 60%, no further testing is recommended. If either is < 60% but > 30%, then a simple exercise test such as stair climbing or SWT is suggested. If either the ppo FEV1 or ppo TLCO is less than 30%, then a CPET should be performed. If patients fail an SWT (25 shuttles) or stair climbing test (<22 m), they should then undergo a CPET. If patients' VO2max is < 10 ml/kg/min or < 35% predicted, then they should be counselled to undergo limited resection or non-operative oncological treatment.

ERS/ESTS

FEV1 and TLCO should be measured in all lung resection candidates. If both are > 80%, no further

testing is required. If either is < 80%, then exercise testing is recommended (either CPET or stair climbing as available). If the VO2max is > 20 ml/kg/min or > 75% predicted, no further testing is required. If VO2max is < 35% predicted or < 10 ml/kg/min, then patients should undergo limited resection or non-operative treatment. If patients perform between 35 and 75% predicted or between 10 and 20 ml/kg/min on CPET, then the ppoFEV1 and ppoTLCO are calculated: if both are > 30%, then the patient can undergo the proposed resection; if one is < 30%, then the ppoVO2max is calculated; if this is > 35% or > 10 ml/kg/min, then the patient can undergo the proposed resection if not lesser resection or non-operative treatment is recommended.

BTS/SCTS

Advocate a tripartite assessment of the patient's risk of operative mortality, a post-operative cardiac event and post-operative dyspnoea. The first two are achieved using an operative risk scoring system such as Thoracoscore[6] and the American College of Cardiologists, American Heart Association Guidelines[7]. Assessment of dyspnoea risk is achieved using ppoFEV1 and ppoTLCO by segment counting or VQ scan. Those where both are > 40% have a low risk; if one or both are < 40%, exercise testing should be considered. An SWT > 400 m or a VO2max > 15 ml/kg/min is considered adequate. Once a patient's risk is determined, the surgeon is then advised to discuss those risks with the patient and determine the best course of action for that specific patient.

Conclusion

The thoracic surgeon having a good understanding of respiratory physiology and the available tests for its assessment can advise patients of the short- and long-term risks of surgery. An understanding of the pathology and natural history of the disease being treated is also vital to help the patient to make an informed decision. Thoracic surgical patients are complex, and as such, while lung function tests give a surgeon a quantitative data, their application is a matter of clinical judgement.

Acknowledgement: Mr Pilling wishes to acknowledge the assistance of Mark Unstead, Chief Respiratory Physiologist, Royal Berkshire Hospital, with the figures in this chapter.

References

1　Bousy SF, Billig DM, North LB, et al. Clinical course related to preoperative and postoperative pulmonary function in patients with bronchogenic carcinoma. *Chest* 1971; 59:383–91.

2　Kearney DJ, Lee TH, Reilly DJ, et al. Assessment of operative risk in patients undergoing lung resection. Importance of predicted pulmonary function. *Chest* 1994; 105:753–9.

3　Ferguson MK, Little L, Rizzo L, et al. Diffusing capacity predicts morbidity and mortality after pulmonary resection. *J Thorac Cardiovasc Surg* 1988; 96:894–900.

4　Brunelli A, Refai MA, Salati M, et al. Carbon monoxide lung diffusion capacity improves risk stratification in patients without airflow limitation: evidence from systematic measurement before lung resection. *Eur J Cardiothorac Surg* 2006; 29:567–70.

5　Brunelli A, Refai M, Monteverde M, et al. Stair climbing tests predict cardiopulmonary complications after lung resection. *Chest* 2002; 121:1106–10.

6　Falcoz PE, Conti M, Brouchet L, et al. The thoracic surgery scoring system (Thoracoscore): risk model for in-hospital death in 15,183 patients requiring thoracic surgery. *J Thorac Cardiovasc Surg* 2007; 133:325–32.

7　Fleisher LA, Beckman JA, Brown KA, et al. ACC/AHA 2007 guidelines on perioperative cardiovascular evaluation and care for non cardiac surgery: a report of the American College of Cardiology/American Heart Association task force on practice guidelines. *J Am Coll Cardiol* 2007; 50:e159–242.

Endobronchial and endoscopic ultrasound for mediastinal staging

Robert C. Rintoul and Nicholas R. Carroll

Endobronchial ultrasound

Endobronchial ultrasound (EBUS) is a broncho-scopic technique that uses ultrasound to visualize structures within and adjacent to the airway wall. There are two forms of endobronchial ultrasound – radial probe and linear (or convex) probe. This chapter will largely focus on the applications of linear probe EBUS.

Radial probe EBUS

Radial probe EBUS provides a 360° image of the airway wall and adjacent structures. It can be used to (a) examine the airway wall layers, (b) localize parenchymal lung nodules or (c) identify the position of parabronchial and paratracheal lymph nodes prior to sequential (non-ultrasound-guided) transbronchial needle aspiration[1]. The latter application has been largely superseded by the development of linear EBUS. Nowadays, radial EBUS is predominantly used to localize a peripheral parenchymal lung lesion to allow placement of a guide sheath through which biopsies can be taken[2]. While radial EBUS helps with the localization of a peripheral lesion, the problem of navigating to a peripheral bronchus remains, and therefore, in recent years considerable effort has been directed at the development of navigation systems to aid guide sheath placement[3]. As navigation systems improve, it is likely that the use of radial EBUS will spread, but for the time being, it is limited to a relatively small number of specialist centres.

Linear Probe EBUS

Linear probe EBUS was first described in 2003 using a convex probe bronchoscope developed by Olympus Medical Systems, Japan[4]. Several models are now available, all of which comprise an electronic curved linear array ultrasound transducer mounted at the distal end of a flexible bronchoscope (Figure 2.1). To provide an ultrasound image, the transducer has to be brought into contact with the airway wall – an inflatable balloon can be placed over the transducer to improve contact. Side-by-side conventional endobronchial and ultra-sound imaging allow lymph node station identification. Ultrasound imaging is undertaken at a frequency of 5–10 MHz, which allows tissue penetration of 10–50 mm. Using EBUS, it is possible to identify and perform transbronchial needle aspiration (TBNA) from medias-tinal lymph node stations 2R, 2L, 3P, 4R, 4L and 7 and hilar and interlobar nodes in stations 10R, 10L, 11R and 11L. With experience, lymph nodes as small as 4 mm in short axis can be sampled using dedicated 21G, 22G or 25G needles (Figure 2.2).

Although EBUS can be performed under general anaesthesia, in most centres it is performed under moderate sedation using a combination of an intravenous

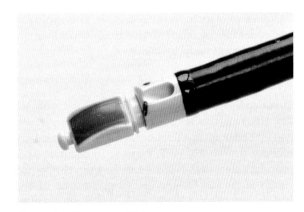

Figure 2.1 Linear probe EBUS.

Core Topics in Thoracic Surgery, ed. Marco Scarci, Aman Coonar, Tom Routledge and Francis Wells. Published by Cambridge University Press. © Cambridge University Press 2016

(a)

(b)

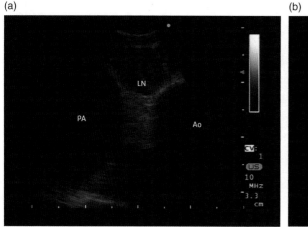
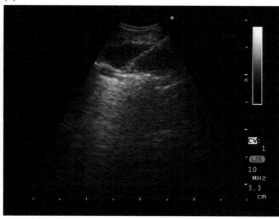

Figure 2.2 Ultrasound imaging using linear probe EBUS.

benzodiazepine and an opiate. Local anaesthetic is applied to the oropharynx using spray, and a cricothyroid injection is often valuable to anaesthetize the trachea.

During the procedure, all lymph node stations should be identified and evaluated in a systematic fashion before beginning to take any biopsies. The technique for identification of each lymph node station has been described previously[5]. On most ultrasound systems, Doppler is available which can help differentiate vascular from non-vascular structures. When staging the mediastinum, it is important to consider which nodes are to be biopsied and in which order. Lymph nodes classified as N3 should be biopsied initially, followed by N2 nodes, then N1 nodes and finally the primary tumour if accessible. This approach minimizes the risk of any sample cross-contamination and inadvertent nodal upstaging.

Endoscopic ultrasound

Linear endoscopic ultrasound (EUS) has been available since 2003 and uses an esophageal approach to evaluate lymph nodes in the inferior and posterior mediastinum – stations 2L, 4L, 7, 8 and 9. In addition, EUS provides access to the left lobe of the liver, the coeliac lymph nodes and the left adrenal gland. Like EBUS, EUS is normally performed under moderate sedation and local anaesthesia. In combination, EBUS and EUS can be used to access all the mediastinal and hilar/interlobar stations bar lymph nodes in the true aorto-pulmonary window (station 5) and pre-vascular nodes (station 6) and anterior mediastinum (station 3A).

Both procedures can be performed under sedation with local anaesthesia, and an experienced team can perform the investigations in about 50 minutes.

Diagnosis and staging of lung cancer

The initial reports concerning the efficacy of EBUS-TBNA were published as small case series between 2003 and 2006[4,6-8]. These were followed by several larger non-randomized, prospective case series drawn together in a meta-analysis in 2009, which showed that the pooled sensitivity of EBUS-TBNA was 0.93 (95% CI 0.91–0.94)[9]. A more recent meta-analysis by Dong et al. (2013) incorporating 1066 patients, all of whom had surgical confirmation of results, showed that the pooled sensitivity was 0.90 (95% CI 0.84-0.96) and pooled accuracy 0.96[10].

In 2011, Yasufuku et al.[11] reported the first prospective, controlled trial comparing EBUS-TBNA (under general anaesthesia) with mediastinoscopy for mediastinal lymph node staging. The sensitivity, negative predictive value and diagnostic accuracy for EBUS-TBNA were 81, 91 and 93%, respectively, and for mediastinoscopy 79, 90 and 93%. No significant differences were found between EBUS-TBNA and mediastinoscopy in determining N stage. Um et al. (2015)[12] undertook a prospective study in which 138 patients underwent sequential EBUS-TBNA (under sedation and local anaesthesia) and cervical mediastinoscopy with the aim of assessing the efficacy of both approaches for mediastinal staging. In those where no mediastinal nodal disease was identified by either modality, surgical resection and lymph node dissection were undertaken. In total, 138 patients underwent EBUS-TBNA and 127 had both EBUS and mediastinoscopy. The prevalence of N2/N3 disease was 59%. The diagnostic sensitivity, negative predictive value and accuracy of mediastinoscopy were 81, 79, and 89%, respectively. For EBUS-TBNA the equivalent values were 88, 85 and 93%, all of which were significantly higher than for mediastinoscopy.

Combined endobronchial and endoscopic ultrasound

Following early reports showing that EBUS had high sensitivity and accuracy for staging the mediastinum, some groups explored whether combined EBUS and EUS could provide even better results. The rationale for this approach is that while EBUS provides excellent coverage of the anterior/superior mediastinum, EUS offers better access to the posterior/inferior mediastinal nodal stations. With the exception of station 5 (which can sometimes be accessed by EUS), station 6, and anterior mediastinum 3A, the entire mediastinum can be covered using a combined approach.

The first study to compare EBUS/EUS with surgical staging was undertaken by Annema et al. (2010) [13]. They performed a randomized, controlled trial in which patients requiring mediastinal staging were randomized to either EBUS/EUS (under sedation and local anaesthesia) or surgical staging. In the EBUS/EUS arm, those with no evidence of malignancy were referred for surgical staging, usually mediastinoscopy prior to thoracotomy. In the endoscopic arm, the sensitivity for detection of malignancy was 85%, which was not significantly different to 79% in the surgical arm. However, if mediastinoscopy was performed following a 'negative for malignancy' EBUS/EUS, the sensitivity for detection of malignancy rose to 94%. However, this 9% increase in sensitivity translates into the need for 11 mediastinoscopies in order to identify one patient with mediastinal nodal disease.

Liberman et al. (2014)[14] have also compared combined EBUS/EUS with surgical staging, albeit using a different approach. They prospectively enrolled 166 patients with confirmed or suspected NSCLC who required mediastinal staging into a study whereby each patient underwent EBUS, EUS and surgical mediastinal staging during a single procedure. Each patient served as his or her own control. Results from EBUS, EUS and combined EBUS/EUS were compared with surgical staging, and those with no evidence of nodal malignancy went on to resection with lymph node sampling. Overall the prevalence of mediastinal nodal disease was 32%. The sensitivity, negative predictive value and diagnostic accuracy of EBUS were 72% (95% CI, 0.58–0.83), 88% (0.81–0.93) and 91% (0.85–0.95), respectively. For EUS the equivalent results were 62% (0.48–0.75), 85% (0.78–0.91) and 88% (0.82–0.92). Combined EBUS/EUS gave 91% (0.79–0.97), 96% (0.90–0.99) and 97% (0.93–0.99), respectively. The authors estimated that combined EBUS/EUS prevented 14% of patients from undergoing inappropriate thoracotomy.

Who should have combined EBUS and EUS?

The selection of patients for combined EBUS and EUS depends upon the clinical scenario. In cases where pre-biopsy imaging studies (CT and/or PET-CT) have shown extensive disease, it may only be necessary to biopsy one or two lymph nodes in order to obtain a histological diagnosis and confirm mediastinal involvement. In these cases we tend to select either EBUS or EUS depending on the position of the target node and the procedure which we feel is most likely to provide the answer. However, if pre-biopsy imaging in conjunction with the clinical scenario suggests that treatment with potential curative intent is possible (surgical resection, radical radiotherapy or chemoradiotherapy), we undertake full systematic mediastinal assessment using combined endobronchial and endoscopic ultrasound aiming to cover all N3, N2 and N1 lymph node stations (barring inaccessible station 5, 6 and 3A nodes). Until recently, most centres have performed EUS and EBUS using separate EUS and EBUS scopes. However, Hwangbo et al. (2010)[15] reported a prospective series of 150 patients with potentially operable (suspected) NSCLC upon whom they performed EBUS initially followed by EUS using the EBUS bronchoscope (termed EUS-B). They found that the sensitivity, negative predictive value and diagnostic accuracy of EBUS-TBNA for the detection of mediastinal metastasis were 84, 93 and 95%, respectively. Performing EUS with an EBUS bronchoscope to assess nodal stations inaccessible by EBUS increased these outcomes to 91, 96 and 97%, respectively. Overall these results are very similar to those obtained using separate EBUS and EUS scopes.

Re-staging of the mediastinum following neo-adjuvant chemotherapy

With the advent of treatment regimens using neo-adjuvant chemotherapy, the need for mediastinal re-staging following chemotherapy is increasing. Re-staging the mediastinum is challenging and traditionally has been undertaken using mediastinoscopy. However, re-mediastinoscopy is technically more difficult to perform on account of adhesions and fibrotic change induced by the initial procedure and induction treatment, and case series reporting sensitivity for detection of residual disease have given widely disparate results[16-18]. Usually the gold standard that is applied in these cases is analysis of mediastinal nodes at thoracotomy, although this can only address the ipsilateral side.

To date, there have only been a few endosonography studies which have addressed this issue. Herth et al. (2008)[19] undertook a retrospective review of 124 patients with tissue-proven Stage IIIA N2 disease who had been treated with induction chemotherapy and who had undergone re-staging using EBUS-TBNA. Surgical verification was performed in all cases. The prevalence of persistent mediastinal disease was 94%. Sensitivity for EBUS-TBNA detection of residual malignancy was 76%. However, the negative predictive value was low at 20%.

Szlubowski et al. (2014)[20] used transcervical extended mediastinal lymphadenectomy (TEMLA) to clarify mediastinal nodal status in a prospective series of 106 patients undergoing combined endobronchial and endoscopic ultrasound for induction therapy for non-small cell lung cancer. The prevalence of persistent mediastinal nodal disease was 52%. Overall, diagnostic sensitivity of endosonography for mediastinal metastases was 67% (95% CI 53–79), specificity 96% (95% CI 86–99) and overall accuracy 81% (95% CI 73–87). The negative predictive value was 73% (95% CI 61–83).

Taken together, these studies suggest that whenever possible, initial staging should be performed using endobronchial and/or endoscopic ultrasound. Initial re-staging should also be performed using endobronchial and/or endoscopic ultrasound. However, given the low negative predictive value of EBUS/EUS, when there are negative findings, there should

be consideration of surgical staging (mediastinoscopy) prior to thoracotomy.

Role of linear EBUS in the diagnosis of isolated mediastinal lymphadenopathy

Isolated mediastinal lymphadenopathy is a common clinical problem for which EBUS is often used as a first-line investigation. Although EBUS can often provide a diagnosis, there are some situations where a surgical biopsy may be required for clarification, and careful consideration as to the probability of the final diagnosis will help selection of the best test or combination of tests.

A number of groups have shown that EBUS has high diagnostic sensitivity in cases of sarcoidosis, *Mycobacterium tuberculosis* and lymphadenopathy due to metastatic extra-thoracic malignancy[21-25]. While EBUS (with transbronchial biopsies) will provide a diagnosis in the majority of cases of sarcoidosis, some cases of 'burnt out' sarcoid will require a surgical biopsy for confirmation because the yield of diagnostic material showing non-caseating granulomas from fibrotic lymph nodes is very low in a fine-needle aspirate. If the pre-test probability of *Mycobacterium tuberculosis* is high, material should always be sent for culture because the bacillary load in intra-thoracic lymph nodes is often low and acid-fast bacilli may not be seen on light microscopy.

The role of EBUS-TBNA in the diagnosis of lymphoma and recurrent lymphoma is unclear. While a presumptive diagnosis of lymphoproliferative disease may be established by EBUS using a combination of cytopathology and flow cytometry, a surgical biopsy is often required to confirm a specific histological subtype and/or grade. To date, the reported literature around the efficacy of EBUS-TBNA for diagnosis of lymphomas is quite variable, and at the present time, in cases of suspected lymphoma, close liaison between bronchoscopists, thoracic surgeons and the lymphoma MDT (multdisciplinary team meeting) is recommended to achieve the optimal approach to diagnosis.

Complications

Overall, EBUS and EUS are very safe techniques. Major complications are rare, and minor complications such as cough, hypoxaemia and self-terminating post procedure pyrexia are similar to those seen with flexible bronchoscopy. As the number of cases performed globally has risen in recent years, large analyses of complications have been undertaken. One review looked at 16 181 cases from 190 studies and reported a serious adverse event rate of 0.05% for EBUS and 0.3% for EUS[26]. However, the authors suspected that under-reporting bias exists in individual studies, and a prospective registry study which evaluated 1317 EBUS-TBNA cases showing a complication rate of 1.44% would support this view[27].

Training

Until now there has been relatively little written about the training requirements for EBUS. Kemp et al. (2010)[28], using cumulative-sum analysis, showed that the learning curve over the first 100 cases performed by five experienced bronchoscopists was quite variable in terms of length of time before competence in EBUS-TBNA was achieved. Bellinger et al. (2014) [29] showed, maybe not surprisingly, that the diagnostic yield of trainees and experienced bronchoscopists improved with increasing experience, with the latter group achieving a 90% yield after 50 procedures. Stather et al. (2014)[30] looked at competency among interventional pulmonary fellows in the United States and Canada. On-going improvements in technical skill were still being seen after 200 procedures, and one-third of participants did not achieve expert-level technical skill during their fellowship training. Currently there are no specific guidelines on training required, and most national societies have avoided stipulating a specific number of procedures to be performed before an individual is deemed competent as such numbers are often arbitrary and rather the focus should be on monitoring an individual's performance and outcomes. It should be remembered that the skill level required for fully assessing and accurately staging the mediastinum including biopsy of sub-centimetre nodes to achieve a high negative predictive value is very different to that required for biopsying a large station 4R or 7 lymph node for diagnostic purposes only. As with many procedures requiring manual dexterity and hand-eye co-ordination, increasing experience is likely to produce better and more consistent results.

The increasing use of EBUS/EUS also has implications for the trainee surgeon learning surgical staging procedures such as mediastinoscopy. Vyas et al. (2013)[31] have noted that the number of mediastinoscopies being performed is decreasing, an effect we have also noted in our own centre. Although the requirement for fewer mediastinoscopies may be seen as a positive step, it should be borne in mind that if surgeons become less skilled in the procedure, it becomes more challenging to undertake, particularly in complex situations such as the re-staging scenario following neo-adjuvant chemotherapy [32].

References and further reading

1 Herth FJ, Becker HD, Ernst A. Ultrasound-guided transbronchial needle aspiration: an experience in 242 patients. *Chest* 2003; 123:604–7.

2 Steinfort DP, Khor YH, Manser RL, et al. Radial probe endobronchial ultrasound for the diagnosis of peripheral lung cancer: systematic review and meta-analysis. *Eur Respir J* 2011; 37:902–10.

3 Ishida T, Asano F, Yamazaki K, Shinagawa N, et al. Virtual Navigation in Japan Trial Group. Virtual bronchoscopic navigation combined with endobronchial ultrasound to diagnose small peripheral pulmonary lesions: a randomised trial. *Thorax* 2011 Dec; 66(12):1072–7. doi: 10.1136/thx.2010.145490. Epub 11 Jul 2011.

4 Krasnik M, Vilmann P, Larsen SS, et al. Preliminary experience with a new method of endoscopic transbronchial real time ultrasound guided biopsy for diagnosis of mediastinal and hilar lesions. *Thorax* 2003; 58:1083–6.

5 Herth FJF, Krasnik M, Yasufuku K, et al. Endobronchial ultrasound–guided transbronchial needle aspiration. *J Bronchology* 2006; 13:84–91.

6 Rintoul RC, Skwarski KM, Murchison JT, et al. Endobronchial and endoscopic ultrasound-guided real-time fine-needle aspiration for mediastinal staging. *Eur Respir J* 2005; 25:416–21.

7 Herth FJF, Eberhardt R, Vilmann P, et al. Real-time endobronchial ultrasound guided transbronchial needle aspiration for sampling mediastinal lymph nodes. *Thorax* 2006; 61:795–8.

8 Yasufuku K, Chiyo M, Sekine Y, et al. Real-time endobronchial ultrasound-guided transbronchial needle aspiration of mediastinal and hilar lymph nodes. *Chest* 2004; 126:122–8.

9 Gu P, Zhao Y-Z, Jiang L-Y, et al. Endobronchial ultrasound-guided transbronchial needle aspiration for staging of lung cancer: a systematic review and meta-analysis. *Eur J Cancer* 2009; 45:1389–96.

10 Dong X, Qiu X, Liu Q, Jia J. Endobronchial ultrasound-guided

transbronchial needle aspiration in the mediastinal staging of non-small cell lung cancer: a meta-analysis. *Ann Thorac Surg* 2013; 96:1502–7.

11 Yasufuku K, Pierre A, Darling G, et al. A prospective controlled trial of endobronchial ultrasound-guided transbronchial needle aspiration compared with mediastinoscopy for mediastinal lymph node staging of lung cancer. *J Thorac Cardiovasc Surg* 2011; 142:1393–1400.e1.

12 Um SW, Kim HK, Jung SH, et al. Endobronchial ultrasound versus mediastinoscopy for mediastinal nodal staging of non small cell lung cancer *J Thorac Oncol.* 2015 Feb; 10(2):331–7. doi: 10.1097/JTO.0000000000000388.

13 Annema JT, van Meerbeeck PJ, Rintoul RC, et al. Mediastinoscopy vs endosonography for mediastinal nodal staging of lung cancer: a randomized trial. *JAMA* 2010; 304:2245–52.

14 Liberman M, Sampalis J, Duranceau A, et al. Chest. *Endosonographic mediastinal lymph node staging of lung cancer.* 2014 Aug; 146(2):389–97. doi: 10.1378/chest.13-2349.

15 Hwangbo B, Lee GK, Lee HS, et al. Transbronchial and transesophageal fine-needle aspiration using an ultrasound bronchoscope in mediastinal staging of potentially operable lung cancer. *Chest* 2010; 138:795–802.

16 De Leyn P, Stroobants S, De Wever W, et al. Prospective comparative study of integrated positron emission tomography-computed tomography scan compared with remediastinoscopy in the assessment of residual mediastinal lymph node disease after induction chemotherapy for mediastinoscopy-proven stage IIIA-N2 non-small cell lung cancer: a Leuven Lung Cancer Group

Study. *J Clin Oncol* 2006; 24:3333–9.

17 Mateu-Navarro M, Rami-Porta R, Bastus-Piulats R, et al. Remediastinoscopy after induction chemotherapy in non-small cell lung cancer. *Ann Thorac Surg* 2000; 70:391–5.

18 Marra A, Hillejan L, Fechner S, et al. Remediastinoscopy in restaging of lung cancer after induction therapy. *J Thorac Cardiovasc Surg* 2008; 135:843–9.

19 Herth FJ, Annema JT, Eberhardt R, et al. Endobronchial ultrasound with transbronchial needle aspiration for restaging the mediastinum in lung cancer. *J Clin Oncol* 2008; 26:3346–50.

20 Szlubowski A, Zielinski M, Soja J, et al. Accurate and safe mediastinal restaging by combined endobronchial and endoscopic ultrasound-guided needle aspiration performed by single ultrasound bronchoscope. Eur J Cardiothorac Surg Published Online First: 12 January 2014. doi:10.1093/ejcts/ezt 570.

21 von Bartheld MB, Dekkers OM, Szlubowski A, et al. Endosonography vs conventional bronchoscopy for the diagnosis of sarcoidosis: the GRANULOMA randomized clinical trial. *JAMA* 2013; 309:2457–64.

22 Gupta D, Dadhwal DS, Agarwal R, et al. Endobronchial ultrasound guided transbronchial needle aspiration vs conventional transbronchial needle aspiration in the diagnosis of sarcoidosis. *Chest* 2014; 146:547–556.

23 Navani N, Molyneaux PL, Breen RA, et al. Utility of endobronchial ultrasound-guided transbronchial needle aspiration in patients with tuberculous intrathoracic lymphadenopathy: a multicentre study. *Thorax* 2011; 66:889–93.

24 Navani N, Nankivell M, Woolhouse I, et al. Endobronchial ultrasound-guided transbronchial

needle aspiration for the diagnosis of intrathoracic lymphadenopathy in patients with extrathoracic malignancy: a multicenter study. *J Thorac Oncol* 2011; 6:1505–9.

25 Tournoy KG, Govaerts E, Malfait T, et al. Endobronchial ultrasound-guided transbronchial needle biopsy for M1 staging of extrathoracic malignancies. *Ann Oncol* 2011; 22:127–31.

26 von Bartheld MB, van Breda A, Annema JT. Complication rate of endosonography (endobronchial and endoscopic ultrasound): a systematic review. Respiration. Published Online First: 16 January 2014 doi: 10.1159/000357066.

27 Eapen GA, Shah AM, Lei X, et al. Complications, consequences, and practice patterns of endobronchial ultrasound-guided transbronchial needle aspiration: results of the AQuIRE registry. *Chest* 2013; 143:1044–53.

28 Kemp SV, El Batrawy SH, Harrison RN, et al. Learning curves for endobronchial ultrasound using cusum analysis. *Thorax* 2010; 65:534–8.

29 Bellinger CR, Chatterjee AB, Adair N, et al. Training in and experience with endobronchial ultrasound. *Respiration* 2014; 88:476–83.

30 Stather DR, Chee A, MacEachern P, et al. Endobronchial ultrasound learning curve in interventional pulmonary fellows. *Respirology.* 2015 Feb; 20(2):333–9. doi: 10.1111/resp.12450. Epub 9 Dec 2014.

31 Vyas KS, Davenport DL, Ferraris VA, Saha SP. Mediastinoscopy: trends and practice patterns in the United States. *Southern Medical Journal* 2013; 106(10):539–44.

32 Rusch V. Mediastinoscopy: an endangered species? *J Clin Oncol* 2005; 23:8283–85.

Chapter 3

Staging of lung cancer

Mediastinoscopy and VATS

Gaetano Rocco and Giuseppe De Luca

Mediastinoscopy and lung cancer

Mediastinoscopy serves the purpose of providing tissue for the diagnosis of masses in the mediastinum. In addition, cervical mediastinoscopy is used to access the lymph nodes located in the middle mediastinum which represent the N compartment of the modern TNM staging for lung cancer[1,2]. In addition, cervical mediastinoscopy represents a valid diagnostic tool for the diagnosis of lymphoma. Less frequently, it is possible to perform an extended mediastinoscopy by which the surgeon gains access to the lymph nodes of a specific area of the anterior mediastinum, namely, the pre- and subaortic ones beyond the reach of cervical mediastinoscopy. A safe and reliable performance of the procedure also in relatively inexperienced hands has been made possible by the implementation of video-assisted mediastinoscopy[1,2]. As a result, tutoring of cervical mediastinoscopy has since become routine as well as recording of the procedure for medico-legal and training purposes. Video-assisted cervical mediastinoscopy for staging requires the patient to be under general anesthesia and the surgeon to perform the procedure according to time-honoured principles.

Surgical anatomy of video-assisted mediastinoscopy. A basic knowledge of the anatomy of the mediastinum is mandatory for the trainee approaching a surgical mediastinal exploration. The corridor where the mediastinoscope needs to be inserted is a parallelepiped.[1] The posterior face of this geometric space is the anterior wall of the trachea, and it is first visualized when the mediastinoscope is first inserted in this corridor. The anterior wall of the

trachea is indeed the pavement of this corridor and represents the landmark always to be kept in sight for orientation during the procedure. Laterally, the superior vena cava and the right paratracheal nodal stations are found. On the left side, lateral to the trachea, are the left carotid artery, the paratracheal nodal stations and the left recurrent nerve. Anteriorly, the innominate artery crosses this space as it emerges from the aortic arch towards the right thoracic inlet. At the carinal level, the pulmonary artery runs anteriorly, partially hidden by the subcarinal nodes. Laterally, on the right-hand side, the azygos vein is found as it encroaches the right main stem bronchus.

1. With the patient supine, a roll must be placed under the shoulder – usually transversally at the level of the angle of the scapula – in order to obtain maximal extension of the neck at the jugular notch ('thyroid position').

2. Surgical draping should include an area ranging from the chin to the umbilicus sagittally and extending from one posterior axillary line to the contralateral transversally. A sternal saw should be made available on the surgical tray for open surgery at all times.

3. As opposed to first-generation rigid videomediastinoscopes, more recent instruments are devised much like a speculum with one dilating blade, which contributes to controlling and 'fixing' the surgical field, making dissection and biopsy more precise. In addition, complete removal of nodes and other operative steps can be facilitated by bimanual handling of endoscopic instruments. At times, also open surgery instruments can be introduced through this single-access approach to the mediastinum.

---

[1] *Parallelepiped* is a three-dimensional figure formed by six parallelograms.

Core Topics in Thoracic Surgery, ed. Marco Scarci, Aman Coonar, Tom Routledge and Francis Wells. Published by Cambridge University Press. © Cambridge University Press 2016

4. The incision must be placed at one fingerbreadth above the jugular notch; careful hemostasis should be obtained by ligating small venous vessels encountered as the dissection proceeds to the pretracheal fascia. Crucial technical details for successful blunt dissection are using the index finger pressing on the linea alba to guide the dissection into the deeper layers, stepwise retraction of the paratracheal muscles with increasingly longer retractor blades and releasing and cranially dislocating the thyroid isthmus by 'hooking' it with the left (right, for the left-handed) index finger prior to inserting the videomediastinoscope under the opened pretracheal fascia. The instrument must slide onto the first phalanx of the index finger into the pretracheal space ('ship launching') previously created upon opening of the fascia. To this respect, the tunnel under this fascia is created with the purpose of enlarging the cylinder for the videomediastinoscope by gently applying a finger dissection in all directions. Forceful movements should be avoided at all times.

5. The videomediastinoscope is supposed to explore potentially blind areas such as the anterior nodal stations (i.e. 1 and 3) which may go unnoticed during the procedure. The need to identify and avoid the course of the recurrent nerve on the left tracheal groove cannot be overemphasized. Probing an unidentified structure, especially if detected in an uncommon anatomic location, represents good practice. As a rule, superb visualization through video-assisted mediastinoscopy, good common sense and a solid knowledge of the anatomy should make routine probing unnecessary.

6. Bleeding from sampling nodes is usually an easily controllable event. Diathermy coagulation, clipping or simple tight packing all represent effective measures to gain time before completing the diagnostic procedure (i.e. stations 2–4R, 7, 2–4L and 3). The diathermy cautery should not be used in the vicinity of the recurrent nerve. Hemostatic powders or foams tend to cover the surgical field, impeding further visualization. Rarely, the surgeon is confronted with the dilemma of whether to proceed to repeated biopsy of anthraco-sclerotic nodes strictly adherent to

major vessels. However, this is often the case with re-staging mediastinoscopy. In this circumstance, there is nothing which can replace experience and a balance between the risks and the potential clinical benefit resulting from the diagnosis (i.e. PET-negative nodes after chemotherapy) should be carefully established.

Recently, modifications of the classic cervical mediastinoscopic approach, aimed at providing lymph node dissection rather than sampling, were introduced in clinical practice due to the refinement of technology providing video-assistance and the availability of maneuverable endoscopic instruments. As an example, video-assisted mediastinal lymphadenectomy (VAMLA) and transcervical extended mediastinal lymphadenectomy (TEMLA) have been added to the armamentarium of thoracic surgeons with the aim of providing one single surgical access for the exploration and complete removal of multiple mediastinal stations located on the same side or opposite to the primary tumour (T). The advantages of a pathological assessment of both ipsilateral and contralateral mediastinal lymph nodes to better select surgical candidates and prospect a neo-adjuvant treatment for those found with clinically undetected metastatic deposits are obvious. Yet, critics of these approaches emphasize the persistent inaccessibility of stations 5/6 on the left for VAMLA and 8–9 for TEMLA. Also, TEMLA would most likely require a separate session under general anesthesia since complete assessment of the numerous nodes would mandate a careful histological and immunohistochemical analysis[3–9].

Mediastinoscopy and EBUS

Already defined 'medical mediastinoscopy', EBUS is being extensively used to stage the mediastinum in view of comparable results to mediastinoscopy in terms of sensitivity and specificity[10,11]. Also, costs have often argued against the use of mediastinoscopy in favour of EBUS[12]. Recent evaluation seems to confute point by point this view. As a result, while some surgeons still consider mediastinoscopy the 'gold standard' for mediastinal staging[13,14], others have conceived a pathway including EBUS for staging and mediastinoscopy for re-staging of lung cancer. Although the extent of the surgical exploration of the N compartment varies with the interpretation of the idea of 'locally advanced NSCLC', the use of mediastinoscopy in a previously intact surgical field may avoid the untoward complications and the reduced accuracy of re-staging mediastinoscopy[15–18].

VATS for lung cancer staging

In the last two decades, video-assisted thoracoscopic surgery (VATS) has radically changed routine general thoracic surgical practice, becoming a fundamental component of minimally invasive thoracic surgery[19]. Indeed, conventional open surgery has been affected by VATS in as much as surgeons have been induced to limit the invasiveness of open thoracotomy and introduced videoassistance in the so-called hybrid approaches to the chest[20]. The techniques of VATS have themselves evolved from the traditional three-port approach to the use of uniportal VATS for the diagnosis and treatment of several intrathoracic conditions[21]. In this context, VATS is currently utilized for accepted indications, one of them being lung cancer staging[22,23].

1. **Pleural effusion suspected for M1a.** This represents the most widely accepted indication for the use of VATS[24]. The British Thoracic Society guidelines recommend thoracoscopy for suspected but unproven effusions, both under general or local anesthesia, given the 90% accuracy and control of recurrence rates reported in the literature[25,26]. Recently, Katlic et al. have reported on 353 patients managed with VATS utilizing local anesthesia and sedation. In this series, 66 patients had malignant pleural effusion from lung cancer in whom the procedure was performed via one port only[27,28]. The concomitant presence of loculations may indicate the addition of another port to facilitate biopsies. Irrespective of the number of ports used during VATS for pleural effusion, pleural nodules represent an obvious target for biopsy. However, a frozen section of the specimen should be obtained to confirm diagnosis and facilitate prompt start of chemotherapy. The presence of endobronchial obstruction may cause concurrent effusion, which might be due to atelectasis of the lung. In addition, the detection of conglomerates with gelatinous consistency ('jellyfish') concomitant to lung cancer should raise suspicion of an M1a effusion and should be sent for frozen section.

2. **Mediastinal nodal disease suspected for multistation N2 or N3 disease.** When cervical mediastinoscopy poses significant technical difficulties or is not deemed feasible (i.e. previous neck dissection, huge goitre) or mediastinal nodal stations unreachable by conventional mediastinoscopy need to be sampled (i.e. for histological confirmation of PET positive nodes), VATS can be a useful alternative. VATS has increasingly been shown as an excellent approach to remove mediastinal nodes[29–30]. Both uniportal and conventional VATS can be used. The patient lies in the lateral decubitus position. Double-lumen tube is needed to ensure lung exclusion. The standard baseball diamond configuration is used to target the nodal station to be biopsied[31]. Conventional endoscopic instrumentation can be utilized. Alternatively, only one incision (2–2.5 cm) is placed in the fifth intercostal space, 1 cm posterior to the scapular line for lesions in the anterior or middle mediastinum (or anterior to the scapular line for lesions in the posterior mediastinum), and the mediastinal pleura is elevated by using an articulating endograsper. When mediastinal nodes in stations L6 or L5 are addressed, caution should be used to use diathermy to avoid phrenic or recurrent nerve injuries. The mediastinal lymph node can be biopsied as in the conventional mediastinoscopic approach or can be removed entirely[31,32]. Irrespective of the clinical stage, the need for biomolecular studies mandates an adequate size of the biopsy specimen. Many surgeons use a standard suction device to dissect the nodes or, alternatively, endokittners. The suction needs to be clamped when not needed for hemostasis to avoid undue lung re-expansion and subsequent obstruction of the surgical field. Endoclip devices are used for unrelenting bleeding from a small arterial vessel; alternatively, energy devices such as Ligasure or Ultracision may be utilized for peribronchial dissection.

3. **VATS pericardial biopsy and window.** Isolated pericardial effusions are quite rare since they are more frequently found in association with pleural effusion. When a tissue diagnosis is necessary and the cytology on previously aspirated fluid was non-diagnostic, the pericardium can be approached thoracoscopically

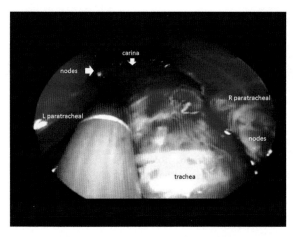

Figure 3.1 Video-assisted mediastinoscopic view: left-sided tracheobronchial node.

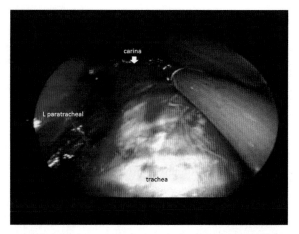

Figure 3.2 Video-assisted mediastinoscopic view: right-sided tracheobronchial node.

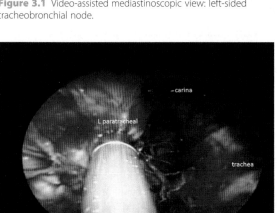

Figure 3.3 Video-assisted mediastinoscopic view: left-sided paratracheal node.

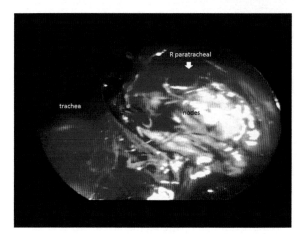

Figure 3.4 Video-assisted mediastinoscopic view: right-sided paratracheal node.

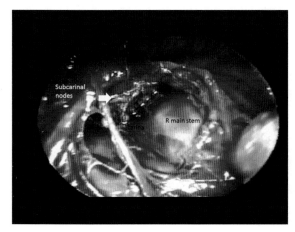

Figure 3.5 Video-assisted mediastinoscopic view: subcarinal nodes.

either by conventional (three-port) or uniportal VATS[33,34]. Interaction with the anesthesiologist is of utmost importance to decide the anesthetic regimen to control alterations of blood pressure related to surgical maneuvers. A chest CT will contribute to the selection of the side with the most prominent pericardial effusion. If the uniportal approach is selected, the incision is placed in the fifth intercostal space, 1 cm behind the scapular line. The area of pericardium to be incised is carefully chosen anterior to the phrenic nerve. If possible, probing of the pericardial effusion with a long spinal needle is feasible both with conventional and with uniportal VATS. By releasing the intrapericardial pressure, the aspiration of small amounts of fluid will make

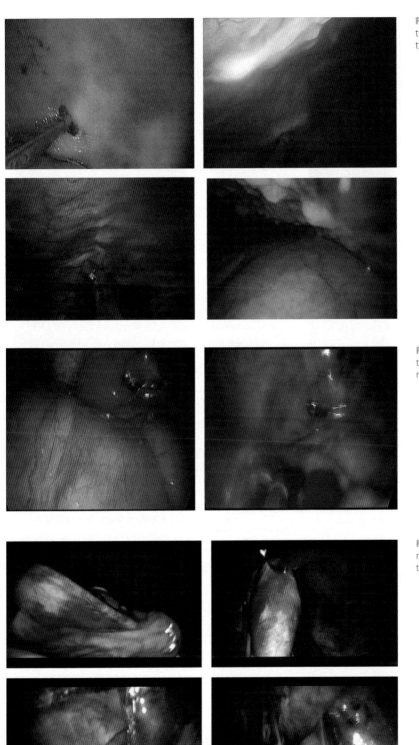

Figure 3.6 Macroscopic appearance of the parietal pleura during video-assisted thoracoscopy. Biopsy of white nodules.

Figure 3.7 Uniportal video-assisted thoracoscopic view: biopsy of mediastinal mass.

Figure 3.8 Wedge resection of a lung metastasis by uniportal video-assisted thoracoscopic approach.

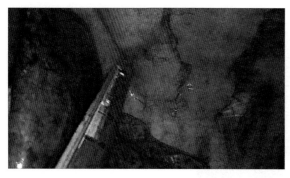

Figure 3.9 Wedge resection of peripheral pulmonary nodule by uniportal video-assisted thoracoscopic approach.

grasping of the target area of the pericardium easier. To this purpose, an Allis clamp is introduced parallel to the thoracoscope during uniportal VATS and through one of the operative ports during conventional VATS. The pericardium is gently suspended, and an incision is performed with endoscissors at the previous puncture site still gushing pericardial fluid.

Once the first incision is placed, the window can be completed under direct thoracoscopic visualization of the pericardial cavity[34].

4. **Wedge resection of peripheral pulmonary nodule.** In the event of a synchronous nodule or ground glass opacity with predominant nodular pattern, either contralateral to or ipsilateral to the primary tumour, the need for histological characterization of the lung lesion may arise. For peripheral nodules, a minimally invasive approach is warranted, either open or VATS. While during the former palpation of the lung usually yields the identification of the lesion, the visualization of the target lesions in the lung may become more challenging, especially if the nodule is not immediately subpleural. Although in select circumstances some degree of lung palpation may still be feasible with conventional, three-port VATS, other techniques of localization (i.e. with dye, hookwire, Tc99, ultrasounds) may be necessary to identify the nodule[35–37].

References

1 Specht G. Erweiterte mediastinoskopie. *Thoraxchir Vask Chir.* 1965; 13:401–7.

2 Ginsberg RJ, Rice TW Goldberg M, et al. Extended cervical medistinoscopy. A single staging procedure for bronchogenic carcinoma of the left upper lobe. *J Thoracic Cardiovasc Surg.* 1987; 94:673–8.

3 Kuzdzał J, Zieliński M, Papla B, et al. The transcervical extended mediastinal lymphadenectomy versus cervical mediastinoscopy in non-small cell lung cancer staging. *Eur J Cardiothorac Surg.* 2007 Jan; 31(1):88–94. Epub 2006 Nov 20.

4 Zieliński M. Transcervical extended mediastinal lymphadenectomy: results of staging in two hundred fifty-six

patients with non-small cell lung cancer. *J Thorac Oncol.* 2007 Apr; 2(4):370–2.

5 Witte B, Hürtgen M. Video-assisted mediastinoscopic lymphadenectomy (VAMLA). *J Thorac Oncol.* 2007 Apr; 2(4):367–9.

6 Hürtgen M, Friedel G, Witte B, et al. Systematic Video-Assisted Mediastinoscopic Lymphadenectomy (VAMLA). *Thorac Surg Sci.* 2005 Nov 9; 2:Doc02.

7 Leschber G, Holinka G, Linder A. Video-assisted mediastinoscopic lymphadenectomy (VAMLA)–a method for systematic mediastinal lymphnode dissection. *Eur J Cardiothorac Surg.* 2003 Aug; 24(2):192–5.

8 Leschber G, Sperling D, Klemm W, Merk J. Does video-

mediastinoscopy improve the results of conventional mediastinoscopy? *Eur J Cardiothorac Surg.* 2008 Feb; 33(2):289–93. Epub 2007 Dec 3.

9 Yendamuri S, Demmy TL. Is VAMLA/TEMLA the new standard of preresection staging of non small cell lung cancer? *J Thorac Cardiovasc Surg.* 2012 Sep; 144(3):S14–7. doi: 10.1016/j.jtcvs.2012.03.038. Epub 2012 Apr 13.

10 Bolton WD, Johnson R, Banks E, et al. Utility and accuracy of endobronchial ultrasound as a diagnostic and staging tool for the evaluation of mediastinal adenopathy. *Surg Endosc.* 2013 Apr; 27(4):1119–23.

11 Zhang R, Mietchen C, Krüger M, et al. Endobronchial ultrasound guided fine needle aspiration

versus transcervical mediastinoscopy in nodal staging of non small cell lung cancer: a prospective comparison study. *J Cardiothorac Surg.* 2012 Jun 6; 7:51.

12 Sharples LD, Jackson C, Wheaton E, et al. Clinical effectiveness and cost-effectiveness of endobronchial and endoscopic ultrasound relative to surgical staging in potentially resectable lung cancer: results from the ASTER randomised controlled trial. *Health Technol Assess.* 2012; 16(18):1–75.

13 Sivrikoz CM, Ak I, Simsek FS, et al. Is mediastinoscopy still the gold standard to evaluate mediastinal lymph nodes in patients with non-small cell lung carcinoma? *Thorac Cardiovasc Surg.* 2012 Mar; 60(2):116–21.

14 Shrager JB. Mediastinoscopy: still the gold standard. *Ann Thorac Surg.* 2010 Jun; 89(6):S2084-9.

15 Zhang R, Ying K, Shi L, et al. Combined endobronchial and endoscopic ultrasound-guided fine needle aspiration for mediastinal lymph node staging of lung cancer: A meta-analysis. *Eur J Cancer.* 2013 May; 49(8):1860–7.

16 Kambartel K, Krbek T, Voshaar T. Comparison of endobronchial ultrasound (EBUS) and mediastinoscopy (MS) for staging lung cancer. *Pneumologie.* 2012 Jul; 66(7):426–31.

17 Medford AR, Bennett JA, Free CM, Agrawal S. Mediastinal staging procedures in lung cancer: EBUS, TBNA and mediastinoscopy. *Curr Opin Pulm Med.* 2009 Jul; 15(4):334–42.

18 Defranchi SA, Edell ES, Daniels CE, et al. Mediastinoscopy in patients with lung cancer and negative endobronchial ultrasound guided needle aspiration. *Ann Thorac Surg.* 2010 Dec; 90(6):1753–7.

19 Rocco G. Operative VATS: the need for a different intrathoracic approach. *Eur J Cardiothorac Surg.* 2005 Aug; 28(2):358.

20 Rocco G, Internullo E, Cassivi SD, et al. The variability of practice in minimally invasive thoracic surgery for pulmonary resections. *Thorac Surg Clin.* 2008 Aug; 18(3):235–47.

21 Rocco G. One-port (uniportal) Video-assisted thoracic surgical resections. A clear advance. *J Thorac Cardiovasc Surg.* 2012 Sep; 144(3):S27-31.

22 Howington JA. The role of VATS for staging and diagnosis in patients with non-small cell lung cancer. *Semin Thorac Cardiovasc Surg.* 2007 Fall; 19(3):212–6.

23 Thomas P, Massard G, Giudicelli R, et al. Role of video-thoracoscopy in the pretreatment evaluation of lung carcinoma. *Rev Med Interne.* 1999 Dec; 20(12):1093–8.

24 Menzies R Charbonneau M. Thoracoscopy for the diagnosis of pleural disease. *Ann Intern Med* 1991; 114:271.

25 Antunes G, Neville E, Duffy J, et al. BTS guidelines for the management of malignant pleural effusions. *Thorax.* 2003 May; 58 Suppl 2:ii29–38.

26 Roberts ME, Neville E, Berrisford RG, et al. Management of a malignant pleural effusion: British Thoracic Society Pleural Disease Guideline 2010. *Thorax.* 2010 Aug; 65 Suppl 2: ii32–40.

27 Katlic MR, Facktor MA. Video-assisted thoracic surgery utilizing local anesthesia and sedation: 384 consecutive cases. *Ann Thorac Surg.* 2010 Jul; 90(1):240–5.

28 Katlic MR. Video-assisted thoracic surgery utilizing local anesthesia and sedation. *Eur J Cardiothorac Surg.* 2006 Sep; 30(3):529–32.

29 Khullar OV, Gangadharan SP. Video-assisted thoracoscopic mediastinal lymph node dissection. *J Thorac Cardiovasc Surg.* 2012 Sep; 144(3):S32–4.

30 Baisi A, Rizzi A, Raveglia F, Cioffi U. Video-assisted thoracic surgery is effective in systemic lymph node dissection. *Eur J Cardiothorac Surg.* 2013 Nov; 44(5):966. doi: 10.1093/ejcts/ezt235. Epub 2013 May 3.

31 Rocco G, Brunelli A, Jutley R, et al. Uniportal VATS for mediastinal nodal diagnosis and staging. *Interact Cardiovasc Thorac Surg.* 2006 Aug; 5(4):430–2.

32 Salati M, Brunelli A, Rocco G. Uniportal video-assisted thoracic surgery for diagnosis and treatment of intrathoracic conditions. *Thorac Surg Clin.* 2008 Aug; 18(3):305–10.

33 Muhammad MI. The pericardial window: is a video-assisted thoracoscopy approach better than a surgical approach? *Interact Cardiovasc Thorac Surg.* 2011 Feb; 12(2):174–8.

34 Rocco G, La Rocca A, La Manna C, et al. Uniportal video-assisted thoracoscopic surgery pericardial window. *J Thorac Cardiovasc Surg.* 2006 Apr; 131(4):921–2.

35 Rocco G. VATS lung biopsy: the uniportal technique. *Multimed Man Cardiothorac Surg.* 2005 Jan 1; 2005(121):

mmcts.2004.000356. doi: 10.1510/mmcts.2004.000356.

36 Rocco G, Martin-Ucar A, Passera E. Uniportal VATS wedge pulmonary resections. *Ann Thorac Surg.* 2004 Feb; 77 (2):726–8.

37 Rocco G, Cicalese M, La Manna C, et al. Ultrasonographic identification of peripheral pulmonary nodules through uniportal video-assisted thoracic surgery. *Ann Thorac Surg.* 2011 Sep; 92(3):1099–101.

Access to the chest cavity
Safeguards and pitfalls

Laura Socci and Antonio E. Martin-Ucar

Introduction

The choice of incision is vital for procedures in the thoracic cavity. The main principle should always be adequate exposure in order to perform a safe and effective procedure without compromise. However, the trauma of entering the chest cavity is particularly severe with impact on pain, muscle performance and respiratory function. As with surgical access in any region of the body, surgeons have always tried to minimize the impact of this trauma in the thoracic wall. As a result, we have at our disposal a myriad of incisions to choose from when facing thoracic procedures, with their own indications and pitfalls. As a general rule, in order to decide our approach, we have to take into account the indication for surgery, the anatomical location of the pathology, the likelihood of encountering difficulties (such as previous surgeries or locally invasive tumours), the pre-operative assessment of the patient, the predicted extent of side effects and also the patient's views in term of cosmesis and recovery.

Common to all techniques are the basic principles: correct positioning of the patient on the operating table, anatomical landmarks to place the incision, correct tissue handling and haemostasis and gradual spread of ribs/sternum to minimize trauma. For the purpose of this chapter, we will divide the incisions into three main groups: open approaches in lateral decubitus position (muscle and non-muscle sparing), open approaches in supine position (sternotomy, anterior thoracotomy, clamshell and their variations) and minimally invasive approaches (VATS and hybrid). We will describe the techniques with points regarding their main indications and their potential pitfalls.

Techniques

Open approaches in lateral decubitus

The majority of the chest wall approaches for thoracic surgery procedures are still performed in the lateral decubitus position. It is crucial that multiple pressure points are padded, with the dependent leg flexed with a pillow between the legs. Ideally, both arms should be flexed 'in the prayer position', although this can vary depending on the surgeon's preference. It is important to widen the intercostal spaces to be entered by hyperextending the chest cavity with a roll positioned under the dependent chest at the level of the tip of the scapula or by 'breaking' the operating table mechanism. We must remember to secure the patient to the operating table by using straps, beanbags or stops not only for safety but also to allow for table movements during the operation.

Posterolateral thoracotomy

The posterolateral thoracotomy is one of the most traditional procedures; however, it is no longer a routine choice because of post-operative pain and the severe impact on the chest muscle. Yet, it is a viable option when a large view is needed, as in the case of major surgery that includes the diaphragm.

The skin incision is performed by joining a point 2–3 cm below the tip of the scapula and the point on the midline between the middle of the spinal border of the scapula and the spinous process of the vertebra. This incision is extended anteriorly until the anterior axillary line (Figure 4.1). The latissimus dorsi muscle is carefully divided with cautery. The serratus anterior muscle was traditionally divided although nowadays is preserved by dividing its attachments to the ribs.

Core Topics in Thoracic Surgery, ed. Marco Scarci, Aman Coonar, Tom Routledge and Francis Wells. Published by Cambridge University Press. © Cambridge University Press 2016

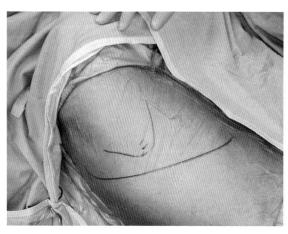

Figure 4.1 Skin marks of a posterolateral thoracotomy. The incision is performed 1–2 cm below the tip of the scapula, from a equidistant point between the thoracic spine and the midpoint of the spinal border of the scapula, then extended anteriorly.

The lateral border of the trapezius is exposed and can be divided in cases where more posterior access is required.

The chosen intercostal space to be entered is identified by counting the ribs from the top (posteriorly) and can be performed by dividing the muscle itself or by lifting the periostium off the rib below. In either case, we aim to minimize damage to the intercostal neurovascular bundle that runs at the inferior border of the ribs. The parietal pleura is then entered so the pleural cavity can be inspected for adhesions and diagnosis. In cases where we suspect the presence of dense adhesions, it is advisable to mobilize a portion of the parietal pleura off the ribs above and below prior to attempting to enter the pleural cavity to reduce the risk of accidental damage to the lungs.

Once the parietal pleura is opened, the rib spreader is inserted. The rib spreader is always opened slowly and progressively, to minimize the risk of accidental rib fracture and maybe to reduce post-operative and long-term pain. In order to facilitate exposure, some surgeons prefer to perform a posterior transection of the rib or a blunt division of the costo-transverse ligaments. Care must be taken during these manoeuvres to avoid damage to the intercostal vessels as bleeding can be difficult to stop due to vessel retraction into the spinal canal.

Indications and advantages: The traditional posterolateral thoracotomy allows the surgeon to perform the vast majority of thoracic procedures both electively and as an emergency. It does provide excellent exposure to all areas of the lungs, the thoracic oesophagus and aorta, and it is very useful for procedures for pleural and diaphragmatic pathologies. Exposure and familiarity with the position are the main advantages of this access.

Another advantage of this approach is that it can be extended cranially at the back if we require more retraction of the scapula (i.e. Pancoast tumours or chest wall invasion) and anteriorly towards the abdomen converting the approach into a thoraco-phreno-laparotomy.

Pitfalls: Posterolateral thoracotomy can be very traumatic, with a known incidence of post-operative and long-term pain as well as an impact on respiratory function following surgery. Division of the latissimus dorsi muscle can cause shoulder movement dysfunction that can delay return to full activities.

Surgeons have to be aware of potential damage to the intercostal vessels during the procedure, the intercostal nerves and ribs while using the rib spreader and the lung while entering the pleural cavity because of adhesions.

Haemostasis is very important during latissimus muscle division and closure to prevent haematomas, especially in younger patients with well-developed muscles.

Because of the morbidity of this approach, surgeons have moved away from division of the serratus anterior muscle and gradually reduced the size of the incision, while still considering it as a posterolateral thoracotomy.

Muscle-sparing posterolateral thoracotomy

A variant of the posterolateral thoracotomy performed via the auscultatory triangle[1–7]. The patient is positioned and prepared in the same fashion, but with the operating table slightly tilted anteriorly (away from the surgeon).

The skin incision will be limited to the initial part of the posterolateral thoracotomy, only we would not need to extend the incision anteriorly from the tip of the scapula. The chest wall muscle layer will be entered via fascia, without division of any muscles. To expose the auscultatory triangle, the posterior border of the latissimus dorsi is mobilized anteriorly, and the lateral border of the trapezius is mobilized posteriorly. These muscles are mobilized by dissecting them off the subcutaneous fat, creating flaps. The intercostal muscle is entered in the same manner as in a posterolateral thoracotomy, with the same precautions and the same length. The surgical field is then secured by the use of two smaller spreaders simultaneously, one retracting the ribs and another one at 90 degrees retracting the trapezius and latissimus muscles creating a square 'window' (Figure 4.2).

In this approach the musculofascial layer is closed very easily as there is no muscle division. Prior to closure of the sub-cutaneous tissues and skin, a tissue drain must be placed under the subcutaneous flaps to prevent seromas or haematomas.

Indications and advantages: As the intercostal incision is of similar size to the one in a posterolateral thoracotomy, the exposure and indications are very similar. In particular, this incision can be very efficient to treat pathologies of the posterior mediastinum (neurogenic tumours, oesophageal cysts, etc.), which don't require exposure to the anterior chest cavity. It provides a good exposure for procedures involving reconstruction of the bronchial tree such as sleeve lobectomies or trauma because of their posterior location. It is a particularly effective approach for anatomical segmentectomies of segment 6.

Another good indication is an initial procedure for pulmonary metastasis as the incision would allow inspection of the entire lung, but it might minimize the adhesions should further procedures be required in the future.

Overall this approach provides good exposure of the thoracic cavity with a perceived improvement in terms of cosmesis due to the smaller skin incision and

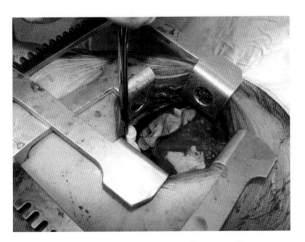

Figure 4.2 Operative view during a muscle-sparing thoracotomy repair of a traumatic rupture of the diaphragm. Two rib spreaders are placed at 90 degrees to secure adequate exposure: the deeper one is separating the ribs and the more superficial one is retracting the preserved muscles.

return to activities due to preservation of muscles. Leaving the latissimus dorsi and serratus muscles intact does allow for these muscles to be used in the future as flaps if complications or further procedures are required[4,8].

Pitfalls: The same possible complications apply as per the posterolateral thoracotomy (damage of intercostal vessels, nerves and lung) with the addition of the more common incidence of seromas due to the creation of subcutaneous flaps (reported incidence of up to 26%). A self-vacuumed subcutaneous drain should be placed and be kept in place for a few days until it stops draining.

In the presence of very central large lung tumours, access to the main pulmonary artery can be difficult, leading to the need to extend the incision anteriorly (especially on right-sided procedures).

Tying knots can be sometimes difficult deep in the thoracic cavity, making surgeons rely on knot pushers; the surgeon should make sure one is available. This is normally not an issue if stapling guns are used. A good tip is to create the chest drain port early during the procedure and use it for insertion of the stapler guns, giving a very comfortable angle for placement and firing. Longer instruments may be needed too.

Muscle-sparing anterolateral thoracotomy

The patient is positioned in lateral decubitus with the same precautions as the posterolateral thoracotomy. The table can be slightly tilted posteriorly to facilitate the surgeon's view (who will be standing in the front of the patient). The skin incision is performed starting from 2 cm below the scapula tip and continuing towards the submammary crease. The subcutaneous layers are divided with cautery; it is important to preserve the intercostal brachial nerve that runs in the superior part of the wound. If dissected, a postoperative numbness of the lateral breast and the nipple area can occur. Posteriorly, the long thoracic nerve is identified and preserved.

The anterior border of the latissimus dorsi is mobilized posteriorly by creating a subcutaneous flap and spared. The 4th or 5th intercostal space is entered in the same manner as per posterolateral thoracotomy. While it is more difficult to divide the costotransverse ligaments to increase rib spreading, the intercostal spaces are wider anteriorly.

The closure will be very similar to the procedure via auscultatory triangle, with the very important subcutaneous drain to prevent seromas or haematomas.

Indications and advantages: The wide anterior intercostal spaces facilitate exposure compared to the more posterior approaches, thus in theory reducing the need for excess rib spreading. It gives a very adequate exposure of lungs, pericardium and diaphragm.

Preservation of the chest wall muscles not only reduces impact on shoulder movements but also allows for their use as flaps should complications (bronchopleural fistula) arise[4,8].

With the increase in the use of the VATS anterior approach, the view is now very familiar for younger thoracic surgeons who recognize promptly this view for access to hilar structures even in central tumours. This might help for this incision to become the preferred 'open' approach in the future.

Pitfalls: Once again the incidence of seromas and haematomas needs to be prevented by self-vacuumed drains post-operatively. While exposure to the hilar structures is improved over posterior approaches, access to the posterior mediastinum can be restricted.

If we have to perform a broncho-angioplasty, it will be easier to perform the bronchial reconstruction first (as it is located more posterior) and then the vascular one.

For posterior anatomical segmentectomies (segments 3 or 6), this access may prove more difficult than using more posterior approaches.

Axillary thoracotomy

The use of the axillary thoracotomy has been less extensive than the other 'lateral' approaches. The lateral decubitus position is slightly altered by tilting the table backwards, increasing exposure of anterior chest wall, and the ipsilateral arm is secured away from the incision by shoulder abduction and elbow flexion at 90 degrees. As always when the arm is secured, care must be taken for it not to be in tension that might result in brachial plexus traction injury.

The axillary approach can be used for access to the high intercostal spaces (2nd) down to 4th or 5th space depending on the indications for surgery. The traditional approach involves a transverse incision at the level of the axillary hairline with the anterior end at the posterior edge of the pectoralis major (anterior axillary line) and the posterior end at the anterior edge of latissimus dorsi (posterior axillary line). Both of these landmarks are easily recognizable due to the bulk of these muscles.

Following the division of the subcutaneous layers, flaps are developed to allow retraction of the latissimus dorsi posteriorly and pectoralis major anteriorly. The extent of this dissection depends on the indication for surgery and the need for exposure. Retraction of the muscles will allow identification of the digitations of the serratus anterior muscles that can either be detached or divided between the digitations. The ribs are then exposed, and entry into the desired intercostal space is then performed according to surgeon's preference. As in other muscle-sparing thoracotomies, normally two small spreaders at 90 degrees of each other are used to create the surgical field.

Indications and advantages: The advent of VATS has reduced the use of these incisions. It does provide a good access for apical procedures: surgery for pneumothorax, sympathectomies and operations at the thoracic outlet[9-12]. As a muscle-sparing thoracotomy, it is well tolerated and has cosmetic results as the incision will remain in a non-exposed area.

Pitfalls: Although it has been used for major procedures, the exposure can be limited, especially in the lower hemithorax. If the procedure is complex, the incision could be extended anteriorly, but it can be quite morbid in the more apical procedures.

Care must be taken with the pressure areas and with the ipsilateral arm to prevent traction or pressure injuries. At the posterior end, the long thoracic nerve should be preserved while dividing the serratus anterior. Due to the creation of the flaps, this incision carries the risk of seromas and haematomas, so care must be taken during closure in terms of haemostasis, approximating the ribs and closure of the serratus anterior.

Open approaches in the supine position
Median sternotomy

As well as being the most used incision for cardiac surgical procedures, median sternotomy has been the incision of choice for large anterior mediastinal tumours and also extensively used for diseases that require access to both pleural cavities (multiple pulmonary metastases, bilateral lung volume reduction surgery, bilateral bullectomies or pleurectomies)[13–18].

The patient is positioned in the supine position with a degree of neck extension to expose the top of the manubrium. The skin incision is performed on the midline from the sternal notch towards the xiphoid process. The length of the incision is mainly dependent on the surgeon's preference. The subcutaneous layers are dissected with cautery towards the pectoralis fascia, and the periostium is 'scored' with the cautery over the midline. The superior end of the incision is retracted towards the neck to allow the identification of the structures in the space of Burns. The interclavicular ligament can be dissected with cautery, paying attention to the innominate vein. Then blunt dissection is commonly used to open the retrosternal space. The xiphoid process is identified and dissected at the caudal end of the incision.

The sternum is divided with a saw along its midline. At that moment usually the surgeon asks the anaesthetist to keep the patient in a transient apnea to minimize the potential risk of entering into the pleural space. Haemostasis is achieved at the periostium with cautery or prothrombotic materials. Persisting sternal bone marrow bleeding can be controlled with bone wax.

A sternal retractor is used to spread the sternal edges. It is important to open the sternal retractor gradually, avoiding injuries to the brachial plexus. The exposure is then adequate to perform the required procedure either in the mediastinum or any of the pleural cavities. At the end of the procedure, sternal wires are normally used to reapproximate the sternum; a median number of six are generally used (two in the manubrium and four in the sternum), although it depends on the patient's height. A good closure of the sternum is important to minimize the risk of non-union, mediastinitis and wound infection. The pectoralis fascia, the subcutaneous layer and the skin are carefully closed by layers.

Indications and advantages: Median sternotomy is the most commonly used incision for cardiac surgical procedures. In non-cardiac thoracic surgery, its use has been extensive in the management of large anterior mediastinal masses, maximal thymectomy for myasthenia and bilateral pathologies such as multiple lung metastases. Median sternotomy was also the incision of choice following the resurgence of lung volume reduction surgery in the 1990s, although more recently bilateral VATS (even as staged procedures) is more commonly used as it might reduce morbidity.

But median sternotomy has also been used very successfully, especially on the right side, in pleuropulmonary diseases such as central primary cancers in which pericardial involvement is suspected and the surgeon is keen to safely access main pulmonary vessels. Another valid indication is in re-do procedures, for example, completion pneumonectomies for central tumours where control of pulmonary vessels may be easier with a sternotomy than via re-do thoracotomy. The authors found that right extrapleural pneumonectomies for mesothelioma were feasible via median sternotomy and indeed reduced the incidence of post-operative complications.

The advantages are clear: great exposure of mediastinal structures (even carina), easy access to control main pulmonary vessels and ability of entering both pleural cavities. From the experience in the post-operative management and analgesia requirements following cardiac surgery, we know that a median sternotomy is very well tolerated by patients with lesser incidence of pain-related complications in the short and the long term than a large posterolateral thoracotomy.

Pitfalls: Although experienced cardiac surgeons could consider median sternotomy a very simple and routine part of the procedure, many potential complications can arise as a result of it. Care must be taken not to damage the anterior jugular veins when dissecting the area at the suprasternal notch or even the innominate vein at that time or when dissecting the thymic tissue or fat (Figure 4.3). It is important to perform the sternotomy in the midline as it is easier than expected to perform a paramedian one, increasing the risk of sternal fractures and non-union. Careful 'scoring' of the periostium in the midline helps to guide the saw. Infective and sternal complications are uncommon (less than 5%) but potentially very morbid.[19–20]

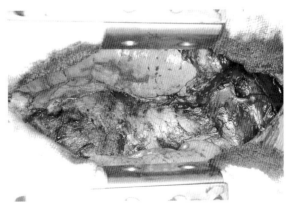

Figure 4.3 Median sternotomy following thymectomy for stage II thymoma. The innominate vein has been exposed to divide the thymic vein. The right pleura has been entered.

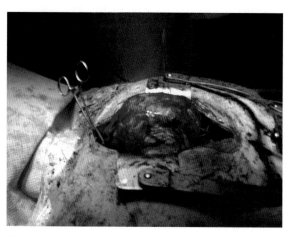

Figure 4.4 A median sternotomy performed to excise a very large mediastinal mass. The size of the mass did require a hemi-clamshell extension towards the right side to perform the dissection safely.

Accidental entry into the pleural cavities during the sternotomy can be prevented by temporary apnea, being more important in patients with hyperinflated lungs with emphysema or bulla.

Poor access to the posterior areas of the lungs, posterior mediastinal structures and left lower lobe are the main pitfalls in terms of exposure (Figure 4.4).

Bilateral thoracosternotomy (clamshell and hemiclamshell)

The clamshell incision consisting of a bilateral anterior thoracotomy with transverse sternotomy has been the choice for bilateral lung transplantation and access to pericardium in the past. Today it is somehow restricted to uncommon indications but is a valuable tool for cardio-thoracic and trauma surgeons[21–25]. A number of modifications such as the hemiclamshell have been described for diverse indications[26].

With the patient in the supine position, the skin incision is made along the inframammary skin creases from the midaxillary/anterior axillary lines. The subcutaneous tissues are divided with cautery, and the pectoralis major muscles are raised from their inferior and sternal attachments. The 4th or 5th intercostal spaces are identified and entered bilaterally. If the skin incision is made from the midaxillary lines, it is important that the intercostal spaces are entered beyond these points to allow for better retraction. Care must be taken to identify and ligate the internal mammary vessels. The sternal body is divided transversally with a saw, and after haemostasis, the ends are spread with two sternal retractors. In the hemi-clamshell approach, the skin incision is performed starting on the sternal notch on the midline and running over the inframammary crease towards the anterior axillary line. The pectoralis major is raised or incised over the 5th rib. The 4th intercostal space is entered. The mammary bundle is ligated. Variants of this incision include a cervical extension of the incision along the medial edge of the sternocleidomastoid muscle and the Dartevelle's approach that includes the sectioning of the medial half of the clavicle.

After the indicated procedure has been performed, the sternal ends are approximated with wires, the intercostal spaces are closed routinely and the pectoralis major muscles are reattached to the lower ribs and sternum.

Indications: The clamshell incision provides better exposure of thoracic cavities, but its comorbidities and the trauma involved have restricted its use to specific indications. Currently, its use is limited to very large mediastinal masses, bilateral lung transplantation and trauma. Its use on bilateral lung metastases or excision of pericardium has declined in favour of other approaches.

Pitfalls: The consequences of this approach in the chest wall can be severe. Transternal division carries a high risk of sternal healing complications, up to 30% compared to 1–2% after median sternotomy. In a comparative series, Macchiarini et al. reported more post-operative pain, deformities, need for surgical revision and more impact on respiratory mechanics following clamshell than median sternotomy after double lung or heart-lung transplant.

Apart from care during closure, one of the important steps is to identify and ligate the internal mammary vessels during the incision as it can lead to post-operative bleeding.

Anterior thoracotomies

The anterior thoracotomy did regain some popularity with the advent of minimal invasive cardiac surgery (mitral valve surgery and MIDCAB)[27], although its use in thoracic surgery remains limited to non-complex procedures.

The patient is positioned supine with a roll under the ipsilateral side of the operation to increase intercostal spaces separation. The skin incision is made from the anterior axillary line curving under the breast towards the sternum for procedures that require access through the 4th or 5th intercostal space[9].

A lower approach of an anterior thoracotomy would be a submammary incision, which can be very useful for insertion of pacemakers or creation of pericardial windows. In procedures for the staging of lung cancer, the incision is placed at the level of the 2nd–3rd intercostal space with or without excision of the sternocostal cartilage.

A limited anterior thoracotomy is a good approach for patients who require a lung biopsy but are not fit enough for a single lung ventilation that could make the VATS approach more difficult, and it can be used as invasive mediastinal staging of lung cancer in the form of an anterior mediastinotomy for biopsy of lymph nodes or to confirm suspected direct mediastinal invasion. A good advantage is the fact that the intercostal spaces are wider anteriorly so less rib retraction is required, even being substituted by soft tissue retractors.

Pitfalls of this incision are the poor exposure that makes it rarely used for major thoracic procedures[28]. If the costal cartilage is excised, there is a risk of seromas or hernias, and the possibility of damage to the internal thoracic arteries.

Minimally invasive approaches
Video-assisted thoracic surgery

Video-assisted thoracic surgery (VATS) implies that the surgeon must perform the entire operation through a number of small incisions, the entire visualization done via the optics, and without the use of any rib spreading (either by a retractor or manually)[29].

The procedures performed via VATS initially were primarily diagnostic, then minor therapeutic procedures; currently, most major operations have been described by a VATS approach. Traditionally, VATS has been performed through three or four ports; in the last decade, the evolution of the technique, instruments and the surgeon's experience has permitted minimization of the number of ports to only one. Previous contraindications (adhesions, central tumours, etc.) and pitfalls are being changed by the increased experience of surgeons. Currently, the indications for VATS surgery are increasing rapidly and include the management of all thoracic diseases except lung transplantation. Good results are being achieved in all areas of pulmonary, pleural, mediastinal and thoracic outlet procedures[30–42]. The advantages are mainly the effect of the limitation of

trauma: shorter hospital stay, less post-operative pain, less impact on post-operative shoulder movements and faster return to activities[35,43–44].

The position of the camera port varies according to the surgeon's experience and training and can be broadly divided into anterior, posterior and uniportal approaches.

Posterior approach

In the posterior approach, the surgeon and the assistant are positioned on the back of the patient normally with one screen positioned at each side of the head of the table. Commonly an optic with 30 or 0 degree angle is used[45].

A 5-cm utility port incision is made in the 6th or 7th intercostal space in front of the anterior border of the latissimus dorsi muscle. The camera is temporarily introduced through this port to facilitate safe creation of a 1.5-cm incision posteriorly in the auscultatory triangle at the point nearest to the upper end of the oblique fissure. A port is inserted to accommodate the camera, which is positioned in this posterior port for the remainder of the procedure. A further 2-cm port can be created in the midaxillary line at the level of the upper third of the anterior utility port. The anterior and posterior ports lie at opposite ends of the oblique fissure. The upper anterior port is converted into a utility incision for major procedures to permit retrieval of large specimens.

Advantages: There is easy access to the posterior hilum including the bronchial branches and the pulmonary arteries. The lymph nodes are better seen, and tips of the instruments are coming towards the camera, which provides safe dissection.

Pitfalls: The position of the camera implies that for major procedures the instruments get moved towards the optics, making it a very difficult technique to learn and thus creating a steep learning curve. The posterior port may contribute to increased pain due to injury to the intercostal nerve at the narrowest part of the intercostal space, especially if a trocar is used.

Anterior approach

In the anterior approach, the surgeon and the assistant are positioned on the anterior (abdominal) side of the patient and with the surgeon cranially. One or two screens are positioned in front of the surgeon. The scrub nurse is positioned at the back of the patient and follows the operation on a separate screen.

Two port incisions of 1 cm are placed at the anterior axillary line (camera port) and posterior axillary line (tissue retractor port) commonly at the 7th intercostal space. A 5-cm anterolateral utility incision is usually performed at the 4th intercostal space for major procedures[46]. This incision is later used for specimen retrieval. This results in a triangle with two approximately 10-cm limbs and the camera positioned at the apex, with a working channel on each side. With the advent of purposely designed VATS instruments, the posterior port can be omitted with probable impact on post-operative pain[47].

Advantages: The position of the lens makes it easier to learn techniques as surgeons are operating away from the lens rather than towards it. The utility incision is placed directly over the hilum and the major pulmonary vessels, so access to main vessels is easier if control is required in case of bleeding or complex procedures. The first structures to be transected during major lung resections are the hilar structures, and most surgeons have adopted a fissure-less technique to minimize post-operative air leaks. Because of the wider intercostal spaces in the front, the trocar for the camera port is not really necessary, so post-operative pain might be reduced.

The anterior approach is proving an approach that can be reproducible and learnt, allowing more procedures to be performed via VATS. Although very complex procedures or those with very large tumours are probably best served with an open approach, there are no major pitfalls for the anterior VATS approach; the only limitation is that of the operating surgeon's experience.

Uniportal approach

Initially designed for diagnostic procedures, small therapeutic operations via the uniportal technique were described[48]. Now, with the improvement in surgeons' skills and the development of curved VATS-designed instruments and articulated staplers, major procedures are performed in an increasing number of centers[49–59].

In the single-port VATS approach, the whole procedure is performed via the utility incision ranging from 2.5 to 6 cm depending of the operation to be performed (Figure 4.5a and 4.5b). The incision is made at the level of the 4th intercostal space along the anterior axillary line, in front of the anterior border of the latissimus dorsi muscle. The surgeon is positioned in front of the patient, cranially; his assistant is positioned at his side, caudally. A screen is positioned in front of the surgeon. The scrub nurse is positioned on the posterior side of the patient. A second screen is positioned in front of the scrub nurse if required. The camera with a 30-degree lens lies on the most posterior end of the wound, and the remaining space is utilized to introduce the instruments (Figure 4.6a). The chest drain is inserted trough this same wound at the end of the procedure (Figure 4.6b).

(a)

(b)

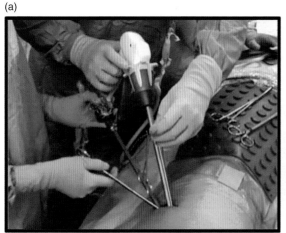
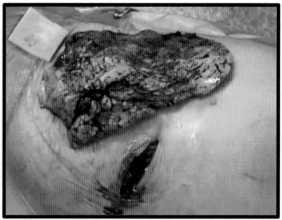

Figure 4.5 Uniportal VATS lobectomy. The anterior incision allows for the placement of multiple instruments and the optics in order to perform the whole procedure (**5a**). The size of the incision has to allow retrieval of the specimen (**5b**).

(a)

(b)

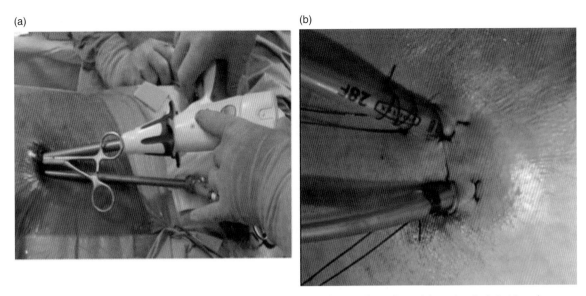

Figure 4.6 Uniportal VATS lung volume reduction surgery. The entire procedure can be performed through a single incision when articulated staplers and VATS-designed instruments are available (**6a**). At the end of the procedure two intercostal drains can be placed in the incision (**6b**).

Advantages: The advantages are the same as the anterior approach, plus the potential for less post-operative pain and better cosmetic results due to a lesser number of incisions[60–61]. Currently, any procedure that can be performed by VATS can be performed with the uniportal technique, and an increasing number of experiences and indications are reported monthly by different surgeons[50–59,62]. The presumed difficulty of performing the whole procedure via a single incision is outweighed by the comfortable view and ergonomics of this approach[63].

Pitfalls: As with any VATS approach, it does require training and carries a learning curve. If performing major pulmonary resections, it is important to place the incision on the 4th intercostal space and not the 5th to allow for division of the pulmonary artery before the superior pulmonary vein to minimize chances of vascular injury during dissection. It does require access to specifically designed VATS instruments and articulated stapler machines, so it might not be universally available.

Hybrid approaches (Figure 4.7)

Ever since the advent of VATS, surgeons have used some of its advantages to assist in open procedures in

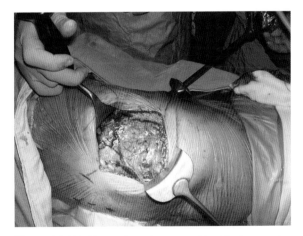

Figure 4.7 Hybrid procedure where an en-bloc lobectomy and chest wall resection was guided by a thoracoscopy.

order to minimize trauma and/or benefit from its view. The size of the incision can be reduced during the use of VATS-assisted thoracotomies with good results[64]. As experience with the use of VATS in more complex procedures grows, the role of combining VATS and open accesses may increase. Authors have described the use of hybrid procedures in lung tumours involving the chest wall by performing the pulmonary resection through VATS and then the chest wall resection and reconstruction via a limited open approach even on superior sulcus tumours[65–67]. We have reported the use of single-port VATS for the confirmation and 'mapping' of the chest wall involvement, thus allowing correct placement of the incision with limitation of trauma to the tissues[68]. Another use of the hybrid techniques is the initial assessment of patients requiring open re-do surgery where dense adhesions are expected and 'blind' re-do thoracotomy could lead to damage to pulmonary parenchyma. With the help of a single-port VATS (whose port will be used for the intercostal drain placement), we can identify the safe area to perform the re-do incision. New hybrid approaches have been described for mediastinal surgery as well [69].

Summary

Thoracic surgery can be performed via a large number of approaches and incisions. All of them do have their advantages and their limitations. The responsibility of the surgeon is to perform the correct procedure for the right indication using the approach that provides the best exposure with the least amount of injury to the patient. For this, important factors to take into account are the surgeon's experience and training, good planning based on the indications for surgery and the patient's status and adequate positioning.

Other approaches such as cervical, supraclavicular or substernal incisions have not been described in this chapter as they are performed less commonly, but they might increase their indications as part of hybrid procedures in the near future[70–72].

References

1   Mitchell R, Angel W, Wuerflein R, Dor V. Simplified lateral chest incision for most thoracotomies other than sternotomy. *Ann Thorac Surg* 1976; 22:284–6.

2   Bethencourt DM, Holmes EC. Muscle-sparing posterolateral thoracotomy. *Ann Thorac Surg* 1988; 45:337–9.

3   Horowitz MD, Ancalmo N, Ochsner JL. Thoracotomy through the ausculatory triangle. *Ann Thorac Surg* 1989; 47:782–3.

4   Ziyade S, Baskent A, Tanju S, et al. Isokinetic muscle strength after thoracotomy: standard vs. muscle-sparing posterolateral thoracotomy. *Thorac Cardiovasc Surg* 2010; 58(5):295–8.

5   Hazelrigg SR, Landreneau RJ, Boley TM, et al. The effect of muscle-sparing versus standard posterolateral thoracotomy on pulmonary function, muscle strength, and postoperative pain. *J Thorac Cardiovasc Surg* 1991; 101(3):394–400; discussion 400–1.

6   Athanassiadi K, Kakaris S, Theakos N, Skottis I. Muscle-sparing versus posterolateral thoracotomy: a prospective study. *Eur J Cardiothorac Surg* 2007;

31(3):496–9; discussion 499–500. Epub 2007 Jan 22.

7   Nazarian I, Down G, Lau OJ. Pleurectomy through the triangle of auscultation for treatment of recurrent pneumothorax in younger patients. *Arch Surg* 1988; 123:11.

8   Li S, Feng Z, Wu L, et al. Analysis of 11 trials comparing muscle-sparing with posterolateral thoracotomy. *Thorac Cardiovasc Surg* 2014 Jun; 62(4):344–52. doi: 10.1055/s-0033-1337445. Epub 2013 Apr 1. Review.

9   Becker RM, Munro DD. Transaxillary minithoracotomy: the optimal approach for certain pulmonary and mediastinal lesions. *Ann Thorac Surg* 1976; 22:254–9.

10 Ochroch EA, Gottschalk A, Augoustides JG, et al. Pain and physical function are similar following axillary, muscle-sparing vs posterolateral thoracotomy. *Chest* 2005; 128(4):2664–70.

11 Freixinet JL, Canalís E, Juliá G, et al. Axillary thoracotomy versus videothoracoscopy for the treatment of primary spontaneous pneumothorax. *Ann Thorac Surg* 2004; 78(2):417–20.

12 Han S, Yildirim E, Dural K, et al. Transaxillary approach in thoracic outlet syndrome: the importance of resection of the first-rib. *Eur J Cardiothorac Surg* 2003; 24(3):428–33.

13 Meng RL, Jensik RJ, Kittle CF, Faber LP. Median sternotomy for synchronous bilateral pulmonary operations. *J Thorac Cardiovasc Surg* 1980; 80(1):1–7.

14 Urschel HC Jr, Razzuk MA. Median sternotomy as a standard approach for pulmonary resection. *Ann Thorac Surg* 1986; 41(2):130–4.

15 Martin-Ucar AE, Stewart DJ, West KJ, Waller DA. A median sternotomy approach to right extrapleural pneumonectomy for mesothelioma. *Ann Thorac Surg* 2005; 80(3):1143–5.

16 Edwards JG, Martin-Ucar AE, Stewart DJ, Waller DA. Right extrapleural pneumonectomy for malignant mesothelioma via median sternotomy or thoracotomy? Short- and long-term results. *Eur J Cardiothorac Surg* 2007; 31(5):759–64.

17 Asaph JW, Handy JR Jr, Grunkemeier GL, et al. Median sternotomy versus thoracotomy to resect primary lung cancer:

analysis of 815 cases *Ann Thorac Surg* 2000; 70(2):373–9.

18 Welti H. Upper median sternotomy in the treatment of mediastinal tumors; 7 personal cases. *Mem Acad Chir (Paris)* 1950 14–21; 76(22–23):638–54.

19 Zacharias A, Habib RH. Factors predisposing to median sternotomy complications. Deep vs superficial infection. *Chest* 1996; 110(5):1173–8.

20 Robicsek F, Daugherty HK, Cook JW. The prevention and treatment of sternum separation following open-heart surgery. *J Thorac Cardiovasc Surg* 1977; 73:267.

21 Bains MS, Ginsberg RJ, Jones WG 2nd, et al. The clamshell incision: an improved approach to bilateral pulmonary and mediastinal tumor. *Ann Thorac Surg* 1994; 58(1):30–2; discussion 33.

22 Germain A, Monod R. Bilateral transversal anterior thoracotomy with sternotomy; indications and technics. *J Chir (Paris)* 1956; 72(8–9):593–611.

23 Bains MS, Ginsberg RJ, Jones II WG, et al. The Clamshell incision: an improved approach to bilateral pulmonary and mediastinal tumor. *Ann Thorac Surg* 1994; 58:30–3.

24 Sarkaria IS, Bains MS, Sood S, et al. Resection of primary mediastinal non-seminomatous germ cell tumors: a 28-year experience at Memorial Sloan-Kettering Cancer Center. *J Thorac Oncol* 2011; 6(7):1236–41.

25 Macchiarini P, Ladurie FL, Cerrina J, et al. Clamshell or sternotomy for double lung or heart-lung transplantation? *Eur J Cardiothorac Surg* 1999; 15(3):333–9.

26 Dartevelle Fg, Chapelier AR, Macchiarini P. Anterior transcervical-thoracic approach for radical resection of lung

tumors invading the thoracic inlet. *J Thorac Cardiovasc Surg* 1993; 105:1025.

27 Lucà F, van Garsse L, Rao CM, et al. Minimally invasive mitral valve surgery: a systematic review. *Minim Invasive Surg* 2013; 179569. Epub 2013 Mar 27.

28 Schuchert MJ, Souza AP, Abbas G, et al. Extended Chamberlain minithoracotomy: a safe and versatile approach for difficult lung resections. *Ann Thorac Surg* 2012; 93(5):1641–5; discussion 1646.

29 Rocco G, Internullo E, Cassivi SD, et al. The variability of practice in minimally invasive thoracic surgery for pulmonary resections. *Thorac Surg Clin* 2008; 18(3):235–47.

30 Onaitis MW, Petersen RP, Balderson SS, et al. Thoracoscopic lobectomy is a safe and versatile procedure: experience with 500 consecutive patients. *Ann Surg* 2006; 244:420–5.

31 Nwogu CE, Yendamuri S, Demmy TL. Does thoracoscopic pneumonectomy for lung cancer affect survival? *Ann Thorac Surg* 2010; 89:S2102–6.

32 McKenna RJ Jr, Houck W, Fuller CB. Video-assisted thoracic surgery lobectomy: experience with 1,100 cases. *Ann Thorac Surg* 2006; 81:421–5.

33 Nagahiro I, Andou A, Aoe M, et al. Pulmonary function, postoperative pain, and serum cytokine level after lobectomy: a comparison of VATS and conventional procedure. *Ann Thorac Surg* 2001; 72:362–5.

34 Demmy TL, Curtis JJ Minimally invasive lobectomy directed toward frail and high-risk patients: a case-control study. *Ann Thorac Surg* 1999; 68:194–200.

35 Atkins B, Harpole D, Mangum J, et al. Pulmonary segmentectomy by thoracotomy or thoracoscopy: reduced hospital length of stay with a minimally-invasive

approach. *Ann Thorac Surg* 2007; 84:1107–13.

36 Nakas A, Klimatsidas MN, Entwisle J, et al. Video-assisted versus open pulmonary metastasectomy: the surgeon's finger or the radiologist's eye? *Eur J Cardiothorac Surg* 2009; 36(3):469–74.

37 Lin JC, Wiechmann RJ, Szwerc MF, et al. Diagnostic and therapeutic video-assisted thoracic surgery resection of pulmonary metastases. *Surgery* 1999; 126(4):636–41; discussion 641–2.

38 Gaunt A, Martin-Ucar AE, Beggs L, et al. Residual apical space following surgery for pneumothorax increases the risk of recurrence. *Eur J Cardiothorac Surg* 2008; 34(1):169–73.

39 Nakas A, Martin Ucar AE, Edwards JG, Waller DA. The role of video assisted thoracoscopic pleurectomy/decortication in the therapeutic management of malignant pleural mesothelioma. *Eur J Cardiothorac Surg* 2008; 33(1):83–8.

40 Tong BC, Hanna J, Toloza EM, et al. Outcomes of video-assisted thoracoscopic decortication. *Ann Thorac Surg* 2010; 89(1):220–5.

41 Loscertales J, Congregado M, Jiménez Merchán R. First rib resection using videothorascopy for the treatment of thoracic outlet syndrome. *Arch Bronconeumol* 2011; 47(4):204–7.

42 Zahid I, Sharif S, Routledge T, Scarci M. Video-assisted thoracoscopic surgery or transsternal thymectomy in the treatment of myasthenia gravis? *Interact Cardiovasc Thorac Surg* 2011; 12(1):40–6.

43 Li WW, Lee RL, Lee TW, et al. The impact of thoracic surgical access on early shoulder function: video-assisted thoracic surgery versus posterolateral

thoracotomy. *Eur J Cardiothorac Surg* 2003; 23:390–6.

44 Paul S, Altorki NK, Sheng S, et al. Thoracoscopic lobectomy is associated with lower morbidity than open lobectomy: a propensity-matched analysis from the STS database. *J Thorac Cardiovasc Surg* 2010; 139(2):366–78.

45 Richards JMJ, Dunning J, Oparka J, et al. Video-assisted thoracoscopic lobectomy: the Edinburgh posterior approach. *Ann Cardiothorac Surg* 2012; 1(1):61–9.

46 Hansen HJ, Petersen RH. Video-assisted thoracoscopic lobectomy using a standardized three-port anterior approach: the Copenhagen experience. *Ann Cardiothorac Surg* 2012; 1(1):70–6.

47 Burfeind WR, D'Amico TA. Thoracoscopic lobectomy – operative techniques. *Thorac Cardiovasc Surg* 2004; 9:98–114.

48 Rocco G, Martin-Ucar A, Passera E. Uniportal VATS wedge pulmonary resections. *Ann Thorac Surg* 2004; 77(2):726–8.

49 Gonzalez-Rivas D, Fernandez R, de la Torre M, Martin-Ucar AE. Thoracoscopic lobectomy through a single incision. *MMCTS* 2012; mms007.

50 Rocco G. Single-port video-assisted thoracic surgery (uniportal) in the routine general thoracic surgical practice. *Op Techn Thorac Cardiovasc Surg* 2009; 14:326–35.

51 Jin CH, Liu K, Yu KZ, et al. The use of single incision thoracoscopic surgery in diagnostic and therapeutic thoracic surgical procedures. *Thorac Cardiovasc Surg* 2014 Aug; 62(5):439–44. doi: 10.1055/s-0032-1327764. Epub 2013 Mar 8.

52 Marra A, Huenermann C, Ross B, Hillejan L. Management of pleural empyema with single-port video-

assisted thoracoscopy. *Innovations (Phila)* 2012; 7(5):338–45.

53 Kilic D, Dursun P, Ayhan A. Single port video-assisted thoracoscopy for the management of pleural effusion in ovarian carcinoma. *J Obstet Gynaecol* 2013; 33(1):98–9.

54 Ng CS, Lau KK, Wong RH, et al. Single port video-assisted thoracoscopic lobectomy for early stage non-small cell lung carcinoma. *Surgical Practice* 2013; 17:35–6.

55 Chen CH, Lee SY, Chang H, et al. Technical aspects of single-port thoracoscopic surgery for lobectomy. *J Cardiothorac Surg* 2012; 7:50.

56 Apiliogullari B, Esme H, Yoldas B, et al. Early and midterm results of single-port video-assisted thoracoscopic sympathectomy. *Thorac Cardiovasc Surg* 2012; 60:285–9.

57 Kang do K, Min HK, Jun HJ, et al. Single-port video-assisted thoracic surgery for lung cancer. *Korean J Thorac Cardiovasc Surg* 2013; 46(4):299–301.

58 Wang BY, Tu CC, Liu CY, et al. Single-incision thoracoscopic lobectomy and segmentectomy with radical lymph node dissection. *Ann Thorac Surg* 2013; 96(3):977–82.

59 Rocco G, Martucci N, La Manna C, et al. Ten-year experience on 644 patients undergoing single-port (uniportal) video-assisted thoracoscopic surgery. *Ann Thorac Surg* 2013; 96(2):434–8.

60 Jutley RS, Khalil MW, Rocco G. Uniportal vs standard three-port VATS technique for spontaneous pneumothorax: comparison of post-operative pain and residual paraesthesia. *Eur J Cardiothorac Surg* 2005; 28:43–6.

61 Tamura M, Shimizu Y, Hashizume Y. Pain following thoracoscopic

surgery: retrospective analysis between single-incision and three-port video-assisted thoracoscopic surgery. *J Cardiothorac Surg* 2013; 12(8):153.

62 Gonzalez-Rivas D, Fernandez R, Fieira E, Rellan L. Uniportal video-assisted thoracoscopic bronchial sleeve lobectomy: first report. *J Thorac Cardiovasc Surg* 2013; 145:1676–7.

63 Bertolaccini L, Rocco G, Viti A, Terzi A. Geometrical characteristics of uniportal VATS. *J Thorac Dis* 2013; 5(Suppl 3): S214–6.

64 Giudicelli R, Thomas P, Lonjon T, et al. Video-assisted minithoracotomy versus muscle-sparing thoracotomy for performing lobectomy. *Ann Thorac Surg* 1994; 58: 712–717; discussion 717–718.

65 Berry MF, Onaitis MW, Tong BC, et al. Feasibility of hybrid thoracoscopic lobectomy and en-bloc chest wall resection. *Eur J Cardiothorac Surg* 2012; 41(4):888–92.

66 Demmy TL, Nwogu CE, Yendamuri S. Thoracoscopic chest wall resection: what is its role? *Ann Thorac Surg* 2010; 89(6):S2142–5.

67 Shikuma K, Miyahara R, Osako T. Transmanubrial approach combined with video-assisted approach for superior sulcus tumors. *Ann Thorac Surg* 2012; 94(1):e29–30.

68 Bayarri CI, de Guevara AC, Martin-Ucar AE. Initial single-port thoracoscopy to reduce surgical trauma during open en bloc chest wall and pulmonary resection for locally invasive cancer. *Interact Cardiovasc Thorac Surg* 2013; 17(1):32–5.

69 Zieliński M, Kuzdzał J, Szlubowski A, Soja J. Transcervical-subxiphoid-videothoracoscopic 'maximal' thymectomy–operative technique

and early results. *Ann Thorac Surg* 2004; 78(2):404–9; discussion 409–10.

70 Chamberlain MH, Fareed K, Nakas A, et al. Video-assisted cervical thoracoscopy: a novel approach for diagnosis, staging and pleurodesis of malignant pleural mesothelioma. *Eur J Cardiothorac Surg* 2008; 34(1):200–3.

71 Zieliński M. Video-assisted mediastinoscopic lymphadenectomy and transcervical extended mediastinal lymphadenectomy. *Thorac Surg Clin* 2012; 22(2):219–25.

72 Leschber G, Holinka G, Linder A. Video-assisted mediastinoscopic lymphadenectomy (VAMLA) – a method for systematic mediastinal lymphnode dissection. *Eur J Cardiothorac Surg* 2003; 24(2):192–5.

Chapter

5

Therapeutic bronchoscopy

Keyvan Moghissi

Background introduction

The celebrated American oto-rhino-laryngologist Chevalier Jackson[1] has been an important player in the field of bronchoscopy since the 1920s. His instrument, with a few modifications, became what is basically the rigid bronchoscope (RB) of today. By the 1950s, bronchoscopy became a well-established procedure, and every trainee thoracic surgeon had to be proficient in diagnostic and therapeutic bronchoscopy, the latter being confined to foreign body (FB) removal, clearing the tracheo-bronchial tree of secretions, cauterization of bleeding tumours and therapeutic bronchial lavage.

The flexible fibreoptic bronchoscope (FFB) was developed in the 1960s, the first instrument being designed by the Japanese, Shigeto Ikeda[2]. Its flexibility allowed examination of segmental bronchi. Until then this had only been possible with the use of straight and right-angled telescopes introduced through the rigid bronchoscope. The ease of FFB bronchoscopy under topical anaesthesia and sedation attracted respiratory physicians, and for thoracic surgeons, the flexible instrument became an important addition to bronchoscopic instrumentation for use independently or in conjunction with the rigid instrument. At present, for the thoracic surgeon, the two instruments are complementary to one another, and skills in both are necessary for the diagnosis of endobronchial lesions and for therapeutic endoscopic interventions.

Instrumentation and general principles of therapeutic bronchoscopy

Rigid bronchoscope (RB)

RB alone, or in conjunction with the FFB, remains the instrument of choice and sine qua non of many therapeutic bronchoscopies. Accessory devices include a range of forceps for grasping, provision of biopsy and/or punching/coring out tumours, dilators and diathermy probes. In addition, operative bronchoscopes have been designed for specific interventions such as lasertherapy[3,4]. Rigid bronchoscopy is performed under general anaesthetic during which ventilation is provided most effectively by hand-operated (Sander's) injectors or jet ventilation. The author's preference is the injector, since it allows effective control by the anaesthetist.

Flexible fibreoptic bronchoscope (FFB)

There are now a number of FFBs available with various accessory devices, such as biopsy forceps, needles for injection, aspirators and dilators.

FFB offers a recording system and monitor for live viewing and storing of bronchoscopic events. It can incorporate a fluorescence imaging system for auto-fluorescence bronchoscopy (AFB), which is several times more sensitive than white light in imaging pre- and early neoplastic endobronchial lesions.

FFB is essentially a diagnostic tool, which can be used under local/topical anaesthetic and sedation. Some models provide facilities for delivery devices for some of the therapeutic endoscopic methods. However, its use alone for interventional bronchoscopy, though publicized by some, can be uncomfortable for both patient and operator. Also, it can prove hazardous if there is bleeding which requires rapid clearance or control, and it can hinder a procedure when there are copious bronchial secretions which, in some patients, make the operation akin to an 'underwater' undertaking. This is because the suction channel is too narrow to be efficient for serious volume and high-viscosity secretions.

Core Topics in Thoracic Surgery, ed. Marco Scarci, Aman Coonar, Tom Routledge and Francis Wells. Published by Cambridge University Press. © Cambridge University Press 2016

For many therapeutic bronchoscopies, the combined use of RB-FFB under general anaesthetic is the ideal method of practice. This allows comfort for patient and operator, efficient visualization of the lesion using white light and fluorescence bronchoscopy, precise targeting and application of the delivery device undisturbed by cough or bronchial secretion. It is important to note that such a method is not incompatible with treatment being undertaken as a day-case procedure.

Therapeutic bronchoscopic methods

This chapter will describe the most frequently used methods of therapeutic bronchoscopy, particularly those for which important experience is available to be relied upon. Nevertheless, mention is made of methods which are less universally employed. (Table 5.1) Available therapeutic bronchoscopic methods include

- Bronchial cleansing and lavage
- Retrieval of foreign bodies (FB)
- Cryotherapy
- Electrocautery
- Argon plasma coagulation
- Radiofrequency ablation
- CO_2 laser
- Neodymium–yttrium aluminium garnet (Nd:YAG) radiation
- Intraluminal radiotherapy/brachytherapy
- Photodynamic therapy (PDT)
- Stent

Table 5.1 Classification of therapeutic bronchoscopy

i	Mechanical	Cleaning of bronchial tree/bronchial lavage Retrieval of FB
ii	Thermal	Cryotherapy Electrocautery Plasma argon coagulator Radiofrequency CO_2 laser Nd:YAG laser
iii	Biological (cancer-specific methods)	Brachytherapy PDT
iv		Stents

The basis for selecting a method for a given patient is governed by

- The morphology of the lesion within the bronchial lumen
- The histopathology of the lesion
- The objective of therapy
- The experience of the operator

Mechanical methods
Bronchoscopic clearing of the airway

This is one of the simplest of procedures, commonly practiced by thoracic surgeons in patients with retention of secretions after pulmonary resection. When seriously tenacious secretions are present, the FFB is often inappropriate and ineffective. Passing a RB down the upper airway of a patient under topical anaesthetic is a simple and easy procedure to master. This is even easier when the patient is sitting up in bed.

Bronchoscopy and suction of copious secretions in patients with collapse (atelectasis) of the residual lobe or even the whole lung is attended by immediate expansion of the lung if sputum retention is recognized early enough before pneumonic consolidation sets in.

Bronchial lavage (synonym: whole lung lavage)

Classically, in this procedure, a large volume (several litres) of normal saline is introduced into the bronchial tree and aspirated. The procedure has been identified for treatment of pulmonary alveolar proteinosis[5,6]. A modification of the technique has also been used for other broncho-pulmonary conditions in which copious purulent secretions teeming with antibiotic-resistant bacteria or fungal organisms cause repeated pulmonary infection (e.g. cystic fibrosis and extensive bronchiectasis). In such cases, lavage, using saline or a suitable aqueous mild antiseptic solution, is instilled into the bronchial tree by repeated injection of 50 ml of solution at body temperature, followed by aspiration. The aim is to thoroughly clear the bronchial tree from debris or purulent and thick secretion.

Foreign-body (FB) retrieval

A variety of FBs have been removed from patients of all ages. The rigid bronchoscope remains the instrument of choice for the purpose, to be used under general anaesthesia. Occasionally, the fibreoptic instrument needs to be used if the FB is in a lobar or segmental bronchi, inaccessible to the rigid instrument.

In theory, the thoracic surgeon should be in a position to introduce a range of rigid scopes which match the size/age of the patient. In practice, however, the contemporary trainee surgeon is not exposed to such a range of patients and should at least be accustomed to adults of either sex, adolescents and teenagers.

Thermal methods

Cryotherapy

Cryotherapy is a treatment which deploys freezing to achieve necrosis of pathological tissues. The method is based on a rapid freeze of less than −40°C, within seconds, followed by a slow thawing, which leads to destruction of the targeted tissue[7].

The mechanism involves the formation of ice crystals both within the cell and in the extracellular compartment.

In addition, there are also vascular effects: vasoconstriction followed by vasodilatation and vascular thrombosis within 6–10 hours. This effect is induced via a probe delivering nitrous oxide (N_2O) which is passed through the bronchoscope.

There are a variety of flexible and rigid cyroprobes to match the FFB or RB.

Indications: Cryotherapy has been used for

- Locally advanced endobronchial tumours, either benign or malignant. In the latter the aim is palliation of symptoms such as dyspnoea or haemoptysis.
- Superficial endobronchial malignant tumours in patients ineligible for surgical resection, where the treatment is undertaken with curative intent.

Cryotherapy can also be used in association with chemo/radiation[8].

Instrumentation/equipment: Bronchoscopic cryotherapy requires

- Bronchoscope: it can be performed under topical anaesthesia using a flexible bronchoscope and flexible cryoprobe[8]. However, many practitioners prefer and advocate the use of general anaesthetic with rigid bronchoscope and a rigid cryoprobe[9].

- Cryotherapy device: This has three components:
  - Cryoprobe: This is the delivery device which targets the tissue to be treated. The rigid probe has an added heating device that the flexible probe does not have.
  - Transfer line: Connects the cryoprobe to the cooling agent (gas cylinder) and the command counsel.
  - The cooling agents: Most often liquid nitrogen (LN_2) or nitrous oxide (N_{20}). The latter is most often used.

Following cryotherapy the patient needs to have repeat bronchoscopy 8–10 days later in order to

- Evaluate the extent of tissue damage/destruction
- Remove debris/slough
- Undertake possible additional treatment cycles

Results: In bulky obstructive endoluminal tumours, subjective and objective improvement is achieved in >70% of patients[10]. In early neoplastic lesions, a long-period complete response has also been reported[9].

Complications: Reactive oedema leading to respiratory complications, haemorrhage and pneumothorax. Overall, it has been reported in 7–10% of cases[10].

Electrocautery/electrodiathermy

This method uses an electric current to generate and deliver heat via a probe in order to coagulate or vaporize the tissue[11]. There are two types of probes: monopolar and bipolar. The later carries high voltage and needs to be used through the RB to achieve vaporization/cutting effect; the monopolar probe can be used through the FFB with a low voltage for hemostasis. The bipolar system can deliver a mixed cutting and coagulation current.

Elecrocautery has been used in patients with haemoptysis; a 70% success rate has been reported[12,13]. It has also been used to vaporize obstructive lesions of the airway. However, the procedure is time-consuming when there is a bulky obstructing tumour within the bronchus.

Argon plasma coagulation (APC)

APC uses high-frequency electric current delivered via ionized argon gas (plasma). The process involves emission of a jet of argon gas which is ionized by a high-voltage discharge (approximately 6 kV). High-frequency electric current is then conducted through the jet of gas resulting in thermal coagulation. There is no physical contact with the lesion, thus enhancing the safety of the procedure. The depth of coagulation is usually only a few millimetres.

Indications: The indication par excellence is coagulation at a distance where the electrodiathermy probe and catheter cannot reach[14]. The second line indication is disposal of superficial and obstructing endoluminal tumours[12,13]. However, for bulky lesions, coagulation needs to be used in conjunction with piecemeal removal. APC is particularly attractive to practitioners wanting to use FFB under topical anaesthetic and sedation.

Equipment: The basic APC system is composed of an argon gas source, a computer-controlled high-frequency electrosurgical generator and the endoscopic probe.

Results: Control of haemoptysis is achieved in over 97% of patients[14]. Recurrence is to be expected in cancer cases, and long-term complete response is rare. Also, the relief of endobronchial obstruction is less effective, requiring a long session and repeat treatment.

Complications: APC is relatively safe and complications are rare. Nevertheless, haemorrhage, perforation, fire and gas embolism have been reported even in some experienced centres.[15]

Radiofrequency ablation (RFA)

Radiofrequency ablation (RFA) is a treatment modality employing an electromagnetic wave with the same frequency band as an electric scalpel commonly used in surgery and a radiofrequency interchange with an electric current. It is a minimally invasive modality. The insertion of the radiofrequency electrode into a tumour generates heat with the effect of tissue heating which induces coagulative necrosis and cell death. The method has been used in hepatic tumours and also peripheral lung tumours under CT guidance[16]. The bronchoscopic use has not had thorough clinical evaluation.

Bronchoscopic laser

The term LASER is an acronym for light amplification by stimulated emission of radiation. In essence, lasers are specific wavelengths of light. However, the term is now more generally used in reference to devices which produce a laser light, which is

- Monochromatic, denoting that the emitted light comprises a single wavelength output;
- Coherent, defining a close phase relationship between all components of the emitted light;
- Collimated, meaning that the radiation propagation is a narrowly confined beam with low divergence.

Different lasers can generate and emit light across a broad range of the electromagnetic spectrum, but it is only those within the ultraviolet, visible light and infrared spectral regions that have found clinical application.

Classification: Lasers may be classified in a number of ways:

- According to wavelength
- Based on their effect on tissue (e.g. thermal/non-thermal)
- Depending on their 'gain medium', that is, the element which generates the laser light

Currently, thermal bronchoscopic laser therapy is performed exclusively with the use of neodimium–yttrium aluminium garnet (Nd:YAG), although CO_2 laser is used by ear nose and throat surgeons for the upper airway.

The basic Nd:YAG laser machine comprises a generator emitting light of 1064 nm (infrared) accommodated within the control console. The emitted light is colourless and, therefore the emission is coupled with a helium-neon aiming beam emitting 630 nm red light. In this way, the Nd:YAG beam can be visibly directed via an appropriate delivery optical fibre. This needs to be coupled with a cooling system.

The mechanism of action is thermal coagulative necrosis and vaporization (ablation) of the tumour using high power at 30–50 watts and pulses of 10–20 seconds.

Indications[17-20]: Bronchoscopic laser is used for

- Benign tumours of major airways, when complete cure can be expected.

- Locally advanced primary endobronchial malignant tumours (i.e. central lung cancer).
- In these, anatomical and functional integrity of the airway is rapidly restored. The method has been, and continues to be, the most important indication in malignant endoluminal obstructive lesions of the airway needing immediate/urgent relief.
- Primary early central lung cancer. This indication has not received general acceptance since the advent of PDT.
- Secondary malignant endoluminal airway lesions.

Method: Nd:YAG laser therapy is best carried out under general anaesthesia using a dedicated rigid instrument, if available. Alternatively, a standard RB-FFB as described previously is employed. After identification of the lesion, its topography and extent, the laser delivery fibre is introduced through the biopsy channel of the FFB instrument. Care is taken to see the distal end of the delivery fibre protruding at least 1 cm beyond the end of the FFB because the intense heat will damage the FFB. The pilot He-Ne beam is activated to show the red circle which is indicative of the firing line of the laser light. Bursts of 4–10 seconds at a power setting of 30–50 watts is delivered over the tumour. The resulting 'soot' and half-burnt tissue are removed using biopsy forceps. The pulses or bursts of energy delivery (power in watts × time in seconds = joules) is continued until all the obstructing lesion is disposed of. When the obstructed lumen of the airway is opened up satisfactorily, the laser radiation is discontinued, and the bronchial tree is thoroughly washed with warm normal saline.

Results: The Nd:YAG laser is the best thermal method for immediate relief of benign and malignant exophytic tumours. It has a long safety and efficacy record. It can easily be used in a day-surgery setting. However, in malignant obstructive lesions it needs to be repeated every 4-6 weeks.[19-21]

Complications are rare in experienced hands. However, rare haemorrhage, perforation and very rarely fire in the airway have been reported[21,22].

Cancer-specific methods (CSM) of therapeutic bronchoscopy

Mechanical and thermal bronchoscopic therapies are designed to eliminate any type of tissue within the lumen of the bronchi, with the objective of relieving obstruction or effecting cure by physical methods. In these methods, the lesion is targeted by the operator with the motto: 'SEE, TARGET, ZAP' (STZ).

CSMs interventional bronchoscopy specifically targets and destroys the malignant tissues. As such, it is endowed with a double targeting mechanism. First is the STZ in which the operator views the lesion and targets it under vision. The second is the ability of the methods and the mechanisms under which they operate to specifically and preferentially target the malignant lesions independent of visual and imaging systems which are operator dependent.

There are two bronchoscopic CSMs, namely, brachytherapy (BT) and photodynamic therapy (PDT). In both of these, patient preparation and lesion assessment, with certain physical measurements, are mandatory prior to treatment in order to plan effective therapy.

Brachytherapy (BT)

BT refers to treatment which places a radioactive source (iridium-192) within the bronchus involved by a malignant tumour, thus providing local radiotherapy[23].

This treatment needs the active participation of a radiotherapist in order to undertake the planning of the radiation dose and number of sessions/fractions to achieve optimal outcome.

The mechanism involved concerns DNA damage resulting in accelerated apoptosis and decrease in cell proliferation.

By convention, BT recognizes three classes which are named according to the level of emitted energy. These are: *low dose rate (LDR), medium dose rate (MDR)* and *high dose rate (HDR)*. The International Commission of Radiation Units defines HDR, which has more advocates than LDR and MDR, as the application of >12 Gy/h with a dose fraction of up to 1,000 cGy.

Patient preparation is an important part of the treatment package, and in stenotic or exophytic lesions, balloon dilatation or preliminary preparation with endoluminal electrodiathermy or laser may become a necessary pre-brachytherapy preparation.

BT can be performed as a day-case procedure using the fibreoptic instrument and with the patient under topical/local anaesthetic.

A wide variety of treatment schedules concerned with number of fractions and total radiation dose have been advocated; each centre will have its own method. In practice, endobronchial brachytherapy is undertaken in many centres by respiratory physicians, in collaboration with a radiation oncologist, who plans the radiotherapy schedule.

Indications and results: Brachytherapy can be used either for palliation or with curative intent. In either of the indications, it is important to evaluate the extent and topography of the tumour, taking account of the previous treatment, particularly External Beam Radiotherapy.

In its palliative role, BT achieves its objective of improving ventilation, cessation of haemoptysis and reduction of dyspnoea[20,23]. In its curative intent role, BT provides long-lasting complete response in over 25% of patients[20,25].

Complications: Brachytherapy under topical anaesthesia is not well tolerated by patients with profuse secretion and in patients with COPD. Temporary pleuritic pain and pneumothorax can occur, the former not infrequently and the latter rarely. Radiation bronchitis, haemoptysis and bronchial fistula are also rare occurrences, with fever and wheeze the usual presentation.

Photodynamic Therapy (PDT)

PDT is a treatment modality which has three components:

- A chemical photosensitizer (the drug)
- An appropriate light whose wavelength matches the absorption bands of the photosensitizer
- Molecular oxygen

The interaction between the drug and the light, in the presence of oxygen, releases cytotoxic species, notably singlet oxygen, which bring about necrosis of the treated cells and tissues.

The mechanism of tissue destruction in PDT involves direct cellular damage, through injury to cell membranes and subcellular structures, and also by vascular ischemic action through vasoconstriction and endothelial damage. In bronchology, PDT is used principally for endo-bronchial malignancies[26].

Bronchoscopic PDT is undertaken as a two-phase process[27]:

1. The first phase: pre-sensitization in which the photosensitizer (PS) is administered intravenously. Time is allowed for the uptake and retention of the PS predominantly in the neoplastic tissue. This 'latent period' is variable according the chemical structure of the PS.

2. The second phase: illumination refers to bronchoscopic exposure of the lesion to light (usually laser light).

At present, the drug commonly used for broncho-scopic PDT is Photofrin (porfimer sodium). This drug is licensed in most countries of the world, including the UK and EU. It is activated by red light in the region of 630 nm.

In practice, pre-sensitization is undertaken using Photofrin at 2 mg/kg/body weight; after a period of between 24 and 72 h, bronchoscopic illumination is undertaken. There are two types of delivery fibres: in one the distal fibre tip is provided with a cylindrical diffuser for interstitial illumination that is inserted into the tumour mass. The other type has an end diffuser (microlens) to allow forward illumination. The method of choice is to carry out bronchoscopic illumination under general anaesthesia using RB-FFB combination (Figure 5.1)[27,28].

Following Illumination, debridement is carried out using the RB's biopsy forceps.

Indications: PDT has been extensively used in a variety of types of lung cancer:

- Locally advanced endobronchial exophytic tumours. The aim in these cases is palliation.
- Early superficial endobronchial carcinoma, with curative intent. This is for patients who are ineligible for surgical resection on account of high co-morbidity and poor general and cardio-pulmonary function.
- Multifocal and metachronous lesions, the latter after major previous resection.
- Salvage PDT in patients unresponsive to chemotherapy.

- Elimination of over- and undergrowth of neoplastic tissue in the airway in patients with an airway stent.

Results: In *locally advanced disease*, PDT achieves the objective of palliation[27,29,30]. Symptomatically, breathing and performance status improve. Anatomically, malignant bronchial obstruction is substantially (>60%) relieved and the lung expands. Physiologically, there is improvement in ventilation and spirometry.

There are very few complications other than photosensitivity skin reaction in bronchoscopic PDT. A review of the literature[29] shows 2% haemorrhage, 3–4% respiratory complications and 11% photosensitivity skin reaction. The latter in centres which are doing PDT fairly routinely is 0–5%[33].

In *early-stage disease*, PDT can achieve total response and clearance for long periods amounting to nearly 60% 5-year survival[28,31-33]. In patients with small superficial or occult bronchial lesions, a figure of 80% 5-year survival has been recorded[31]. Such early and occult cancers often require AFB for their detection[35,36].

Stents

Stents are devices which are fitted within the airway to maintain their luminal opening. Their only function is as an internal splint, and as such, they have no effect on the pathology of the lesion. There are now many different stents, which, at times, makes difficult the choice of stent for a given case. However, this difficulty is rewarded by the availability of a stent for every kind of situation.

Indications: The cardinal indication for stenting is stenosis of the major airway, caused by extrinsic compression by malignant tumour. Other secondary indications highlighted by some authors are

- Endoluminal benign and malignant obstruction.
- Bypassing malignant fistula or covering bronchial dehiscence in cases of bronchopleural fistula. In the opinion of this author, stenting in such cases is only valid when the method is used for short-term palliation, in other words, for malignant cases.

Their more recent use has been in emphysema.

The pathology, topography of the lesion and the objectives of stenting have important consideration in selecting a device prior to embarking on stenting.

Instrumentation and methods: Most, if not all, practitioners concede that the RB is the instrument of choice for use in stenting of trachea and main stem bronchi. The Gianturco stent is designed to be inserted by FFB. General anaesthesia is used with rigid bronchoscopy for insertion of many stents. However, the bronchial stent can be inserted quite easily using FFB under topical anaesthetic.

Types of stent: Basically there are three types of stents:

1. Plastic, most commonly silicone
2. Metallic
3. Combination of plastic and metal

From the topographical point of view, stents are either tracheal, tracheo-bronchial or bronchial. Stents can be life-savers, particularly in an emergency situation and when the trachea and its bifurcation are the start of the obstruction, but unfortunately they have many drawbacks such as migration, obstruction, ulceration and extrusion. There is no ideal stent; a good stent should be selected based on the following criteria:

- Remain in place with no or low migration potential
- Be flexible yet have firmness to maintain the lumen
- Tissue friendly
- Be designed to prevent tumour ingrowth and granulation tissue
- Not be easily blocked by inspicated secretions
- Not cause ulceration and not cause perforation
- Be easily removable and re-insertable

The commonly used stents are

- Montgomery type (T-tube) and its variants[37,38] which are for the trachea and its bifurcation; it is tissue friendly and easy to maintain its position.
- Dumon stent, and its modified subtypes,[39,40] with external studs for major airway; the studs reduce the chance of migration.

45

- Expandable metallic stents (Gianturco) with a single zigzag loop of stainless steel coil[41,42] of which both covered and uncovered types are available. Also, it is possible to place these stents using FFB[43].
- An interesting stent was one developed by Frietag in plastic with loops of metal anterolaterally[44].

Aftercare and complications: All patients with stents of any kind need regular follow-up and check bronchoscopy, inspection and cleaning. Migration, extrusion, granulation tissue formation, bleeding, ingrowth (in particular) and undergrowth by neoplastic tissue have been reported with variable frequency.

References

1 Jackson C. Bronchoscopy, past, present, and future. *New Engl J Med* 1928; 199:759–63.

2 Ikeda S, Tsuboi E. ONO R flexible bronchofiberscope JPN. *J Clin Oncol* 1971; 1:55–65.

3 Bryan-Dumon Rigid Bronchoscope; www.Bryancorp.com/ therpeutic-endoscopy.cfm.

4 Moghissi K, Jessop T, Dench M. A new bronchoscopic set for laser therapy *Thorax* 1986; 41:485–6.

5 Ramirez-Rivera J, Schultz RB, Dutton RE. Pulmonary alveolar proteinosis: a new technique and rationale for treatment. *Archives of Internal Medicine* 1963; 112:173–85.

6 Lippmann M, Mok MS. Aesthetic management of pulmonary lavage in adults. *Anesth Analg* 1977 Sep-Oct; 56(5):661–8.

7 Homasson JP, Renault P, Angebaut M, et al. Bronchoscopic cryotherapy for airway stricture caused by tumours. *Chest* 1986; 90:159–64.

8 Vergnon JM. Cryotherapie endobronchique technique et indication. *Rev Mal Resp* 1999; 16:619–23.

9 Vergnon JM, Huber RM, Moghissi K. Place of cryotherapy, brachytherapy and photodynamic therapy in therapeutic bronchoscopy of lung cancers. *Eur Respir J* 2006; 28:200–18.

10 Maiwand MO, Homasson JP. Cryotherapy for trachea-bronchial

disorders. *Clin Chest Med* 1995; 16:427–43.

11 Hooper RG, Jackson FN. Endobronchial electrocautery. *Chest* 1985; 87:712–14.

12 Sutedja T. Bolliger CT. Endobronchia, elecrocautery and argon plasma coagulation, in Bolligher CT, Mathur PN, Eds., *Interventional Bronchoscopy*, Basel: Karger, 2000, pp 120–32.

13 Bolliger CT, Sutedja TG, Strausz J, Freitag L. Therapeutic bronchoscopy with immediate effect: laser, electrocautery, argan plasma coagulation and stents. *Eur Respir J* 2006; 27:1258–71.

14 Morice RC, Ece T, Ece F, Keus L. Endobronchial argon plasma coagulation for treatment of hemoptysis and neoplastic airway obstruction. *Chest* 2001; 119:781–7.

15 Feddy C, Majid A, Michaud G, et al Gas embolism following bronchoscopic argon plasma coagulation: a case series. *Chest* 2008; 134:1066–9.

16 Carrafiello G, Mangini M, Fontana F, et al. Radiofrequency ablation for single lung tumours not suitable for surgery: seven years experience. *Radiol Med* 2012; 117:1320–32.

17 Shah H, Garbe L, Nussbaum E, et al. Benign tumours of the tracheobronchial tree: endoscopic characteristics and role of laser resection. *Chest* 1995; 107:1744–51.

18 Toty L, Personne C, Colchen A, Vourch G. Bronchoscopic

management of tracheal lesions using Nd:YAG laser. *Thorax* 1981; 36(3):175–8.

19 Cavaliere S, Foccoli P, Farina P. Nd:YAG laser bronchoscopy: a 5 years experience with 1,396 applications in 1,000 patients. *Chest* 1988; 94:15–21.

20 Moghissi K, Dixon K. Bronchoscopic Nd:YAG laser treatment in lung cancer, 30 years on: an institutional review. *Lasers Med Sci* 2006; 2:186–91.

21 Personne C, Colchen A, Leroy M, et al. Indications and technique for endoscopic laser resections in bronchology: a critical analysis based upon 2284 resections. *J Thorac Cardiovasc Surg* 1986; 91:710–5.

22 Casey KR, Fairfax WR, Smith SJ, Dixon JA. Intratracheal fire ignited by the Nd:YAG laser during treatment of tracheal stenosis. *Chest* 1983; 84:295–6.

23 Macha HN, Freith GL, The role of brachytherapy in the treatment of central bronchial carcinoma. *Monaldi Arch Chest Dis* 1996; 151:325–8.

24 Macha HN, Wahlers B, Relchele G, von Zwehl D . Endobronchial radiation therapy for obstructing malignancies; ten years experience with irridium-192 high-dose. *Lung* 1995: 173:871–80.

25 Saito M, Yokoyama A, Kurita Y, et al. Treatment of roengenologically occult endobronchial carcinoma with external beam radiotherapy and Intraluminal low dose

brachytherapy. *Int J Radiat Oncol Bio Phys* 1996; 34:1029–35.

26 Castano AP, Demidova TN, Hamblin MR. Mechanisms in photodynamic therapy: 2. Cellular signalling, cell metabolism and mode of cell death. *Photodiagn Photodyn Ther* 2005; 2:1–23.

27 Moghissi K, Dixon K, Stringer MR, et al. The place of bronchoscopic photodynamic therapy in advanced unresectable lung cancer: experience with 100 cases. *Eur J Cardiothorac Surg* 1999; 15:1–6.

28 Moghissi K, Dixon K, Thorpe JA, et al. Photodynamic therapy in early central lung cancer: a treatment option for patients ineligible for surgical resection. *Thorax* 2007; 5:391.5.

29 Moghissi K, Dixon K. Is bronchoscopic photodynamic therapy a therapeutic option in lung cancer? *Eur Resp J* 2003; 22:535–41.

30 Moghissi K, Dixon K, Thorpe JAC, et al. Photodynamic therapy (PDT) for lung cancer: the Yorkshire Laser Centre experience. *Photodiagn and Photodyn Ther* 2004; 1:49–55.

31 Hayata Y, Kato H, Furuse K, et al. Photodynamic therapy of 169 early stage cancer of the lung and oesophagus: a Japanese multi-centre study. *Laser Med Sci* 1996; 11:255–9.

32 Cortese DA, Edell ES, Kinsey JH. Photodyanmic therapy for early stage squamous cell carcinoma of the lung. *Mayo Clin Proc* 1997; 72:595–602.

33 Moghissi K, Dixon K. Update on the current indications, practice and results of photodynamic therapy (PDT) in early central lung cancer. *Photodiagn Photodyn Ther* 2008; 5:10–16.

34 Endo C, Myamato A, Sakurada A, et al. Results of long term follow up of photodynamic therapy for roentergenologically occult bronchogenic squamous cell carcinoma. *Chest* 2009; 136:369–75.

35 Lam S, MacAulay C, Huang J, et al. Detection of dysplasia and carcinoma in situ with lung imaging fluorescence endoscopy device. *J Thorac Cardviocasc Surg* 1993; 105:1035–40.

36 Moghissi K, Dixon K, Stringer MR. Current indications and future prospective of fluorescence bronchoscopy: a review study. *Photodiagn Photodyn Ther* 2008; 5:238–46.

37 Montgomery WW. T-tube tracheal stent. *Arch Otolaryngol* 1965; 82:320–1.

38 Westaby S, Jackson JW, Pearson FG. A bifurcated silicone rubber stent for relief of tracheobronchial obstruction. *J Thorac Cardiovasc Surg* 1982; 83:414–17.

39 Dumon JF. A dedicated tracheobronchial stent. *Chest* 1990; 97:328–32.

40 Tayama K, Eriguchi N, Futamata Y, et al. Modified Dumon stent for the treatment of a bronchopleural fistula after pneumonectomy. *Ann Thorac Surg* 2003; 75:290–2.

41 Wallace MJ, Charnsasavey C, Osawaka K, et al. Tracheo-bronchial tree: expandable metallic stents used in experimental and clinical application. *Radiology* 1986; 309–12.

42 Ushida BT, Putman JS, Rasch J. Modification of Gianturco expandable wire stent. *Am J Roentergenol* 1988; 150:1185–7.

43 Saad CP, Murthy S, Krizmanich G, Mehta AC. Self-expandable metallic airway stents and flexible bronchoscopy: long-term outcomes analysis. *Chest* 2003; 124:1993–9.

44 Freitag L, Ekolf E, Stamatis G, Greschuchna D. Clinical evaluation of a new bifurcated dynamic airway stent: a five-year experience in 135 patients. *Thorac Cardiovasc Surgeon* 1997; 45:6–12.

Further reading

Bolliger CT, Mathur PN, Beamis JF, et al. ERS/EACTS statement on interventional pulmonary. Eur Resp Society/American Thoracic Society. *Euro Respir J* 2002; 19:356.

British Thoracic Society guideline for advanced diagnostic and therapeutic flexible bronchoscopy in adults. November 2011; Vol 66 Supple 3.

Chhajed PN, Malouf MA, Tamm M, Glanville AR. Ultraflex stents for the management of airway complications in lung transplant recipients. *Respirology* 2003; 8:59–64.

Ibrahim E. Bronchial stents. *Ann Thorac Med* 2006; 1:92–7.

Wood DE, Liiu YH, Vallieres E, et al. Airway stenting for malignant and benign tracheobronchial stenosis. *Ann Thorac Surg* 2003; 76:167–72.

Chapter

6

Tracheal stenosis, masses and tracheoesophageal fistula

Timothy M. Millington and Douglas J. Mathisen

Like any hollow viscus in the face of untreated pathology, the trachea can over time develop either symptomatic obstruction or fistula into an adjacent space. Tracheal lesions can be divided according to these two mechanisms.

Obstructive lesions of the trachea (stenosis and masses)

A narrowing of greater than 50% of the cross-sectional area of the trachea by a mass or stricture is necessary before a patient experiences dyspnea at rest. The typical presentation of chronic or subacute tracheal obstruction is the insidious onset of wheezing and shortness of breath that may evolve to stridor and respiratory distress. The finding of tracheal narrowing may not be seen on chest radiographs. Many patients initially receive incorrect diagnoses of asthma or chronic obstructive pulmonary disease and are often treated unsuccessfully with bronchodilators or steroids. Patients with malignant tracheal tumours may report associated hemoptysis and hoarseness, often with a more rapid onset of symptoms.

Axial imaging by computed tomography has superseded linear tracheal tomograms as the imaging study of choice. Three-dimensional reconstruction of images obtained by CT allows virtual bronchoscopy to identify and localize tracheal lesions. Inspiratory and expiratory CT scans are useful to demonstrate tracheomalacia. Pulmonary function testing demonstrating an obstructive pattern may help to suggest the diagnosis but is of limited use in operative planning. Patients with a central airway obstruction will benefit from treatment regardless of pre-operative pulmonary function tests (PFTs).

Bronchoscopy is the mainstay of diagnosis. Relative to flexible bronchoscopy, rigid bronchoscopy with

general anaesthesia provides better visualization and control of the airway, precise measurement of laryngotracheal pathology and improved access for biopsy. Rigid bronchoscopy also permits debulking of tracheal lesions and improves tracheal dilatation. Flexible bronchoscopy without the availability of rigid bronchoscopy should be undertaken with caution because of the risk that endoscopic manipulation may lead to abrupt worsening of critical airway stenosis.

Obstructive lesions

Obstructive lesions of the trachea may be extrinsic, intramural or intraluminal. *Extrinsic lesions* causing tracheal compression include thyroid masses, congenital vascular rings and mediastinal masses. Inflammatory diseases of the mediastinum including tuberculosis, histoplasmosis, sarcoidosis and Wegener's granulomatosis may also lead to extrinsic tracheal obstruction due to lymphadenopathy and fibrosis. Treatment of the underlying cause of extrinsic compression is necessary and usually sufficient to relieve symptoms.

Intramural lesions

Replacement of the normal architecture of the trachea by scar tissue may be post-traumatic (including iatrogenic), inflammatory or idiopathic.

Post-intubation stenosis

Stenosis as a late complication of endotracheal intubation was reported after the widespread use of plastic endotracheal tubes from the 1960s. Use of high-volume, low-pressure cuffs (20–25 mmHg) and tolerance for small cuff leaks in adequately ventilated patients have reduced but not eliminated this complication. Endotracheal tubes may ultimately create

Core Topics in Thoracic Surgery, ed. Marco Scarci, Aman Coonar, Tom Routledge and Francis Wells. Published by Cambridge University Press. © Cambridge University Press 2016

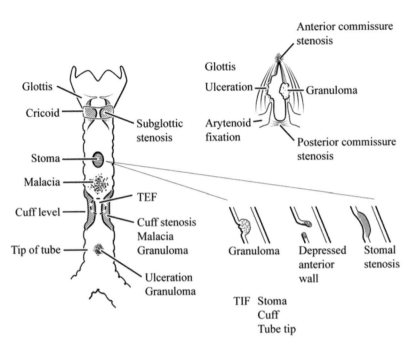

Figure 6.1 Post-intubation tracheal stenosis may occur at various points in the airway, from the point where an orotracheal tube passes through the vocal cords to the contact point between the tube tip and the distal trachea. [From Grillo H (Ed.), *Surgery of the Trachea and Bronchi*. 2004: BC Decker, Inc, Hamilton, Ontario.]

stenoses at various levels including the larynx, the inflatable cuff and the tip of the tube (Figure 6.1).

Laryngeal stenosis
The prolonged presence of an orotracheal tube passing through the vocal cords causes mucosal irritation, which can lead to edema, ulceration, granulation tissue formation and ultimately subglottic stenosis. Tracheostomy generally prevents this complication, although in kyphotic patients pressure on the anterior cricoid may still occur. Laryngeal stenosis in patients with tracheostomy may occur due to infection. Smaller-sized tubes should be used to avoid excessive pressure on the larynx and subglottis.

Obstruction at the site of a stoma
Formation of bulky granulation tissue at the site of a stoma may occur unrecognized while a tracheostomy tube is in place and lead to airway obstruction immediately after tube removal. Later, the defect through which the tube was placed heals by scarring and contraction. This process converts the cross section of the trachea at the site of the stoma from a C to an A shape with resultant narrowing. This phenomenon is magnified by the presence of an excessively large stoma, either from technical error at the time of surgery or excessive traction from the tube.

Infrastomal lesions
Cuff stenosis is the most common complication of prolonged intubation. Pressure necrosis of the tracheal mucosa leads to ulceration and tracheitis and ultimately

to erosion of the underlying cartilaginous rings and dense fibrosis of the airway. Prior to the introduction of low-pressure cuffs, the incidence of symptomatic tracheal stenosis was as high as 20% following prolonged intubation. Prolonged high cuff pressure may also lead to tracheoesophageal fistula (described later) or tracheo-innominate fistula.

Tracheal narrowing may occur due to granulation tissue deposition at the site of contact between the tip of the endotracheal tube and the trachea. This complication is less common with modern, concentrically expanding cuff balloons because contact between the tube tip and tracheal wall is limited.

Management
Because many survivors of prolonged intubation have complex medical problems, conservative management of post-intubation stenosis is often initially favored. Repetitive dilatation or laser ablation may be successful in some patients. Airway patency can be maintained indefinitely by creating a new tracheostomy and using a T-tube to splint the airway open. The sidearm of the T-tube is kept closed and used to access the trachea for cleaning and for periodic T-tube changes as necessary. In placing a T-tube, the stoma should be created through the most damaged part of the trachea to preserve viable trachea for future reconstruction.

Carefully selected patients can be managed by tracheal resection and reconstruction (described later) with a success rate exceeding 95%. Expandable stents are generally contraindicated in benign stenosis. Stents can

49

lead to the deposition of granulation tissue proximal and distal to the stent, potentially converting a short, resectable lesion into a long, unresectable one.

Traumatic tracheal stenosis

Blunt injury to the trachea, carina or bronchi may initially go unrecognized. There is usually a history of pneumothorax, frequently bilateral, requiring tube thoracostomy. Tracheostomy below the level of injury may have been performed. Over time the injured segment of trachea becomes stenotic, and if a tracheostomy is present, the upper airway may become totally occluded. Treatment is by surgical repair several months after injury when local inflammation has subsided.

Stenosis due to inhalation injury

Chemical or thermal injury due to the upper airway is challenging to manage. Injury is usually confined to the subglottic and tracheal mucosa, sparing the tracheal rings. Whereas the pharynx and supraglottic larynx often heal without functional deficit, the subglottic airway may develop fibrosis that is difficult to distinguish from intubation-related stenosis. Protecting the airway carefully with silicone T-tubes permits resection and reconstruction, if needed, to be deferred until inflammation has resolved – often many months later.

Post-therapeutic

Recurrent tracheal stenosis may be a late complication of tracheal resection and reconstruction. This can be caused by interruption of the blood supply, excessive anastomotic tension, granulation tissue or recurrence of primary disease. Reconstruction following radiotherapy should be approached with great caution but is feasible in highly selected patients. Careful assessment of the tracheal architecture is essential. The anastomosis should be covered with well-vascularized tissue – either muscle or omentum – to buttress and aid healing.

Stenosis due to infection

Tuberculous infection of the upper airways may lead to ulcerative tracheitis that progresses to long-segment circumferential fibrosis. Surgical treatment is complicated by the length of the lesion and the presence of ongoing inflammation. Complete eradication of infecting organisms and repeated dilation is the usual treatment. Infection with *Histoplama capsulatum* can lead to fibrotic replacement of mediastinal structures, including the trachea and bronchial tree. Enlarged, fibrotic mediastinal lymph nodes due to histoplasmosis may lead to extrinsic airway compression.

Other causes of tracheal stenosis

Relapsing polychondritis is a systemic condition in which cartilaginous structures become inflamed and fibrotic. When the cartilaginous rings of the trachea are affected, the result is progressive stenosis. Wegener's granulomatosis, sarcoidosis and amyloidosis may also affect the trachea. Because of the diffuse, systemic nature of these diseases, surgical resection and reconstruction are is frequently impossible, and palliative management with a silicone T-tube may be preferable.

Idiopathic tracheal stenosis

Stenosis of the trachea may occur without an antecedent history of trauma, intubation or inflammatory disease. The majority of affected patients are women in the third to fifth decades of life. Symptoms may develop rapidly over a few months or insidiously over years. Most lesions of idiopathic tracheal stenosis are short (1–3 cm), circumferential and centred at the junction between cricoid cartilage and trachea. The subglottic location of these lesions frequently mandates complex laryngotracheal resection (described later). High lesions may require resurfacing of the posterior cricoid plate with a membranous wall tracheal flap.

Intraluminal obstruction (tracheal masses)

Primary neoplasms of the trachea are rare, comprising 1% of bronchial tumours and 2% of upper respiratory tract tumours. In adults, malignant tumours are significantly more common that benign lesions, whereas in children the reverse is true.

Malignant tracheal tumours

Malignant tumours of the trachea are roughly evenly divided between squamous cell carcinoma and adenoid cystic carcinoma. Other primary malignant masses have been described including carcinoid tumours, adenocarcinoma, malignant fibrous histiocytomas and

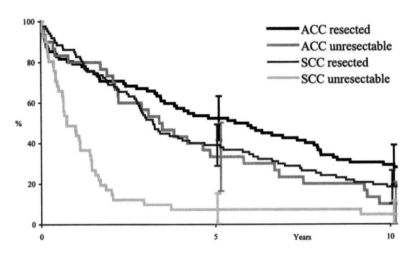

Figure 6.2 Long-term survival after operative and non-operative treatment of adenoid cystic carcinoma (ACC) and squamous cell carcinoma (SCC) of the trachea. [Gaisssert H, Grillo H, Shadmehr M, Wright C, Gokhale M, Wain J, Mathisen D. Long-term survival after resection of primary adenoid cystic and squamous cell carcinoma of the trachea and carina. *Ann Thorac Surg* 2004; 78:1889–1997.]

various sarcomas. Locally invasive extrinsic cancers (thyroid, esophagus, larynx, lung, lymphoma) may also lead to tracheal obstruction.

Squamous cell carcinoma

Squamous cell carcinoma of the trachea is primarily a disease of older male tobacco users. Synchronous primary cancers of the larynx or lung are common. Lesions are typically exophytic or ulcerating and occur in the distal third of the trachea. Local invasion and cervical lymph node metastasis at the time of presentation are common. Staging of regional lymph nodes and careful determination of the length of tumour extension are is important prior to attempts at resection and intraoperatively prior to reconstruction. Post-operative radiation therapy is recommended in almost all patients to improve local control. Survival of up to 47% at 5 years and 36% at 10 years has been reported (Figure 6.2).

Adenoid cystic carcinoma

Adenoid cystic carcinoma is not linked to cigarette smoking and has no age predilection. It is more likely to occur in the proximal third of the trachea than squamous cell carcinomas and is slower growing. Compression of adjacent structures in the mediastinum may occur, but true invasion is uncommon. Although lymphatic spread is rare, hematogenous metastases to the lung are frequently seen. A complete surgical resection is preferable, but because of the relatively indolent nature of adenoid cystic carcinoma, a positive resection margin is preferable to an anastomosis under tension.

All patients should receive post-operative radiation therapy. Survival of 73% at 5 years and 57% at 10 years is described (Figure 6.3).

Benign tracheal tumours

Squamous papilloma

In most series, squamous papillomas are the most common benign neoplasms of the trachea. They are attributed to mucosal infection with human papillomavirus and can occur as solitary lesions or diffuse papillomatosis. Malignant degeneration into squamous cell carcinoma occurs in 10–30% of adult patients and is more common with cigarette smoking and radiation exposure. Bronchoscopic excision is the preferred treatment, although segmental excision is preferable when the suspicion of malignancy exists.

Chondroma

Chondroma is the most common benign tracheal mesenchymal tumour. Chrondromas may arise as submucosal masses projecting into the lumen of the trachea. The possibility of local recurrence and malignant degeneration make segmental tracheal resection the preferred treatment.

Other benign tracheal tumours

The remainder of benign tracheal tumours are described in small cases series or individual case reports. Examples include pleomorphic adenoma, leiomyoma, lipoma and benign nerve sheath tumours.

51

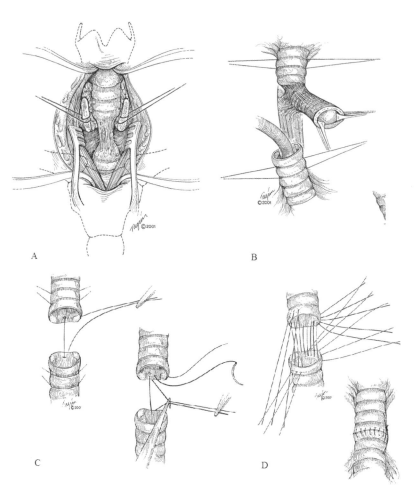

Figure 6.3 Technique of tracheal resection and reconstruction. The affected portion of the trachea is carefully dissected (**A**), and cross-field ventilation is used following division of the airway (**B**). Reconstruction is performed using interrupted absorbable sutures (**C**), and a tension-free anastomosis is created (**D**). [From Grillo H (Ed.), *Surgery of the Trachea and Bronchi*. 2004: BC Decker, Inc., Hamilton, Ontario.]

A

B

C

D

Nonsurgical treatment of tracheal stenosis and masses

Endoscopic treatment

Acutely symptomatic tracheal masses can be palliated via rigid bronchoscopy and coring out of the tumour with biopsy forceps. This procedure permits control of a bleeding lesion, treatment of post-obstructive pneumonia and symptomatic relief prior to radiation or resection. Laser resection with Nd:YAG, cryotherapy and photodynamic therapy have also been used to debride symptomatic lesions. Short-term placement of an endobronchial stent can be used as a bridge to definitive treatment, although this technique should be employed with caution due to the risk of formation of granulation tissue outside the stented region. Stenotic lesions of the trachea may be palliated with a silicone T-tube, as described earlier.

Radiation therapy

Primary radiation therapy is an acceptable alternative to surgical resection and reconstruction only in those patients unable to undergo operative treatment. Long-term survival with radiation therapy alone has occasionally been reported in both squamous cell carcinoma and adenoid cystic carcinoma. Radiation doses from 50 to 70 Gy have been described, although there does not appear to be a survival advantage to doses above 60 Gy, and dose-dependent toxicities including esophagitis, tracheitis and stricture favor a lower radiation dose.

Operative treatment of tracheal stenosis and masses

Initial reports of tracheal resection and reconstruction by Belsey placed the maximum length of trachea that could be safely resected at 2 cm or four tracheal rings.

Subsequent refinements by Grillo at the Massachusetts General Hospital led to the realization that up to half the length of the trachea could be removed with extensive mobilization techniques. These maneuvers include cervical flexion, suprahyoid laryngeal and hilar release. Resection of tracheal segments greater than 4 cm may require release maneuvers. Resection remains contraindicated with long-segment lesions and tumours involving nonresectable mediastinal organs. In the presence of distant metastases, palliative resection is occasionally undertaken.

Bronchoscopy is performed immediately prior to surgery. A tracheal resection should not be performed in the face of unexpected excessive airway secretions or untreated post-obstructive pneumonia. Rigid bronchoscopy and dilatation may be necessary prior to placement of an endotracheal tube.

A cervical collar incision is typically used, sometimes in conjunction with a partial sternotomy. A sternotomy or right thoracotomy may be preferred for distal lesions. Once the trachea has been transected, cross-field ventilation is employed via a sterile endotracheal tube. In combination with periods of hyperventilation, this tube may be removed for short periods to permit construction of an anastomosis. The anastomosis is constructed using interrupted absorbable sutures placed through the cartilaginous rings (anterior) or the membranous wall (posterior). The importance of creating a tension-free anastomosis cannot be overstated.

In cases of subglottic stenosis, the proximal extent of resection may include the anterior cricoid and the mucosa of the posterior cricoid, which is then covered using a flap of the membranous wall of the distal trachea.

Patients are extubated in the operating room and spared a tracheostomy unless concern exists about the status of the airway. The neck is secured in gently flexed position using a 'guardian stitch' placed from the chin to the chest. A routine bronchoscopy is performed on the seventh post-operative day, and the guardian stitch is typically removed at that time.

Tracheoesophageal fistula (TEF)

The clinical presentation of acquired fistula between the esophagus and trachea depends on whether patients are breathing spontaneously and taking food orally or being mechanically ventilated and fed via a tube into the stomach or small intestine.

In patients who are being fed orally, symptoms are similar to poorly controlled aspiration. Forceful coughing after swallowing, recurrent pneumonias and hemoptysis may be seen.

In mechanically ventilated patients, insufflation of the gut through a fistula may occur, leading to abdominal distension and triggering of the ventilator's leak alarm. In addition, frequent pneumonias may occur, and tube feeds may be suctioned via the patient's endotracheal tube.

Radiographs of the chest will frequently reveal diffuse infiltrates, focal pneumonia or a dilated, air-filled esophagus. Dilute barium swallow should demonstrate the fistulous track between esophagus and trachea. Gastrografin should be avoided when TEF is suspected because of the risk of causing pneumonitis. CT may be helpful in defining the TEF but is not the study of choice in making the diagnosis.

Bronchoscopy is more reliable than esophagoscopy in detecting and characterizing small fistulae. Both procedures should be performed, however, as simultaneous bronchoscopy and esophagoscopy are sometimes needed to detect small defects.

Etiologies of TEF

Acquired TEF can originate as a tracheal lesion that penetrates the esophagus or an esophageal lesion that penetrates the trachea or a mediastinal lesion that perforates both.

Tracheal origin

Iatrogenic – In the era of high-pressure, low-volume endotracheal tube cuffs, erosion of the membranous wall of the trachea into the esophagus was a frequent complication. The problem is exacerbated by presence of a rigid nasogastric tube in the esophagus (Figure 6.4). Although the incidence has declined in the modern era, it remains the most common benign cause of TEF.

Infectious – Granulomatous infection of the membranous wall of the trachea related to tuberculosis or histoplasmosis may proceed to TEF.

Malignant – Invasion of airway tumours into the esophagus may occur but is less frequent than the converse (see later).

Esophageal origin

Malignant – Squamous cell cancer of the upper third of the esophagus is most likely to result in

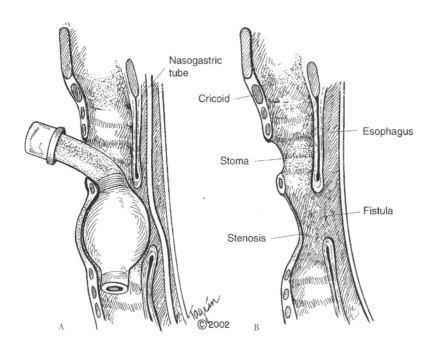

Nasogastric tube

Cricoid

Esophagus

Stoma

Fistula

Stenosis

A   ©2002   B

Figure 6.4 Mechanism of post-intubation tracheoesophageal fistula due to pressure necrosis between a rigid nasogastric tube and the balloon of a tracheostomy tube. [From Grillo H (Ed.), *Surgery of the Trachea and Bronchi*. 2004: BC Decker, Inc., Hamilton, Ontario.]

malignant TEF. In a series of 207 malignant TEFs, 78% derived from esophageal cancer compared to 16% from lung cancer and 1.5% from primary tracheal cancer. The incidence of fistula formation in esophageal cancer approaches 5%.

Anastomotic complication – Following esophagectomy, early anastomotic leak or delayed erosion of a stapled anastomosis may lead to development of acute or chronic TEF. Late dilatation of an anastomotic stricture can also cause a late fistula.

Stent-related – Balloon-expandable metallic stents in the esophagus (and less frequently the trachea) may cause TEF either through erosion or from trauma due to difficulties with removal.

Extrinsic

Trauma – Traumatic TEF may be extrinsic (penetrating injury) or intrinsic (aspirated or swallowed foreign body).

Iatrogenic – Anterior approach to cervical spine fusion may be complicated by iatrogenic injury to the trachea and/or esophagus, leading to TEF formation.

Malignant – Extrinsic mediastinal or cervical malignancies that may lead to TEF

include lymphoma, thyroid cancer and metastatic breast cancer.

Treatment of TEF

Principles of operative treatment

Patients with TEF frequently have additional complex medical problems that must be addressed prior to definitive repair. In particular, the nutritional status must be maximized and any pulmonary infection treated. Contamination of the respiratory tract by gastrointestinal secretions can be minimized prior to surgery by repositioning the cuff of the endotracheal tube below the level of the fistula, optimizing pulmonary toilet, decompressing the stomach with a gastrostomy tube and providing enteral nutrition via a jejunostomy.

Exposure for TEF is usually achieved via a cervical collar incision. The incision may be extended into the mediastinum via partial sternotomy if necessary. A supracarinal fistula requires right thoracotomy for exposure and repair. In cases of benign disease the esophageal defect is closed in two layers, and a pedicle of healthy muscle is placed between the trachea and esophagus (Figure 6.5). Typically, the segment of trachea containing the fistula is resected

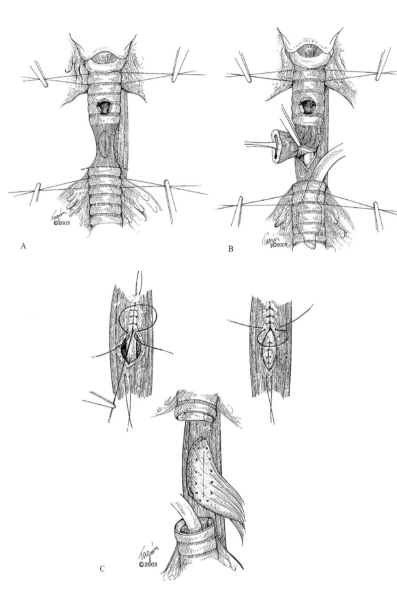

A

B

C

Figure 6.5 Resection and closure of tracheoesophageal fistula. After resection of the portion of trachea containing the defect (**A**, **B**), the esophageal defect is carefully closed in two layers and a buttress of vascularized tissue applied (**C**). Tracheal reconstruction then proceeds in the standard fashion. [From Grillo H (Ed.), *Surgery of the Trachea and Bronchi.* 2004: BC Decker, Inc., Hamilton, Ontario.]

and reconstructed with a tension-free anastomosis. In cases of malignancy or extensive mediastinal soilage, esophagectomy and/or diversion may be necessary.

Special cases
Malignant TEF

Primary malignancies leading to TEF, whether originating in the esophagus or the airway, are seldom curable by combined airway and esophageal resection. Palliative stenting of the trachea, esophagus or both may help to control respiratory infection and allow swallowing. Operative palliation involves isolating the affected segment of esophagus with cervical esophagostomy and gastrostomy. Regardless of the means of palliation, survival is 5–10 weeks.

In cases of TEF occurring later after esophageal resection, the first step is to determine whether residual or recurrent cancer is present. If the fistula is attributable to an anastomotic complication, then the gastric conduit may be resected and an esophageal diversion created to permit treatment of infectious sequelae of the fistula. Reconstruction with colonic or jejunal interposition may subsequently be required. In patients with recurrent or metastatic disease, conservative management with stenting may be more appropriate.

Post-intubation TEF

Attempts to repair an intubation-related fistula in patients who remains mechanically ventilated are likely to fail. Once the patient's pulmonary and nutritional status have been optimized, a single-stage repair is usually possible. Successful fistula repair in 94% of patients, with freedom from tracheal appliance in 71% and resumption of oral nutrition in 83%, has been described.

Traumatic TEF

Successful management of traumatic TEF depends on accurately identifying and repairing the esophageal injury. We prefer a primary two-layered repair of the esophagus using interrupted sutures buttressed with a flap of healthy tissue. Once the esophageal defect has been controlled, repair of the trachea proceeds as described for reconstruction.

Further reading
Tracheal anatomy

Minnich D, Mathisen D. Anatomy of the Trachea, Carina and Bronchi. *Thor Surg Clin* 2007; **17**:571–85. *Summary of tracheobronchial anatomy and relationships to adjacent structures and their role in the advancement of airway surgery.*

Tracheal stenosis

Ashiku S, Kuzucu A, Grillo H, et al. Idiopathic laryngotracheal stenosis: effective definitive treatment by laryngotracheal resection. *J Thorac Cardiovasc Surg* 2004; **127**:99–107. *Reports on the outcome of 73 patients treated for undergoing laryngotracheal resection at the Massachusetts General Hospital between 1971 and 2002, with no perioperative mortality and excellent long-term results in 91%.*

Donahue D, Grillo H, Wain J, et al. Reoperative tracheal resection and reconstruction for failed repair of postintubation stenosis. *J Thorac Cardiovasc Surg* 1997; **1114**:934–9. *Discussion of 75 patients operated on at the Massachusetts General Hospital between 1966 and 1997 after initially failed repairs with further resection ranging from 1 to 5.5 cm, with good or satisfactory outcomes in 82%.*

Tracheal tumour

Gaissert H, Grillo H, Shadmehr B, et al. Laryngotracheoplastic resection for primary tumors of the proximal airway. *J Thorac Cardiovasc Surg* 2005; **129**:1006–9. *Reports on the results of 25 patients undergoing laryngotracheal resection for primary airway tumours close to the vocal cords with median follow-up of 101 months and overall 5- and 10-year survival of 79% and 64%.*

Gaissert H, Grillo H, Shadmehr B, et al. Uncommon primary tracheal tumors. *Ann Thorac Surg* 2006; **82**:268–73. *Retrospective analysis of treatment and outcomes of 360 benign and malignant tracheal tumours other than squamous cell and adenoid cystic carcinoma over a 40-year period.*

Gaisssert H, Grillo H, Shadmehr M, et al. Long-term survival after resection of primary adenoid cystic and squamous cell carcinoma of the trachea and carina. *Ann Thor Surg* 2004; **78**:1889–997. *Retrospective analysis of 270 patients with adenoid cystic or squamous cell carcinoma treated between 1962 and 2002 comparing 5- and 10-year survival in resected and unresected patients by histology.*

Gaissert H, Honings J, Grillo H, et al. Segmental laryngotracheal and tracheal resection for invasive thyroid Carcinoma. *Ann Thorac Surg* 2007; **83**:1952–9. *Retrospective study of 82 patients demonstrating that thyroid cancer invading the airway can be safely and effective managed by segmental airway resection.*

Tracheoesophageal fistula

Muniappan A, Wain J, Wright C, et al Surgical treatment of nonmalignant tracheoesophageal fistula: a thirty-five year experience. *Ann Thorac Surg* 2013 Apr; **95**(4):1141–6. doi: 10.1016/j.athoracsur.2012.07.041. Epub 2012 Sep 20. *Retrospective study of 36 patients undergoing various surgical repairs of tracheoesophageal fistula between 1992 and 2010, reporting successful fistula closure in 94%.*

Complications

Wright C, Grillo H, Wain J, et al. Anastomotic complications after tracheal resection: prognostic factors and management. *J Thorac Cardiovasc Surg* 2004; **128**:731–9. *Describes anastomotic complications in 9% of 901 patients with reoperation, diabetes, resection > 4 cm, age < 17 years, and pre-operative tracheostomy as independent risk factors.*

Congenital and developmental lung malformations

Naziha Khen-Dunlop, Guillaume Lezmi, Christophe Delacourt and Yann Revillon

Landmarks

- There are three main congenital lung malformations: cystic forms also named congenital pulmonary airway malformation (CPAM), broncho-pulmonary sequestrations (BPS) and congenital lobar emphysema also named congenital alveolar overdistension. Among them, cystic lung malformations are the most frequent.

- Cystic lung malformations are focal and occur sporadically, suggesting they result from a defect in normal lung development rather from a genetic abnormality.

- The description of hybrid malformation, associating CPAM and sequestration features and the observation of microcystic elements in about half of extralobar sequestrations reflect the complex status of pulmonary malformations.

- Prenatal mediastinal shift is observed in 50% of CPAM and polyhydramnios in 20% of cases; both of these signs do not have to be interpreted as complications and do not lead to impaired lung development or fetal distress. On the opposite, hydrops is present in about 10% of cases and is associated to fetal or neonatal death in more than 95%.

- The 'disappearance' of congenital malformations of the lung on last prenatal ultrasound was classically described and interpreted as a complete regression of the malformation, but such evolution is exceptional and only documented for sequestrations. Post-natal thoracic imaging (MRI or CT scan) is required to check the persistence of congenital lung malformations regardless of prenatal evolution.

- Cystic lesions are congenital lung malformations for which complications are most often reported. Respiratory impairment and lung infection are the two main symptoms but, although exceptional, they are associated to malignant degeneration. If non-operated, asymptomatic cystic lesions have to be followedup into adulthood.

- Over 90% of bronchopulmonary sequestrations are found in the thorax, and less than 10% are located in the abdomen. As respiratory symptoms are rare and no malignancy reported, expectance can then be proposed, provided that there is no cystic component.

- Progressive respiratory signs, secondary to lobar overinflation, are the most common symptoms in congenital lobar emphysema. Signs may have a favourable evolution with clinical and ventilatory parameter improvements. In case of respiratory distress, surgical excision of the malformation is necessary.

Important publications in the speciality

- Morrisey E, Hogan B. Preparing for the first breath: genetic and cellular mechanisms in lung development. *Dev Cell* 2010; 18:8–23.

- Sekine K, Ohuchi H, Fujiwara M, et al. FGF10 is essential for limb and lung formation. *Nat Genet* 1999; 21:138–41.

- Adzick NS. Open fetal surgery for life-threatening fetal anomalies. *Semin Fetal Neonatal Med* 2010 Feb; 15:1–8.

Core Topics in Thoracic Surgery, ed. Marco Scarci, Aman Coonar, Tom Routledge and Francis Wells. Published by Cambridge University Press. © Cambridge University Press 2016

- Langston C. New concepts in the pathology of congenital lung malformations. *Semin Pediatr Surg* 2003; 12:17–37.
- Stocker JT. Cystic lung disease in infants and children. *Fetal Pediatr Pathol* 2009; 28:155–84.
- Bush A. Prenatal presentation and postnatal management of congenital thoracic malformations. *Early Hum Dev* 2009; 85:679–84.

Introduction

Advances in antenatal imaging over the past 10 years have dramatically changed diagnosis and management of congenital lung disease, especially for the two lesions most commonly detected: congenital cystic adenomatoid malformations (CCAM), also named congenital pulmonary airway malformation (CPAM), and bronchopulmonary sequestrations (BPS). If early surgical excision is required for all symptomatic malformations, management of asymptomatic cases is still controversial. The natural evolution and consequences of late complications of lung malformations still need to be compared with the benefits of elective resection and surgical morbidity. Complete regression of sequestrations or clinical and morphological improvement in congenital lobar emphysema (also named congenital alveolar overdistension) plead for clinical watching. On the other hand, resection is advocated for cystic malformations because of an increased risk of acute respiratory distress, later infections and the possibility of malignant transformation. Further studies and long-term follow-up are still needed to understand the natural history of congenital lung malformations and help to define the optimal way to manage them.

Lung morphogenesis and congenital malformations

Lung development begins at embryonic day 28 when the primary lung buds evaginate from a domain expressing TTF-1 within the ventral foregut endoderm[1]. Once formed, the primary lung buds extend and undergo branching. Branching morphogenesis is a developmental process that occurs during the pseudoglandular stage of lung development (6–16 weeks), and leads the primary lung buds to form the conducting airways. Branching morphogenesis results from interactions between epithelium and underlying mesenchyma[2]. Such interactions are mediated by diffusible factors, mainly members of the fibroblast growth factor (FGF) family[1]. In particular, FGF10 plays a key role in lung development. FGF10 is secreted by fibroblasts of the mesenchyma and may act on epithelium through its receptor FGFR2b to induce branching morphogenesis. When FGF10 or FGFR2b are absent, the primary buds are present but are unable to branch[3-5].

Cystic lung malformations are focal and occur sporadically, suggesting that they result from a defect in normal lung development rather from a genetic abnormality. This is supported by studies reporting that many molecules involved in normal lung development remain overexpressed in CCAM/CPAM. Markers of early lung development such as HOXb-5 and TTF-1 have been found to remain overexpressed in fetal mesenchyma and epithelium of cysts, respectively, when compared with controls[6]. Platelet-derived growth factor-B, which stimulates lung growth by increasing proliferation, remains overexpressed in severe fetal CCAM/CPAM complicated of hydrops when compared with age-matched control lungs[7], and conditional overexpression of the cell fate regulator NOTCH-Ic within lung epithelium of fetal transgenic mice results in cystic-like lesions instead of normal saccules[8]. Several animal models have recently highlighted the relevance of FGF10 overexpression in CCAM/CPAM pathogenesis. In vitro studies showed that excess of FGF10 in cultured fetal lung explants from mice and rats induces a cystic-like enlargement of lung buds[9-10]. In vivo, the overexpression of FGF10 in proximal and distal airways of fetal transgenic mice induces marked adenomatoid malformation[11], whereas localized injection of the rFGF10 transgene in the lungs of rats during gestation results in cystic lung lesions resembling CCAM/CPAM[12]. Although animal models support that an FGF10 overexpression may lead to the formation of CCAM/CPAM, this hypothesis has yet never been confirmed in humans[10,13]. These discrepancies point the difficulties in understanding developmental disease mechanisms in humans and support the development of in vivo animal models to provide new insights in their pathogenesis. Moreover, the description of hybrid malformation, associated CPAM and sequestration features and the observation of microcystic elements in about half of extralobar sequestrations reflect the complex status of pulmonary malformations[14,15].

Prenatal diagnosis

Fetal lung malformations are present in about 1/20 000 pregnancies and are classified into two major types based on their sonographic appearance: cystic or echogenic. Cystic lesions are in the vast majority of cases CPAM (previously named CCAM). Hyperechogenic lesions may correspond to CPAM, bronchopulmonary sequestrations, congenital emphysema or bronchial atresia. CPAM is one of the most frequent lesions visualized during prenatal ultrasound[16]. Mediastinal shift is observed in 50% of cases and polyhydramnios in 20% of cases because of a mass effect on mediastinum or oesophageal compression. Both of these signs do not have to be interpreted as complications and do not lead to impaired lung development or fetal distress. On the other hand, hydrops is present in about 10% of cases and is a sign of poor cardiac tolerance either by decreased venous return or by direct myocardial compression. Hydrops is associated in more than 95% of cases to fetal or neonatal death[17,18].

Bronchopulmonary sequestrations are the second malformations diagnosed prenatally. The aspect is the same as the microcystic forms of CPAM or congenital lobar emphysema, and only visualization of a feeding systemic artery can affirm the diagnosis. Despite their volume, bronchopulmonary sequestrations are usually well tolerated by the fetus and do not lead to prenatal nor post-natal symptoms. However,

complications such as hydrothorax and hydrops are reported but stay exceptional[19]. If persistent, they can also lead to pre- or post-natal death.

Because of their reduced size during fetal life, bronchogenic cysts are rarely diagnosed prenatally, and compressive effects in the fetus are very uncommon[17,20]. Prenatal diagnosis of lobar emphysema is rare and unspecific[21,22].

Two indications for prenatal intervention are identified: hydrops, due to the significant risk of death, and persistent mediastinal compressive effect, because of the risk of pulmonary hypoplasia. However, a decrease in the volume of the malformations is usually observed during pregnancy after the thirtieth week of gestation, resulting in an improvement in the appearance of the lung parenchyma and fetal tolerance[18,20]. Given the importance of spontaneous regression in the third trimester of pregnancy, procedures are usually performed after the thirtieth week and after a first test of maternal corticosteroids. In cystic lesions, a simple puncture has little interest because of the high risk of secondary recurrence. Provided that there is a large or dominant cyst, drainage into the amniotic cavity achieves a survival rate of 70% when hydrops regresses and the drainage is effective, with a collapse of the cyst and a shift of the mediastinum (Figure 7.1). A second drainage may be required due to exclusion of the drain, which occurred in one-third of the cases[23]. Drains can also

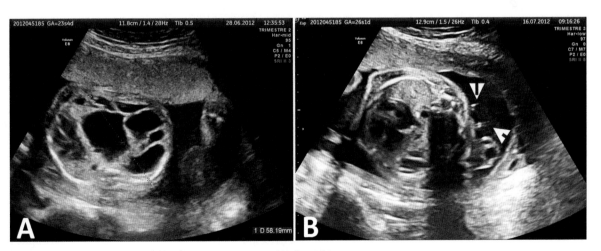

Figure 7.1 Prenatal imaging of compressive CPAM (courtesy of Prof. Y. Ville).
A. Prenatal ultrasound exam of a compressive CPAM of the left lung at 23 WG. The heart is displaced to the right by a macrocystic lesion of 58-mm diameter with compression of both lungs and secondary polyhydramnios but without hydrops. Prenatal thoracoamniotic shunting was decided.
B. Prenatal ultrasound exam at 26 WG, 2 weeks after the CPAM drainage by two catheters (white arrows) placed in the predominant cysts. The cysts are well subsided, and the mediastinal shift is corrected. The drainage will remain functional until birth.

be placed to evacuate pleural effusion compressions, which can complicate pulmonary sequestration[24,25].

Prenatal treatment of hyperechogenic lesions is still debated. Sclerosis of the mass or coagulation of vascular pedicles has been proposed by some teams with mixed results[17]. Similarly, interventions by open surgery after hysterotomy and maternal fetal thoracotomy were performed for solid malformations. Series from Scott Adzick's team are the largest to date, with 24 cases of in utero fetal thoracotomy within 15 years, carried out between 21 and 34 weeks. The fetal survival rate was about 50%. Half the deaths occurred intraoperatively during resection of the lesion and the other half in the hours following the intervention secondary to fetal bradycardia, uterine contractions or uncontrolled chorioamnionitis[26].

The decrease in prenatal volume of the malformations was estimated between 15 and 65%. This regression accounts for almost half of CPAM when the volume of the lesion is reported to total lung volume[26,27]. The 'disappearance' of congenital malformations of the lung on last prenatal ultrasound was classically described and interpreted as a complete regression of the malformation. This evolution, although exceptional, was documented for sequestrations[28] but not for cystic malformations, for which the ultrasound disappearance is attributed to changes in prenatal morphological feature at the third trimester. Thus, post-natal thoracic imaging

(MRI or CT scan) is required to check the persistence of congenital lung malformations regardless of the prenatal evolution.

Post-natal diagnosis

Cystic lung malformations

Cystic lesions are congenital lung malformations for which complications are most often reported. In the neonatal period, respiratory distress secondary to compression of the lung parenchyma is the main symptom and leads to an emergency operation in the first month of life in about 20% of the children[21] (Figure 7.2).

On the other hand, bronchogenic cysts are small in the neonatal period and thus remain asymptomatic long after birth. Gradually, intracystic secretions lead to cystic growth and tensioning. This increase can be rapid and significant with symptoms related to the compression of adjacent structures: the trachea in most cases, more rarely the oesophagus or the vena cava and the myocardium. Cysts located just under the carena are particularly at risk and life threatening because of the simultaneous compression of both bronchi[29,30,31]. Although exceptional, symptoms can also be secondary to a fistula in the tracheobronchial tree, oesophagus or lung tissue[32,33].

After the neonatal period, infection is the most common complication of cystic malformations. It can

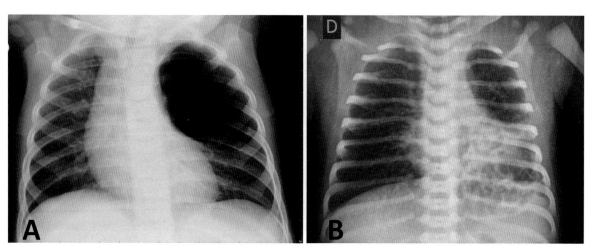

Figure 7.2 Neonatal imaging of CPAM.
A. Macro-cystic malformation of the upper lobe of the left lung leading to post-natal respiratory distress. Chest X-ray shows cardiac shift with left mediastinal compression and tracheal deviation to the right.
B. Multicystic malformation of the lower lobe of the left lung without respiratory symptoms (prenatal diagnosis). The chest X-ray did not show mediastinal or lung compressive effect.

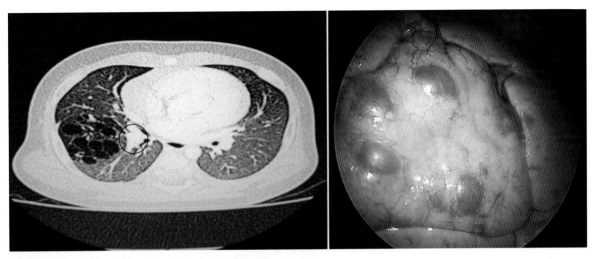

Figure 7.3 CPAM with multiple cysts: imaging and perioperative correlation.
Cystic malformation of the middle lobe of the right lung diagnosed after two episodes of pulmonary infection and abnormal chest X-ray. CT scan (left) shows numerous cysts with some thick dividing walls and proximal bronchocele (grey circle) leading to the diagnosis of associated bronchial atresia. Thoracoscopic per-operative view (right) shows the cysts at the surface of the middle lobe and the absence of lesions in the two other lobes.

be manifested by febrile episodes but also by recurrent respiratory symptoms that are usually diagnosed and treated as asthma[32]. Chronic inflammation may remain latent or be complicated by hemoptysis or pneumothorax[34,35]. In all theses cases, the diagnosis of the malformation, if undetected prenatally, or the confirmation of the complication is made on the chest CT scan (Figure 7.3).

To date, 50 cases of malignant degeneration of cystic malformations have been reported in children; the youngest age at diagnosis was 1 year[36,37]. Three kinds of tumours are described: pleuropneumoblastoma, bronchioloalveolar carcinoma and rhabdomyosarcoma. These tumours have been mainly described in CPAM but also, even though exceptional, in bronchogenic cysts[38,39]. In CPAM, the risk seems to depend on the type of cystic malformation: clearly associated to type 1 and type 4 CPAM when type 2 CPAM seems not involved[40,41]. Intracystic mucinous cell clusters, with K-ras mutations, have been described in type 1 CCAM, making these lesions potential precursors of bronchoalveolar carcinoma[42]. These concordant data strongly suggest that CPAM (at least type 1 CCAM) may predispose to malignant transformation. But the incidence of malignant transformation is still difficult to estimate: on systematic histological analyses, it was evaluated up to 4% in children's CPAM and 20% in adults'

CPAM[43,44] and such differences may be reflecting the evolution with time of cystic congenital malformations[45,46].

Solid lung malformations

Solid malformation corresponds to bronchopulmonary sequestration (BPS). Two sub-types are described (i) intralobar sequestrations which share common visceral pleura with the normal lung and (ii) extralobar sequestrations which have their own pleura. Extralobar sequestrations account for 20% of prenatally detected BPS (Figure 7.4). Over 90% of sequestrations are found in the thorax, and less than 10% are located in the abdomen (all extralobar forms), typically described in the left suprarenal area. Because of this particular location, differential diagnoses such as neuroblastoma, adrenal hematoma, hemolymphangioma and teratoma have to be excluded[47]. BPS is characterized by a systemic vasculature that most commonly arises from the descending thoracic aorta, less frequently from the upper abdominal aorta (or celiac and splenic branches) and in rare cases from intercostal, subclavian or coronary arteries[48]. The existence of intradiaphragmatic locations is rare but is of embryological interest. The presence of abnormal tissue embedded within the diaphragm suggests that the sequestration forms prior to embryologic closure

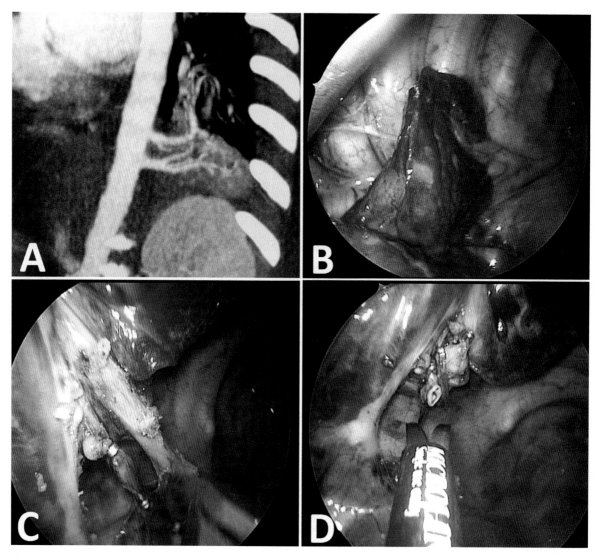

Figure 7.4 Bronchopulmonary sequestration: imaging and perioperative correlation.
A. CT scan showing left basal bronchopulomonary sequestration with two feeding arteries arising from aorta. The malformation appears as a dense lesion without cystic component.
B. Thoracoscopic perioperative view confirming an extralobar sequestration with two feeding vessels.
C. Dissection of the vessels and ligation by thoracoscopic clips.
D. Section of the vessels and mobilization of the BPS.

of the diaphragm, which is before the eighth week of gestation, and thus pleads for the origin from an early ectopic pulmonary bud. BPS with gastric duplications is also described[49]. The term is gastric duplication was proposed due to the fusion between the sequestration and the stomach, even in the absence of identified intestinal mucosa, considering that histological overlaps can occur because of the primitive digestive origin of lung tissues[50].

In the post-natal period, symptoms are common to other malformations: respiratory discomfort and infection but more specifically, although exceptional, vascular complications, such as intralesional bleeding or heart failure[51,52]. Diagnosis appears earlier in extralobar sequestrations as 60% are recognized in the first 6 months of life, whereas intralobar sequestrations are most often diagnosed after the age of 2 years[50]. Sequestrations may also completely disappear in the pre- and post-natal periods, presumably by spontaneous thrombosis of the vascular pedicle, although histological data are not available to confirm the diagnosis. Expectant management can then be proposed for BPS, especially when the size of the lesion is small and if it is an extralobar form[34]. Percutaneous embolization could then be a good therapeutic alternative because of less morbidity, but it is reserved for BPS with a single artery and in the absence of associated cystic structures[53,54].

Emphysema

Emphysema is typically diagnosed in the neonatal period due to respiratory distress, acute or progressive effect by trapping and overinflation of the segment or the pulmonary lobe[55] (Figure 7.5). Although bronchus malformations were described at histological analysis in only half the cases, emphysema is attributed to abnormal bronchial cartilage without malformations of the lung parenchyma but secondary alveolar overdistension[56].

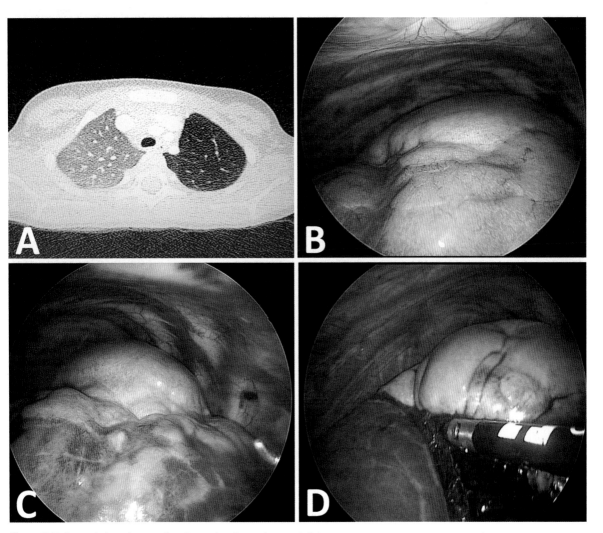

Figure 7.5 Congenital emphysema: imaging and perioperative correlation.
A. CT scan showing parenchymal hyperlucency of the upper left lobe.
B. Thoracoscopic perioperative view. The upper part of the lung is discreetly clearer with very small superficial bubbles. The malformative zone can, however, be continuously delineated.
C. After ventilation exclusion of the left lung, the normal lower part is collapsed when the malformative upper part stays overinflated.
D. Thermal fusion parenchymal section at the edge of the emphysematous part.

Functional respiratory signs, with or without associated infection, are also common symptoms at diagnosis after the neonatal period. They occur in the majority of cases within the first 6 months of life[57]. In older children, it is sometimes difficult to tell the difference between late symptomatic congenital lobar emphysema and emphysematous lesions secondary to extrinsic bronchial compression or post-infectious lung damage[58,59].

Difficulty in breathing may also remain moderate with a favourable evolution and a regression of the lesions, provided there is not a local mechanical cause. Clinical improvements are associated to changes in ventilatory parameters[60].

Post-natal treatment

The principles of surgery in newborns are identical to those in older children, but the thoracoscopic approach, even if feasible as it was assessed by numerous publications, is difficult because of the limited space in the thorax at this age. As infants remain asymptomatic in the majority of cases, it allows an initial follow-up and avoids intervention and general anaesthesia in the first months of life; consensus seems to be emerging for intervention after 6 months[16,34].

At birth, chest X-ray is performed before discharge from hospital to assess the impact of the malformation once the lung is ventilated. CT scan or MRI, realized between 2 and 3 months of life, can precisely evaluate the morphological characteristics and the local impact of pulmonary malformation. The early term for this imaging, in the absence of planned surgery, has the advantage to still be performed at this age without general anaesthesia, which will not be the case in babies older than 3 months. In our experience, in the aim to limit irradiation, MRI provides a good pulmonary, mediastinal or vascular evaluation but fails to give a good evaluation of cystic components and can thus be completed by a low-dose scanner. This evaluation allows us to define precisely the type of malformation: strictly cystic (CPAM), entirely solid malformation (BPS) or cystic and solid components (i.e. hybrid malformation) in case of prenatal malformation with systemic pedicle; CPAM, BPS, emphysema or bronchial atresia in case of prenatal hyperechogenic malformations.

The surgical resection of lung congenital malformations is consensual when they become symptomatic:

dyspnea, tachypnea, acute respiratory distress, discomfort in food intake, etc.[16,34]. For asymptomatic malformations (prenatally diagnosed), the main argument of the wait-and-see attitude is the possible disappearance of lesions over time. Disappearance was also documented for BPS[28,61], but there were no clear evidences of such evolution in cystic malformations.

The second argument for the expectative attitude is the poor knowledge of the natural history of congenital lung malformations, particularly with regard to delayed symptoms. Lobar emphysema may remain asymptomatic with little risk of major complications, and clinical and morphological improvements were even shown, justifying a long-term surveillance[60]. But even in the absence of functional symptoms, resection of cystic lesions is proposed. Although the evaluation of secondary infection is variable (from 10 to 85%), they were associated to higher perioperative complications with longer operativetimes, increased blood loss or higher rates of conversion when performed thoracoscopically[62]. Post-operative morbidity was also increased with longer lengths of stay and more frequent post-operative complications (pulmonary fistulae, secondary haemorrhage, reoperation, etc.)[14,63].

Early surgery is also recommended in cystic malformations because of the risk of malignant transformations[41,43]. Unlike bronchopulmonary carcinoma (cf supra), it is most likely that CPAM and pulmonary pleuroblastoma (PPB) are two separate lesions without natural evolution between them; chromosomal abnormalities that are identified in PPB cases are not found in CPAM cases[64,65]. Without complete resection, low-grade cystic PPB (type I) is likely to progress over 2–4 years to a high-grade solid disease (type III)[41]. Delayed recognition or failure to resect type I PPB significantly worsens prognosis. Overall survival rate in PPB ranges from 80–85% for type I to 45–50% for type III[66,67]. As these two entities share similar clinical and radiological features, pathologic examination is the only means to establish the final diagnosis[68]. Although some clinical features associated with cystic lung lesions can be helpful to suspect a type I PPB, they lack specificity and are often misinterpreted[66,67]. In their retrospective analysis of 51 patients with type I PPB, Hill et al. found that type I PPB was never suspected pre-operatively despite the high rate of pneumothorax at presentation and/or multiple lesions in the lung[67]. Thus, only systematic surgical removal of congenital cystic lung lesions, associated with a thorough pathologic study by a trained team, can formally exclude the diagnosis of PPB.

Cystic malformations (CPAM) with systemic vascularization or a predominantly solid lesion (BPS) but containing cystic structures, now defined as hybrid malformations, are thus to be considered for surgical resection.

Surgical procedure

The optimal period for lung resection seems to be between 6 months and 2 years. Surgery in the first 6 months for asymptomatic forms seems not necessary nor useful regarding the increased anaesthetic risk in the neonatal period compared to the incidence/consequences of complications. Moreover, the growth and development of the chest offer better technical conditions for thoracoscopic surgery after the first year. If resections are decided, interventions should be realized before the onset of complications, considering the data on increased morbidity, that is, in the first 3 years.

Progress in the miniaturization of equipment offers instruments of 3- or 5-mm diameters and 5-mm optics, perfectly suited for the thorax of infants. Lung resections, either thoraco-assisted or entirely thoracoscopic, are possible in the vast majority of cases, with an advantage (vs thoracotomy) on postoperative pain and costal healing[68]. In children, their low weight does not allow the use of a doublelumen endotracheal tube for transient pulmonary exclusion work, and the pulmonary exposure is more difficult than in adults. When the lesion is on the left lung, right selective intubation can be performed, if tolerated. When the lesion is on the right lung, a good collaboration with the anaesthesia team, providing a high-frequency and low-volume ventilation, is the key of this surgery.

The optical port is placed at the tip of the blade, on the mid-axillary line, and insufflation is performed at a maximum of 4–5 mmHg. Two 5-mm ports are positioned in triangulation location, and a third port may be necessary to improve the exposure. For parenchymal sections we used preferentially thermal tissue fusion (LigaSure) that provides both control of the haemostasis and a good pneumostasis. Vascular controls, if necessary, are obtained by clips, endoloops or only by thermal tissue fusion, depending on the size of the pedicles. In children, the bronchi are flexible, and endoloop ligation is often sufficient without complementary stapling. In sequestrations, systemic arteries are controlled from the start of the intervention, venous return can be variable and there is no connection with the bronchial tree.

One or two chest tubes are left in place for an average of 48–72 hours. They are removed after ensuring the absence of bubbling and our usual test without prior clamping. Because of the lack of scholarship skin, a compression bandage is left for 48 h. The return home is made the day after the drains are removed after a final chest X-ray control.

Conclusion

Because histological overlaps are described between the four classical types of congenital lung malformations, the classical classification now seems imperfect. Last works on pathogenetic mechanism plead for a malformation sequence based on fetal airway obstruction events that lead to lung parenchymal maldevelopment.

There is general agreement in favour of resecting lung congenital malformations when symptomatic. The optimal period for lung resection of congenital cystic malformation diagnosed prenatally seems to be between 6 months and 2 years. If resection is decided, intervention should be realized before the onset of complications, considering the data on increased morbidity. A European Task Force stated that unoperated stable cystic lesions should be followedup into adulthood, but the optimal frequency of repeated evaluations is not given. As post-natal natural history of congenital lung malformations remains a mystery, long-term observation of patients is still needed.

References

1   Morrisey E, Hogan B. Preparing for the first breath: genetic and cellular mechanisms in lung development. *Dev Cell* 2010; 18:8–23.

2   Alescio T, Cassigni A. Induction in vitro of tracheal buds by pulmonary mesenchyme grafted on tracheal epithelium. *J Exp Zool* 1962; 150: 83–94.

3   Min H, Danilenko DM, Scully SA, et al. FGF-10 is required for both limb and lung development and exhibits striking functional similarity to *Drosophila*

branchless. *Genes Dev* 1998; 12:3156–61.

4 Sekine K, Ohuchi H, Fujiwara M, et al. FGF10 is essential for limb and lung formation. *Nat Genet* 1999; 21:138–41.

5 Peters K, Werner S, Liao X, et al. Targeted expression of a dominant negative FGF receptor blocks branching morphogenesis and epithelial differentiation of the mouse lung. *EMBO J* 1994; 13:3296–301.

6 Jancelewicz T, Nobuhara K, Howgood S. Laser microdissection allows detection of abnormal gene expression in cystic adenomatoid malformation of the lung. *J Pediatr Surg* 2008; 43:1044–51.

7 Liechty KW, Crombleholme TM, et al. Elevated platelet-derived growth factor-B in congenital cystic adenomatoid malformations requiring fetal resection. *J Pediatr Surg* 1999; 34:805–9.

8 Guseh JS, Bores SA, Stanger BZ, et al. Notch signaling promotes airway mucous metaplasia and inhibits alveolar development. *Development* 2009; 136:1751–9.

9 Bellusci S, Grindley J, Emoto H, et al. Fibroblast growth factor 10 (FGF10) and branching morphogenesis in the embryonic mouse lung. *Development* 1997; 124:4867–78.

10 Jesudason EC, Smith NP, Connell MG, et al. *Am J Respir Cell Mol Biol* 2005; 32:118–27.

11 Clark JC, Tichelaar JW, Wert SE, et al. FGF-10 disrupts lung morphogenesis and causes pulmonary adenomas in vivo. *Am J Physiol Lung Cell Mol Physiol* 2001; 280:L705–15.

12 Gonzaga S, Henriques-Coelho T, Davey M, et al. Cystic adenomatoid malformations are induced by localized FGF10 overexpression in fetal rat lung.

Am J Respir Cell Mol Biol 2008; 39:346–55.

13 Wagner AJ, Stumbaugh A, Tigue Z, et al. Genetic analysis of congenital cystic adenomatoid malformation reveals a novel pulmonary gene: fatty acid binding protein-7 (brain type). *Pediatr Res* 2008; 64:11–6.

14 Langston C. New concepts in the pathology of congenital lung malformations. *Semin Pediatr Surg* 2003; 12:17–37.

15 Carsin A, Mely L, Chrestian MA, et al. Association of three different congenital malformations in a same pulmonary lobe in a 5-year-old girl. *Pediatr Pulmonol* 2010; 45:832–5.

16 Davenport M, Warne SA, Cacciaguerra S, et al. Current outcome of antenatally diagnosed cystic lung disease. *J Pediatr Surg* 2004; 39:549–56.

17 Witlox RS, Lopriore E, Oepkes D. Prenatal interventions for fetal lung lesions. *Prenat Diagn* 2011; 31:628–36.

18 Hadchouel A, Benachi A, Delacourt C. Outcome of prenatally diagnosed bronchial atresia. *Ultrasound Obstet Gynecol* 2011; 38:119.

19 Yoshitomi T, Hidaka N, Yumoto Y, et al. Grayscale and Doppler sonographic evaluation of response to in utero treatment of hydrops fetalis caused by extralobar pulmonary sequestration. *J Clin Ultrasound* 2012; 40:51–6.

20 Wilson RD, Hedrick HL, Liechty KW, et al. Cystic adenomatoid malformation of the lung: review of genetics, prenatal diagnosis, and in utero treatment. *Am J Med Genet A* 2006; 140:151–5.

21 Stanton M, Njere I, Ade-Ajayi N, et al. Systematic review and meta-analysis of the postnatal management of congenital cystic lung lesions. *J Pediatr Surg* 2009 May; 44:1027–33.

22 Lecomte B, Hadden H, Coste K, et al. Hyperechoic congenital lung lesions in a non-selected population: from prenatal detection till perinatal management. *Prenat Diagn* 2009; 29:1222–30.

23 Deprest JA, Devlieger R, Srisupundit K, et al. Fetal surgery is a clinical reality. *Semin Fetal Neonatal Med* 2010; 15:58–67.

24 Kitano Y, Sago H, Hayashi S, et al. Aberrant venous flow measurement may predict the clinical behavior of a fetal extralobar pulmonary sequestration. *Fetal Diagn Ther* 2008; 23:299–302.

25 Salomon LJ, Audibert F, Dommergues M, et al. Fetal thoracoamniotic shunting as the only treatment for pulmonary sequestration with hydrops: favorable long-term outcome without postnatal surgery. *Ultrasound Obstet Gynecol* 2003; 21:299–301.

26 Adzick NS. Open fetal surgery for life-threatening fetal anomalies. *Semin Fetal Neonatal Med* 2010 Feb;15:1–8.

27 Sauvat F, Michel JL, Benachi A, et al. Management of asymptomatic neonatal cystic adenomatoid malformations. *J Pediatr Surg* 2003; 38:548–52.

28 Lababidi Z, Dyke PC 2nd. Angiographic demonstration of spontaneous occlusion of systemic arterial supply in pulmonary sequestration. *Pediatr Cardiol* 2003; 24:406–8.

29 De Baets F, Van Daele S, Schelstraete P, Asphyxiating tracheal bronchogenic cyst. *Pediatr Pulmonol* 2004; 38:488–90.

30 Mawatari T, Itoh T, Hachiro Y, et al. Large bronchial cyst causing compression of the left atrium. *Ann Thorac Cardiovasc Surg* 2003; 9:261–3.

31 Turkyilmaz A, Aydin Y, Ogul H, Eroglu A. Total occlusion of the superior vena cava due to bronchogenic cyst. *Acta Chir Belg* 2009; 109:635–8.

32 Sarper A, Ayten A, Golbasi I, et al. Bronchogenic cyst. *Tex Heart Inst J* 2003; 30:105–8.

33 Pages ON, Rubin S, Baehrel B. Intra-esophageal rupture of a bronchogenic cyst.*Interact Cardiovasc Thorac Surg* 2005; 4:287–8.

34 Laberge JM, Puligandla P, Flageole H. Asymptomatic congenital lung malformations. *Semin Pediatr Surg* 2005; 14:16–33.

35 Pelizzo G, Barbi E, Codrich D, et al. Chronic inflammation in congenital cystic adenomatoid malformations; an underestimated risk factor? *J Pediatr Surg* 2009; 44:616–9.

36 Ozcan C, Celik A, Ural Z, et al. Primary pulmonary rhabdomyosarcoma arising within cystic adenomatoid malformation: a case report and review of the literature. *J Pediatr Surg* 2001; 36:1062–5.

37 Adirim TA, King R, Klein BL. Radiological case of the month. Congenital cystic adenomatoid malformation of the lung and pulmonary blastoma. *Arch Pediatr Adolesc Med* 1997; 151:1053–4.

38 Murphy JJ, Blair GK, Fraser GC, et al. Rhabdomyosarcoma arising within congenital pulmonary cysts: report of three cases. *J Pediatr Surg* 1992; 27:1364–7.

39 Jakopovic M, Slobodnjak Z, Krizanac S, Samarzija M. Large cell carcinoma arising in bronchogenic cyst. *J Thorac Cardiovasc Surg* 2005; 130:610–2.

40 Stocker JT. Cystic lung disease in infants and children. *Fetal Pediatr Pathol* 2009; 28:155–84.

41 Priest JR, Williams GM, Hill DA, et al. Pulmonary cysts in early childhood and the risk of malignancy. *Pediatr Pulmonol* 2009; 44:14–30.

42 Lantuejoul S, Nicholson AG, Sartori G, et al. Mucinous cells in type 1 pulmonary congenital cystic adenomatoid malformation as mucinous bronchioloalveolar carcinoma precursors. *Am J Surg Pathol* 2007; 31:961–9.

43 Nasr A, Himidan S, Pastor AC, et al. Is congenital cystic adenomatoid malformation a premalignant lesion for pleuropulmonary blastoma? *J Pediatr Surg* 2010; 45:1086–9.

44 MacSweeney F, Papagiannopoulos K, Goldstraw P, et al. An assessment of the expanded classification of congenital cystic adenomatoid malformations and their relationship to malignant transformation. *Am J Surg Pathol* 2003; 27:1139–46.

45 Ioachimescu OC, Mehta AC. From cystic pulmonary airway malformation, to bronchioloalveolar carcinoma and adenocarcinoma of the lung. *Eur Respir J* 2005; 26:1181–7.

46 Stacher E, Ullmann R, Halbwedl I, et al. Atypical goblet cell hyperplasia in congenital cystic adenomatoid malformation as a possible preneoplasia for pulmonary adenocarcinoma in childhood: a genetic analysis. *Hum Pathol* 2004; 35:565–70.

47 Laje P, Martinez-Ferro M, Grisoni E, Dudgeon D. Intrabdominal pulmonary sequestration: a case series and review of the literature. *J Pediatr Surg* 2006; 41:1309–12.

48 Osaki T, Kodate M, Takagishi T, et al. Unique extralobar sequestration with atypical location and aberrant vessels. *Ann Thorac Surg* 2010; 90:1711–2.

49 Carrasco R, Castañón. M, San Vicente B. Extralobar infradiaphragmatic pulmonary sequestration with a digestive communication. *J Thorac Cardiovasc Surg* 2002; 123:188–9.

50 Corbett HJ, Humphrey GM. Pulmonary sequestration. *Paediatr Respir Rev* 2004; 5(1):59–68.

51 Hofman FN, Pasker HG, Speekenbrink RG. Hemoptysis and massive hemothorax as presentation of intralobar sequestration. *Ann Thorac Surg* 2005; 80:2343–4.

52 Millendez MB, Ridout E, Pole G, Edwards M. Neonatal hyperreninemia and hypertensive heart failure relieved with resection of an intralobar pulmonary sequestration. *J Pediatr Surg* 2007; 42:1276–8.

53 Curros F, Chigot V, Emond S, et al. Role of embolisation in the treatment of bronchopulmonary sequestration. *Pediatr Radiol* 2000; 30:769–73.

54 Tokel K, Boyvat F, Varan B. Coil embolization of pulmonary sequestration in two infants: a safe alternative to surgery. *AJR Am J Roentgenol* 2000; 175:993–5.

55 Olutoye OO, Coleman BG, Hubbard AM, Adzick NS. Prenatal diagnosis and management of congenital lobar emphysema. *J Pediatr Surg* 2000; 35:792–5.

56 Andersen JB, Mortensen J, Damgaard K, et al. Fourteen-year-old girl with endobronchial carcinoid tumour presenting with asthma and lobar emphysema. *Clin Respir J* 2010; 4:120–4.

57 Mani H, Suarez E, Stocker JT. The morphologic spectrum of infantile lobar emphysema: a study of 33 cases. *Paediatr Respir Rev* 2004; 5 (Suppl A):S313–20.

58 Kanamori Y, Iwanaka T, Shibuya K. Congenital lobar emphysema caused by a very rare great vessel anomaly (left aortic arch, right descending aorta and left ligamentum arteriosum). *Pediatr Int* 2008; 50:594–6.

59 Carrol ED, Campbell ME, Shaw BN, Pilling DW. Congenital lobar

emphysema in congenital cytomegalovirus infection. *Pediatr Radiol* 1996:900–2.

60 Kennedy CD, Habibi P, Matthew DJ, Gordon I. Lobar emphysema: long-term imaging follow-up. *Radiology* 1991; 180:189–93.

61 Adzick NS, Harrison MR, Crombleholme TM, et al. Fetal lung lesions: management and outcome. *Am J Obstet Gynecol* 1998; 179:884–9.

62 Seong YW, Kang CH, Kim JT, et al. Video-assisted thoracoscopic lobectomy in children: safety, efficacy, and risk factors for conversion to thoracotomy. *Ann Thorac Surg* 2013 Apr; 95:1236–42.

63 Conforti A, Aloi I, Trucchi A, et al. Asymptomatic congenital cystic adenomatoid malformation of the lung: is it time to operate? *J Thorac Cardiovasc Surg* 2009; 138:826–30.

64 de Krijger RR, Claessen SM, van der Ham F, et al. Gain of chromosome 8q is a frequent finding in pleuropulmonary blastoma. *Mod Pathol* 2007; 20:1191–9.

65 Vargas SO, Korpershoek E, Kozakewich HP, et al. Cytogenetic and p53 profiles in congenital cystic adenomatoid malformation: insights into its relationship with pleuropulmonary blastoma. *Pediatr Dev Pathol* 2006; 9(3):190–5.

66 Hill DA, Jarzembowski JA, Priest JR, et al. Type I pleuropulmonary blastoma: pathology and biology study of 51 cases from the international pleuropulmonary blastoma registry. *Am J Surg Pathol* 2008; 32:282–95.

67 Priest JR, Hill DA, Williams GM, et al. Type I pleuropulmonary blastoma: a report from the International Pleuropulmonary Blastoma Registry. *J Clin Oncol* 2006; 24:4492–8.

68 Rothenberg SS. First decade's experience with thoracoscopic lobectomy in infants and children. *J Pediatr Surg* 2008; 43:40–5.

Lung volume reduction surgery for the treatment of advanced emphysema

Nathaniel Marchetti and Gerard J. Criner

Introduction

Chronic obstructive pulmonary disease (COPD) is a common worldwide problem associated with morbidity and mortality that, unlike other diseases, is increasing. Recently, COPD has become the third leading cause of death in the United States, an event that was not predicted to occur until the year 2020[1]. Therapy for COPD focuses on smoking cessation, bronchodilators, oxygen therapy, pulmonary rehabilitation, lung volume reduction surgery (LVRS), transplantation and treatment of comorbidities[2]. While many of these interventions may improve dyspnea and quality of life, only oxygen supplementation in those with hypoxemia at rest[3,4], smoking cessation[5] and LVRS[6,7] have been associated with improved mortality in COPD. This chapter will review the role of LVRS in the treatment of patients with advanced COPD, and also examine the current status of minimally invasive bronchoscopic techniques for lung reduction that are approved overseas but are currently under study in the United States.

Rationale for lung reduction in COPD

COPD is an inflammatory disease that leads to airflow obstruction secondary to a combination of airway disease and emphysema, primarily in the distal small airways of the lung. The small airways become narrowed due to airway inflammation, smooth muscle hypertrophy, peribronchial fibrosis and mucus plugging. In emphysema, the destruction of alveolar walls leads to a loss of tethering of distal small airways, predisposing the airway to expiratory collapse. Most individuals with COPD will have a mixture of small airways obstruction and emphysema, but some will have a predominance of one abnormality or the other.

Lung emptying is determined by the expiratory time constant, which is the product of airway resistance and lung compliance. Because subjects with emphysema have both increased lung compliance and airways resistance, they have impaired lung emptying and are prone to hyperinflation. As emphysema progresses, total lung capacity (TLC) and residual volume (RV) both increase as a result of decreased lung compliance and unopposed chest wall recoil causing hyperinflation and gas trapping, respectively. During exertion, the respiratory rate increases, reducing the time available for lung emptying, and the end-expiratory lung volume (EELV) rises even further, leading to dynamic hyperinflation[8]. Figure 8.1 demonstrates the rise in lung volumes that occurs during exercise in severe COPD. EELV rises during exercise, thereby limiting the normal increase in tidal volume that occurs during exercise. Static and dynamic hyperinflation are recognized as the main contributions to dyspnea development in COPD, which leads to increased work of breathing and places the inspiratory muscles at a mechanical disadvantage. Furthermore, extreme static hyperinflation has been linked to increased mortality in patients with COPD[9]. While it is intuitive to realize that lowering lung volumes would improve respiratory muscle function and exercise performance, it is less intuitive to understand how LVRS could improve forced expiratory volume in 1 second (FEV_1). Initially it was felt that LVRS improved lung function (FEV_1) primarily by increasing lung elastic recoil, but while LVRS does improve the lung recoil, it fails to totally explain the increase in FEV_1 following lung reduction, since preoperative lung recoil fails to significantly correlate with increases in post-LVRS FEV_1[10]. LVRS may improve lung function by "resizing" the lungs to better match thoracic dimensions[11,12]. As a

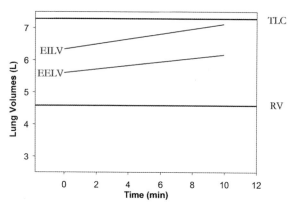

Figure 8.1 Lung volumes measured during exercise demonstrating development of dynamic hyperinflation. The EELV rises throughout exercise until a critical point is reached and tidal volume can no longer be increased. (EILV = end-inspiratory lung volume, EELV = end-expiratory lung volume, TLC = total lung capacity, RV = residual volume).

result of resizing, vital capacity (VC) increases post LVRS due to a greater reduction in RV than TLC. If the VC increases then the FEV_1 should increase, since $FEV_1 = FEV_1/FVC \times FVC$ (forced expiratory vital capacity)[11,12]. It has been postulated that if only cysts and bullae were removed with LVRS, the lung compliance would not change, since these empty spaces (cysts and bullae) do not contribute to lung elasticity. In this scenario, RV would fall by the volume of the cysts and bullae, and TLC would decrease. However, due to resizing of the lung relative to the thoracic cavity, the respiratory muscles would be at a more optimal precontraction length to produce force generation and increase TLC. Thus RV would fall more than TLC, resulting in a larger VC. This theory may explain why LVRS appears to be more effective in heterogeneous disease[11,12].

History of LVRS

Brantigan[13] was the first to resect emphysematous tissue in an attempt to reduce lung volumes in severe hyperinflated emphysema. While many of the surviving patients reported subjective improvement, the perioperative mortality was 18%, and postoperative lung function was not measured in a systematic manner. The procedure was not widely accepted because of high operative mortality without objective outcomes to document efficacy. The procedure was reintroduced in 1995 after Cooper reported the results of 20 cases of bilateral LVRS demonstrating dramatic improvements in pulmonary physiology

and 6-minute walk distances[14]. Shortly thereafter, the same group published their outcomes in 150 consecutive cases of LVRS and reported a 90-day operative mortality of 4%. Postoperative FEV_1 (0.70 L [25% predicted] to 1.0 L [38% predicted], $p < 0.0001$), RV (6.0 L [288% predicted] to 4.3 L [205% predicted], $p < 0.001$), TLC (8.4 L [143% predicted] to 7.2 L [125% predicted]) all significantly improved when compared to preoperative values[15]. Subsequent to these reports, other uncontrolled series and case reports suggested that LVRS could be beneficial in selected emphysematous patients. The first randomized, controlled trial evaluating the effectiveness of LVRS was published by Criner et al. in 1999[16]. In this study, 37 subjects were randomized to either LVRS or continued pulmonary rehabilitation and optimized medical care, and subjects in the nonsurgical arm could cross over to surgery following the period of continued pulmonary rehabilitation. The authors found that LVRS significantly improved FEV_1, TLC, RV, Pa_{CO2} (partial pressure of carbon dioxide), 6-minute walk distance, VO_2 (oxygen consumption) on cardiopulmonary exercise testing, and quality of life 3 months following surgery compared to medical therapy[16]. A subsequent randomized, controlled trial comparing LVRS to maximal medical therapy in 48 patients also demonstrated an improvement in FEV_1, TLC, RV, and shuttle walk distance[17]. Five of the surviving surgical patients did not have improvement following surgery, and all of these subjects were noted to have diffuse emphysema present on computed tomographic (CT) imaging. Neither of these studies was powered to evaluate survival with LVRS. The Centers for Medicare and Medicaid Services (CMS) noted increased utilization of this procedure code between October 1995 and January 1996; there were 711 LVRS procedures performed with a 1-year mortality of 26%, which was much higher than that being reported in the literature[18]. Both the Agency for Healthcare Research and Quality (AHRQ) and CMS recognized that some patients did benefit from LVRS, but they recommended that a prospective trial be conducted in order to study the effect of LVRS in subjects with comprehensive, long-term postoperative follow-up.

National Emphysema Treatment Trial (NETT) design

The majority of the data regarding LVRS originated from the NETT, a multicenter prospective randomized, controlled trial comparing optimal medical therapy, including pulmonary rehabilitation, to optimal medical therapy plus LVRS[19]. The trial was designed to examine the effect of LVRS on the coprimary endpoints of survival and exercise performance. Secondary outcomes included the effects of LVRS on lung function, patient symptoms, and quality of life compared to maximal medical therapy. NETT sought to enroll patients with moderate to severe bilateral emphysema on high-resolution CT (HRCT) imaging who were free from other diseases that would interfere with either data collection or the subject's ability to complete the trial. Inclusion and exclusion criteria are listed in Tables 8.1 and 8.2, respectively, but essentially investigators sought to enroll subjects with either heterogeneous or homogeneous disease who were not at high risk for perioperative morbidity and mortality and who were likely to complete the trial[19]. All subjects were optimally medically treated and underwent pulmonary rehabilitation prior to randomization. Pulmonary rehabilitation was conducted in three different phases of the trial including prerandomization (16–20 sessions over 6–10 weeks), postrandomization (10 sessions over 8–9 weeks), and maintenance therapy for study duration.

Surgical and anesthetic procedures

All centers performed surgical LVRS; 8 of the 17 centers performed median sternotomy (MS), 3 of the 17 centers used video-assisted thorascopic surgery (VATS) approach, and the remaining 6 centers randomized subjects to MS or VATS. Surgeons removed 25 to 30% of the total lung tissue from each lung targeting the most diseased regions, and they were permitted to use buttress suture material to reinforce staples lines at their discretion to minimize postoperative air leaks. All MS subjects received a thoracic epidural catheter for perioperative pain management, and all subjects were expected to be extubated within 2 hours. Additionally, everyone received chest respiratory therapy and physical therapy on the first postoperative day to enhance mobility[19].

Data analysis

The investigators used an intention-to-treat analysis and reported the outcomes of the entire cohort. The NETT steering committee determined *a priori* that a 10-watt change in exercise performance and an 8-point change in St George's Respiratory Questionnaire (SGRQ) were clinically meaningful changes

Table 8.1 Inclusion criteria for enrollment in NETT

History and physical exam consistent with emphysema

CT scan evidence of bilateral emphysema

Prerehabilitation postbronchodilator TLC $\geq$ 100% predicted

Prerehabilitation postbronchodilator RV $\geq$ 150% predicted

Prerehabilitation FEV$_1$ (maximum of pre- and postbronchodilator values) $\leq$ 45% of predicted and, if age $\geq$ 70 years, prerehabilitation, FEV$_1$ (maximum of pre- and postbronchodilator values) $\geq$15% of predicted

Prerehabilitation room air, resting PaCO$_2$ $\leq$ 60 mmHg ($\leq$ 55 mmHg in high altitude)

Prerehabilitation room air, resting PaO$_2$ $\geq$ 45 mmHg ($\geq$ 30 mmHg in high altitude)

Prerehabilitation plasma cotinine $\leq$ 13.7 ng/ml (if not using nicotine products) or prerehabilitation arterial carboxyhemoglobin $\leq$ 2.5% (if using nicotine products)

Bodymass index $\leq$ 31.1 (males) or $\leq$ 32.3 (females) as of randomization

Nonsmoker (tobacco products) for 4 months prior to initial interview

Approval for surgery by cardiologist if any of the following: unstable angina, left ventricular ejection fraction cannot be estimated from the echocardiogram, left ventricular ejection fraction < 45%, dobutamine-radionuclide cardiac scan indicates coronary artery disease or ventricular dysfunction, > 5 premature ventricular beats/minute (rest), cardiac rhythm other than sinus or premature atrial contractions noted during resting EKG, S$_3$ gallop on physical examination

Completion of all prerehabilitation assessments

Judgment by study physician that patient is likely to be approved for surgery upon completion of the rehabilitation program

Completion of NETT rehabilitation program

Completion of all postrehabilitation and all randomization assessments

for a surgical procedure with significant morbidity and mortality. Because one of the main goals of NETT was to define which subjects would benefit from LVRS *a priori*, the investigators identified the following prognostic factors prior to initiation of the

Table 8.2 Exclusion criteria for enrollment in NETT

CT scan evidence of diffuse emphysema judged unsuitable for LVRS

Previous LVRS (laser or excision)

Pleural or interstitial disease which precludes surgery

Giant bulla ($\geq$ one-third of the volume of the lung)

Clinically significant bronchiectasis

Pulmonary nodule requiring surgery

Previous sternotomy or lobectomy

Myocardial infarction within 6 months of interview and ejection fraction < 45%

Congestive heart failure within 6 months of interview and ejection fraction < 45%

Uncontrolled hypertension (systolic > 200 mmHg or diastolic >110 mmHg)

Pulmonary hypertension: mean PPA on right heart catheterization $\geq$ 35 mmHg ($\geq$ 38 mmHg in high altitude) or peak systolic PPA on right heart catheterization $\geq$ 45 mmHg ($\geq$ 50 mmHg in high altitude); right heart catheterization is required to rule out pulmonary hypertension if peak systolic PPA on echocardiogram > 45 mmHg

Unplanned, unexplained weight loss > 10% usual weight in 90 days prior to interview or unplanned, explained weight loss > 10% usual weight in 90 days prior to interview

History of recurrent infections with daily sputum production judged clinically significant

Daily use of > 20 mg of prednisone or its equivalent

History of exercise-related syncope

Resting bradycardia (<50 beats/min), frequent multifocal PVCs (premature ventricular contractions) or complex ventricular arrhythmia or sustained SVT (supraventricular tachycardia)

Cardiac dysrhythmia that poses a risk to the patient during exercise testing or training

Oxygen requirement during resting or oxygen titration exceeding 6 L/min to keep saturation $\geq$ 90%

Evidence of systemic disease or neoplasia that is expected to compromise survival

Any disease or condition which may interfere with completion of tests, therapy, or follow-up

6 MWD (maximum walking distance) $\leq$ 140 m postrehabilitation

Inability to complete successfully any of the screening or baseline data collection procedures

trial: age, FEV_1 percent predicted, Pa_{CO2}, RV percent predicted, distribution of perfusion on radionuclide lung scanning, homogeneity or heterogeneity of emphysema distribution on HRCT, and the presence of hyperinflation on chest X-ray[19,20]. During the trial, but well before data collection was completed, the Data and Safety Monitoring Board (DSMB) and steering committee additionally identified the following factors: diffusion capacity of carbon monoxide (DL_{CO}), maximal exercise capacity, RV/TLC ratio, ratio of expired ventilation in 1 minute to carbon dioxide excretion in 1 minute, presence or absence upper lobe predominant emphysema, degree of dyspnea, quality of life, race or ethnic group, and sex.

National Emphysema Treatment Trial (NETT) outcomes

Primary NETT outcomes for all patients

In 2003 the first report of NETT outcomes was published after patients were followed for a mean of 29.2 months[20]. A total of 3,777 subjects were screened and 1,218 were randomized to optimal medical therapy (610 subjects) or LVRS (608) subjects. Nearly all the subjects randomized to LVRS (580/608 [5.4%]) underwent LVRS (406 [70%] by median sternotomy, 174 [30%] by video-assisted thoracoscopic surgery), 21 [3.5%] declined LVRS, and 7 (1.2%) were considered unsuitable by the surgeon for LVRS after randomization. The 90-day mortality rate was significantly higher in the LVRS group (7.9% [95% CI 5.9–10.3] vs. 1.3% [95% CI 0.6–2.6]; $p < 0.001$) compared to the medical group. During follow-up (mean of 29.2 months) the overall mortality in all patients was not different between LVRS and medical therapy (relative risk [RR] 1.01, $p < 0.90$) despite an increased early mortality (90-day) in the surgical group[20].

Exercise performance at 6, 12, and 24 months improved by more than 10 watts in 28, 22, and 15% of the subjects undergoing LVRS, respectively, whereas the proportion improving with medical therapy alone was 4, 5, and 3% at the same time points ($p < 0.001$ for all time points). Patients who underwent LVRS were much more likely to improve FEV_1, 6-minute walk distance, dyspnea, and quality of life than those who received medical therapy alone[20].

Identification of the high risk for death with LVRS subgroup

The NETT steering committee predefined a 30-day mortality rate greater than 8% as a stopping endpoint for either group. The investigators found a subgroup of patients who had LVRS with an $FEV_1 \leq 20\%$ predicted and either a $DL_{CO} \leq 20\%$ predicted or homogeneous emphysema on HRCT imaging who had a 30-day mortality rate of 16% compared to 0% in the medical group ($p < 0.001$). Furthermore, those that had survived LVRS had a low likelihood of achieving predefined significant changes in exercise performance and quality of life. Therefore, patients with an $FEV_1 \leq 20\%$ predicted who have either a $DL_{CO} \leq 20\%$ or a homogeneous disease should not undergo LVRS due to high morbidity and mortality[21]. After excluding the high-risk group, there were 1,078 remaining subjects in whom the 30-day mortality was 2.2 and 0.2% in the LVRS and medical therapy groups, respectively ($p < 0.001$). The 90-day mortality rates were also significantly different in LVRS group (5.2%) vs medical therapy (1.5%). The non-high-risk subjects who had LVRS were significantly more likely to have improved 6-minute walk distance, maximal exercise performance, FEV_1 percent predicted, and quality of life compared to medical therapy alone[21].

Predicting LVRS outcomes in non-high-risk NETT patients

One of the stated goals of the NETT was to determine which groups of patients with advanced emphysema would benefit from LVRS. NETT demonstrated that the only factors that discriminated mortality differences were the craniocaudal distribution of emphysema on CT imaging and postrehabilitation prerandomization exercise performance differences, while the only factor to discriminate an improvement in maximal exercise performance at 24 months was the craniocaudal distribution of emphysema. Patients were divided into four subgroups based on exercise performance (high vs low) and emphysema distribution (upper lobe predominant vs non–upper lobe predominant).

A maximal workload on cardiopulmonary exercise testing was defined as < 25 watts for women and < 40 watts for men. The group with upper lobe predominant emphysema and low exercise performance had a mortality benefit with LVRS compared to medical therapy alone ($p = 0.005$). Those that had LVRS in this group were more likely to achieve > 10-watt improvement in maximal exercise performance at 24 months (30% vs 0%, $p < 0.001$) and > 8-point improvement in SGRQ score at 24 months (48% vs 10%, $p < 0.001$). In the group with upper lobe predominant emphysema and high exercise performance there was no survival advantage with LVRS, although LVRS afforded this group a better chance at a > 10-watt improvement in exercise performance at 24 months (15% vs 3%, $p = 0.001$) and > 8-point improvement in SGRQ (41% vs 11%, $p < 0.001$)[20].

Those that underwent LVRS with non–upper lobe predominant emphysema and low baseline exercise performance did not have a survival advantage ($p = 0.49$) or improved exercise performance at 24 months (12% vs 7%, $p = 0.50$), but they were more likely to have improved SGRQ at 24 months (37% vs 7%, $p = 0.001$). Those that underwent LVRS with non–upper lobe predominant emphysema and high baseline exercise performance had increased risk of death ($p = 0.02$), no difference in exercise performance (3% both groups, $p = 1.0$), and no difference in SGRQ (15% vs 12%, $p = 0.61$) at 24 months[20].

In summary, the NETT demonstrated that at a mean follow-up time of 29.2 months, LVRS did not offer a survival advantage compared to optimal medial therapy alone even when the high-risk group was excluded. However, LVRS did result in improved exercise performance, reduction in dyspnea, and improvements in quality of life. Data from NETT suggest that in those with upper lobe predominant emphysema and low baseline exercise performance, LVRS did offer a survival advantage compared to optimal medical therapy alone. The NETT investigators realized that the mean follow-up time of only 2.4 years may not have been long enough and proposed that the group continued to be followed in order to establish the long-term effect of LVRS in this group with advanced emphysema.

Long-term follow-up of NETT subjects

Subjects enrolled in NETT continued follow-up with the clinical centers through June 2004 with scheduled clinic visits, annual testing, and completion of quality-of-life questionnaires. Long-term survival was updated by the clinical centers and through review of the Social Security death file[6]. In all, 1,218 subjects enrolled in NETT with a median follow-up time of 4.3 years, those treated with LVRS demonstrated a long-term survival advantage (Figure 8.2a). The mortality rate was 0.11 deaths per person-year with LVRS and 0.13 medical therapy (RR = 0.85, p = 0.02). Overall, long-term survival improved despite the expected early increase in surgical mortality immediately following LVRS[6]. The survival advantage was similar when the high-risk subjects were excluded from the analysis (RR = 0.82, p = 0.02, Figure 8.2b). Exercise capacity improved by > 10 watts in 23, 15, and 9% following LVRS at 1, 2, and 3 years, respectively, compared to 5, 3, and 1% with medical therapy alone (p < 0.001 at each time point). There was a > 8-point improvement in SGRQ in 40, 32, 20, 10, and 13% following LVRS at 1, 2, 3, 4, and 5 years, respectively, compared to 9, 8, 8, 4, and 7% with medical therapy alone. These differences in SGRQ were significant through 4 years (p < 0.001 years 1 to 3 and p = 0.005 for year 4). In those with upper lobe predominant emphysema and baseline low exercise performance, LVRS markedly decreased mortality (RR = 0.57, p = 0.01, Figure 8.2c) and produced > 10-watt improvement in exercise performance and > 8-point improvement in SGRQ measured quality of life that persisted for 3 years. In the group with upper lobe predominant emphysema and high exercise capacity, there was no survival advantage with LVRS (RR = 0.86, p = 0.19, Figure 8.2d), but more subjects had an increase in exercise performance of > 10 watts and > 8-point improvement in SGRQ during the long-term follow-up period with LVRS[6].

LVRS did not confer a survival benefit or improve exercise performance in the non–upper lobe predominant emphysema and low exercise group. While subjects who had LVRS were more likely to have had > 8-point improvements in the SGRQ score compared to medical therapy, this advantage dissipated by year 3. Subjects in the non–upper lobe predominant emphysema and high exercise group undergoing LVRS did not have a survival benefit and were not more likely to have significant improvements in either exercise (>10-watt change) or quality of life (>8-point increase in SGRQ) compared to medical therapy alone[6].

Not only did the long-term follow-up of the NETT reaffirm that LVRS is beneficial to subjects with advanced emphysema that have upper lobe predominant emphysema, but it demonstrated that these benefits are durable. Benefits include clinically important improvements in exercise and quality of life, dyspnea, lung function, and in those with baseline low exercise, a survival advantage. Individuals with non–upper lobe dependent emphysema did not have a survival advantage with LVRS (regardless of baseline exercise performance), and although there was improved quality of life in subjects with upper lobe disease and low exercise, it was not durable. Most experts would agree that the risk/benefit ratio in this group is not justified, and those with non–upper lobe predominant disease should not receive LVRS.

In addition to the primary and secondary outcomes that were part of the NETT protocol, there were many other analyses that provided insight into LVRS and the pathophysiology of emphysema.

Operative mortality and cardiopulmonary morbidity following LVRS

Investigators examined data from 511 of the non-high-risk subjects who underwent LVRS and found a 5.5% 90-day mortality rate. The only predictor of operative mortality was the existence of non–upper lobe predominant emphysema with a relative odds (RO) of 2.99 (p = 0.009). During the intraoperative period, 91% of subjects had no complications, 2.2% had transient hypoxemia, and 1.2% developed arrhythmias. Also, 58.7% of LVRS subjects had at least one postoperative complication in the 30-day postoperative time frame, with cardiac arrhythmia being the most common (23.5%). Pneumonia developed in 18.2%, 21.8% required intubation at least once, 11.7% were readmitted to the ICU, and 8.2% required tracheostomy. Only 5.1% of subjects undergoing LVRS were not extubated within 3 days postoperatively[22].

Major pulmonary and cardiovascular 30-day morbidity occurred in 29.8 and 20% of subjects, respectively. Multivariate logistic regression determined that pulmonary morbidity was greater in older patients (RO = 1.05, p = 0.02), lower FEV_1 (RO = 0.97, p = 0.05), and lower DL_{CO} (RO = 0.97, p = 0.01). Cardiovascular morbidity was higher with age (RO = 1.07, p = 0.004), preoperative steroid use (RO = 1.72, p = 0.04), and presence of non–upper lobe predominant emphysema (RO = 2.67, p < 0.001)[22].

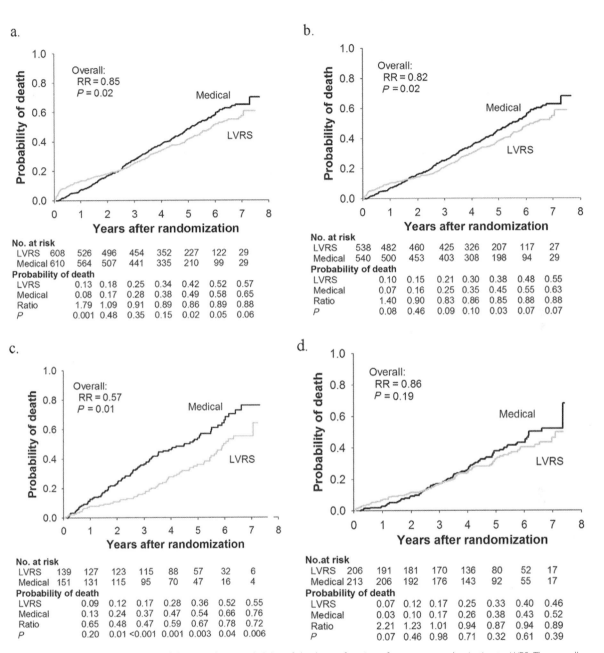

Figure 8.2. Kaplan-Meier estimates of the cumulative probability of death as a function of years post randomization to LVRS. The overall relative risk (RR) and p value represent the 4.3 years median follow-up. Shown below each plot is the number of subjects at risk in each arm, probability of death in each arm, and the RR (LVRS: Medical) for each year and the p value for difference in the probability. (a) All patients (n = 1,218) (b) Non-high-risk patients (n = 1,078) (c) Upper lobe predominant and low baseline exercise performance (n = 290) (d) Upper lobe predominant and high exercise capacity (n = 419). (Reprinted with permission from Naunheim et al., *Ann Thorac Surg* 2006).

Air leak following LVRS

Within the 30-day postoperative period, 90% of patients undergoing LVRS had an air leak with a median duration of 7 days, although 12% had an air leak ≥ 30 days. The choice of buttressing technique, stapler brand, or intraoperative adjunctive procedures (tenting or pleurodesis) did not alter either the incidence or duration of air leaks post LVRS. Risk factors for postoperative air leaks were lower DL_{CO}, presence of upper lobe predominant disease, and most important, the presence of pleural adhesions. Air leaks were more prolonged in Caucasians, patients with lower FEV_1 or DL_{CO}, presence of upper lobe predominant emphysema, use of inhaled corticosteroids, and presence of pleural adhesions[23]. Subjects having air leaks were more likely to have postoperative complications (57 vs 30%, $p = 0.0004$) and a longer hospital stay (11.8 ± 6.5 vs 7.6 ± 4.4 days, $p = 0.0005$). The presence of air leak was not associated with increased mortality and only 4.4% of subjects with an air leak required reoperation.

Median sternotomy (MS) vs video-assisted thorascopic (VATS) approach to LVRS

As mentioned previously, the approach to LVRS was not uniform with MS performed at 8 of the 17 centers, VATS approach used at 3 of the 17 centers and subjects randomized to MS or VATS at the remaining 6 centers. There was no difference in 90-day mortality between the two approaches (5.9% for MS and 4.6% for VATS, $p = 0.42$)[24]. Intraoperative blood loss and the need for subsequent transfusion of blood products were not different between the two groups either. The mean operating time was 21.7 minutes shorter in the MS group. There were fewer episodes of intraoperative hypoxemia in the MS group (0.8 vs 5.3%, $p = 0.004$) and overall fewer intraoperative complications in the MS group as well (93.0 vs 86.2%, $p = 0.02$). There were not any statistically significant differences in postoperative complications between the MS or VATS approaches. Air leak duration was not different between MS and VATS subjects, but median hospital length of stay was shorter with VATS (10 vs 9 days, $p = 0.01$). At 30 days post LVRS, 70.5% of MS patients and 80.9% of VATS patients were living independently ($p = 0.02$), but by 4 months post randomization there was no difference in the number of subjects living independently. There were no differences in functional outcomes following LVRS at 12 and 24 months between the two approaches. Total hospital costs at 6 months post LVRS were about $10,000 less with VATS compared to MS ($61,481 \pm 3,189$ vs $51,053 \pm 4,502$, $p = 0.005$)[24]. Overall outcomes, morbidity, and mortality were similar for both MS and VATS, but recovery time and associated costs were lower with VATS.

Effects of LVRS in α-1 antitrypsin-deficient subjects in NETT

There were 16 subjects (1.3%) with severe α-1 antitrypsin (AAT) deficiency (serum AAT level < 80 mg/dL) randomized in NETT, and 10 underwent LVRS. The 2-year mortality was higher with LVRS compared to medical therapy (20 vs 0%) in subjects with AAT deficiency. AAT-deficient subjects also had less improvement in FEV_1 and exercise capacity, and the benefits were not as durable[25]. Based on these data and the fact that many AAT-deficient patients have non–upper lobe predominant disease, most centers do not offer LVRS to AAT-deficient patients.

Perfusion scintigraphy and patient selection for LVRS

In NETT 1,045 of the 1,218 subjects had complete perfusion scintigraphy performed at baseline, and a post hoc analysis was performed to determine if perfusion scintigraphy could predict outcome following LVRS[26]. The investigators decided a priori to focus on upper lobe perfusion, and they defined low perfusion to the upper third as being < 20% of total lung perfusion. Among the 248 subjects with upper lobe predominant emphysema and low exercise in NETT, the 202 who had low perfusion to the upper lung zone had decreased mortality with LVRS vs medical therapy (RR = 0.56, $p = 0.008$) as opposed to the 82 patients with high perfusion to the upper lung zone in whom mortality was unchanged (0.97, $p = 0.62$). Among the 404 subjects with upper lobe predominant emphysema and high exercise performance, the 278 with low perfusion to the upper lung zone had a reduction in mortality with LVRS compared to medical therapy (RR = 0.70, $p = 0.02$). In the remaining 126 subjects with upper lobe predominant emphysema and high exercise performance who had high perfusion to the upper lung zone, there was no difference in mortality between LVRS and medical therapy (RR = 1.05, $p = 1.0$)[26]. In subjects who had non–upper lobe predominant emphysema the perfusion to the upper lung zones did not predict outcomes from LVRS. These data suggest that in those with upper lobe predominant emphysema the presence of low perfusion to the upper lung zone will have improved survival following LVRS. The most likely explanation for this finding is that lung scintigraphy assesses regional lung function in addition to purely anatomic CT imaging.

Lung function and prediction of LVRS outcome

A small subset of 115 subjects who were randomized to LVRS in NETT had measurements of static lung recoil at total lung capacity (SR_{TLC}) and inspiratory resistance (RI) at baseline. A post hoc analysis of the subjects who had LVRS in NETT was conducted to determine if CT measurements of emphysema (% lung attenuation) and airway wall thickness, ratio of upper to lower zone emphysema, RV/TLC, SR_{TLC}, and RI at baseline could help predict LVRS outcome. The investigators found that SR_{TLC}, RI, and CT measures of airway wall thickness did not predict improvements in either FEV_1 or exercise performance post LVRS. The RV/TLC and CT measures of emphysema were only weakly predictive of postoperative improvements in FEV_1 and exercise performance[10].

Reduction of acute exacerbation of COPD (AECOPD) in NETT

The effect of LVRS on AECOPD was examined in 1,204 subjects enrolled in NETT who had Medicare claims data available pre and post randomization[27]. There were 601 subjects randomized to LVRS and 603 to medical therapy, and subjects were followed up to 3 years post randomization. Subjects undergoing LVRS had a 30% reduction in the rate of COPD emergency department visits and hospitalizations (0.27 vs 0.37 per person-year; $p = 0.0005$) compared to optimal medical therapy. LVRS also delayed the time to the first AECOPD, but this effect did not become apparent until 150 days following randomization to treatment. The change in FEV_1 6 months following LVRS was a significant predictor of an increased time to first AECOPD (HR = 3.2; $p = 0.002$)[27].

Effects of LVRS on oxygenation

The effects of LVRS on oxygenation were evaluated in 1,078 NETT subjects utilizing arterial blood gases, the need for supplemental oxygen during treadmill testing, and the self-reported use of oxygen during rest, exertion, and sleep. Subjects undergoing LVRS required less oxygen at 6 months (33 vs 49%, $p < 0.001$), 12 months (50 vs 36%, $p < 0.001$), and 24 months (52 vs 42%, $p = 0.02$) compared to medical controls. Additionally, self-reported oxygen use was lower with LVRS compared to medical therapy at the same time points. Not surprisingly, multivariate analysis of preoperative characteristics showed that baseline oxygenation was the best predictor for needing postoperative supplemental oxygen[28].

Effect of LVRS on pulmonary hemodynamics

A group of patients from NETT underwent right heart catheterization at baseline and then 6 months post randomization to determine if LVRS altered pulmonary hemodynamics[29]. The mean pulmonary artery pressure was elevated in this group with severe emphysema at baseline (mean pulmonary artery pressure 24.8 ± 5.0 mmHg). The changes from baseline to 6 months post randomization were not significantly different except for a decrease in the pulmonary capillary wedge pressure at end-expiration in the LVRS group compared to medical therapy (–1.8 mmHg vs 3.5 mmHg, $p = 0.04$). These data suggest that postoperative pulmonary hypertension is an unlikely occurrence in patients undergoing LVRS using NETT criterion[29].

The effects of LVRS on breathing pattern during exercise

A NETT substudy involving 238 patients examined the effect of LVRS on breathing pattern, gas exchange, and dyspnea during maximal exercise testing. At 6 months, LVRS subjects had higher maximum minute ventilation (32.8 vs 29.6 L/min, $p = 0.001$), carbon dioxide production (0.923 vs 0.820 L/min, $p = 0.0003$), tidal volume (1.18 vs 1.07 L, $p = 0.001$), heart rate (124 vs 121 beats/min, $p = 0.02$) and workload (49.3 vs 45.1 W, $p = 0.04$), but less breathlessness (4.4 vs 5.2 Borg dyspnea scale, $p = 0.0001$) and were less likely to have a ventilatory limitation to exercise (49.5 vs 71.9%, $p = 0.001$) than medical controls. Following LVRS, patients breathed slower and deeper during exercise at 6 and 12 months with reduced dead space at 6 and 24 months. Patients with upper lobe predominant emphysema showed a downward shift in the partial pressure of carbon dioxide (PCO_2) vs amount of carbon dioxide produced as a result of metabolism (VCO_2) relationship during restful breathing and throughout exercise ($p = 0.001$). These data show that following LVRS, patients breathe slower and deeper during exercise and have improved CO_2 elimination and less dyspnea and dead space ventilation[30].

Effect of LVRS on body mass index (BMI)

A low BMI has been associated with increased mortality in COPD[31]. A posthoc analysis was performed on NETT subjects to examine the effect of this intervention on BMI; subjects who were underweight (BMI < 21) who underwent LVRS were more likely to increase BMI ≥ 5% 6 months post randomization compared to medical therapy alone (37.97 vs 17.65%, $p = 0.02$)[32]. Those subjects with normal weight (BMI 21–25) who underwent LVRS also were more likely to increase BMI ≥ 5% 6 months post randomization (23.67 vs 3.57%, $p < 0.001$), but subjects who were overweight (BMI 25–30) or obese (BMI > 30) did not have significant weight gain[32]. In subjects who underwent LVRS and had ≥ 5% increase in BMI compared to those did not have an increase ≥ 5%, the percent predicted FEV_1 (11.53 ± 9.31% vs 7.55 ± 14.88%, $p < 0.0001$), 6-minute walk distance (38.70 ± 69.57 m vs 7.57 ± 73.37 m, $p < 0.0001$) and SGRQ (−15.30 ± 14.08 vs −9.15 ± 14.44, $p < 0.0001$) had greater change at 6 months. Furthermore, the V_E/V_{CO2} ratio (ventilator equivalent ratio for oxygen and carbon dioxide), a marker of ventilatory efficiency, was lower in the LVRS group, who had ≥ 5% increase in BMI compared to those who did not have the 5% increase in BMI. These data suggest that subjects undergoing LVRS who are underweight or normal weight preoperatively can expect to gain weight following the procedure. Another study suggested that LVRS results in an 8% decrease in resting energy expenditure (REE) that is also associated with a decrease in respiratory muscle oxygen consumption following LVRS[33]. The reduction in V_E/V_{CO2} (i.e. improved ventilatory efficiency) is likely related to reduction in lung volumes, which leads to a lowered REE leading to weight gain.

Cost-effectiveness of LVRS in NETT

The NETT investigators conducted a parallel prospective cost analysis of LVRS compared to medical therapy which estimated costs involved in caring for subjects including medical goods and services, transportation, subject time receiving treatment and even time family spent caring for the subjects. A cost-effectiveness ratio was calculated by taking the cost difference between LVRS and medical therapy divided by the difference in quality-adjusted life-years gained between the two groups[34]. This analysis excluded the high-risk group identified in NETT.

The mean total cost per patient was higher in the LVRS subjects compared to medical therapy in the first 12 months ($71,515 vs $23,371, $p < 0.001$) due to increased costs associated with the surgery and postoperative care. However, the mean cost was lower in LVRS subjects during the second year post randomization ($13,222 vs $21,319, $p < 0.001$). During the third year post randomization, the costs were lower in the LVRS group, but the difference was not statistically significant ($14,215 vs $17,870, $p = 0.08$). From months 7 to 36 post randomization the mean total cost was nearly $10,000 lower in LVRS as compared to medical therapy alone ($36,199 vs $49,628, $p < 0.001$), mainly due to fewer hospitalization days following LVRS. Subjects receiving LVRS had more hospitalization days during the first year post randomization compared to medical therapy (24.9 vs 4.9, $p < 0.001$), but during the second year LVRS subjects had fewer hospitalization days (3.2 vs 6.1, $p < 0.001$). During the third year LVRS subjects still had fewer hospitalization days, but the difference was not statistically significant (4.0 vs 5.2, $p = - 0.08$)[34].

The mean number of quality adjusted life-years was higher in LVRS subjects compared to medical therapy (1.46 vs 1.27, $p < 0.001$) during the first post randomization year, and this difference remained significant during years 2 and 3 post randomization. The cost-effectiveness ratio for LVRS subjects compared to medical therapy was $190,000 per quality-adjusted life year at 3 years post randomization. The investigators projected the cost-effectiveness ratio to be $53,000 per quality-adjusted life year at 10 years post randomization. The cost-effectiveness ratio for LVRS compared to medical therapy in the upperlobe predominant low-exercise subgroup was $98,000 per quality-adjusted life-year at 3 years post randomization and was projected to be $21,000 per quality-adjusted life-year at 10 years[34]. The cost-effectiveness analysis was repeated using data obtained on patients during the extension of NETT, and the cost-effectiveness ratio at 5 years post randomization decreased to $140,000 per quality-adjusted life-year. The projected 10-year cost-effectiveness ratio was similar at $54,000 per quality-adjusted life-year[35].

LVRS: an underutilized therapy

Despite evidence from randomized and controlled clinical trials in well-characterized emphysema subjects demonstrating benefit, there have been relatively few LVRS surgeries performed since CMS approval for the procedure in 2004. Initially in 2004 there were 254 LVRS procedures performed in Medicare beneficiaries, and more recent data suggest that even fewer are being performed. The most recent data available for the years of 2009, 2010, and 2011 demonstrate that only 104, 92, and 93 LVRS procedures were performed in Medicare beneficiaries in the United States, respectively[36].

A retrospective analysis at a single center examined a database of 413 patients who had full pulmonary function data, CT imaging, and a primary diagnosis of emphysema to determine what percentage would benefit from LVRS using NETT criteria[37]. They found that 195 did not meet clinical criteria, with the most common exclusions being malignancy with an expected survival of < 2 years, prior lobectomy, prior sternotomy, and presence of pulmonary hypertension. Twelve more subjects had CT findings such as pleural plaques or extensive pulmonary fibrosis. The investigators found that 61 of the 413 subjects (15%) had evidence of upper lobe predominant disease on CT imaging that would make them good candidates for LVRS[37]. These data suggest that there is a large population of subjects who would benefit from a proven surgical intervention. Although the reasons for underperformance of LVRS are not known, the NETT investigators proposed some possible reasons, which are listed in Table 8.3[38].

Table 8.3 Possible explanations for underperformance of LVRS in the United States

Restriction of LVRS to NETT centers, lung transplant centers, or those with JCAHO-approval limits to patient access

Preoperative testing is overly complicated

Limited availability of outpatient pulmonary rehabilitation centers

Physicians remain unaware of LVRS benefits

Misinterpretation of the report on the group at high risk for mortality in NETT that all patients with severe emphysema are at high risk for death due to LVRS

LVRS is perceived as being too costly

LVRS = lung volume reduction surgery, NETT = National Emphysema Treatment Trial, JCAHO = Joint Commission on Accreditation of Healthcare Organizations

Another reason why some physicians may be reluctant to send patients for LVRS is that even in the NETT subgroup with the most benefit from LVRS (upper lobe predominant emphysema/low exercise) physiologic outcomes can be highly variable. This variability may be secondary to the presence of unrecognized small airway disease that cannot be detected using current preoperative testing[39,40].

Nonsurgical investigative approaches to lung volume reduction (LVR)

Recently, there have been efforts to achieve lung reduction without the morbidity associated with thoracic surgery. Bronchoscopic techniques include placement of one-way endobronchial valves in the airway, self-activating coils placed in the airway, targeted destruction and remodeling of emphysematous tissue, and bypass airway stenting. While these techniques are investigative in the United States, some of them are approved for routine clinical use in other countries. An additional technique, transpleural ventilation, is achieved with a minithoracotomy.

Endobronchial one-way valves

Of all the bronchoscopic techniques, one-way endobronchial valves have been studied more than any other technique. These valves are placed at the segmental or lobar level to block inspiration but permit expiration of air and secretions, and are thought to work by promoting atelectasis of the region distal to the valve. Currently, there are two types of endobronchial valves (EBV) under evaluation. The Spiration intrabronchial valve (Spiration Incorporated, Redmond, WA) system has an umbrella design where an occlusive cover is stretched over a titanium wire frame, which allows expired air and secretions to escape around the outer edges. The Zephyr valve (Pulmonx, Redwood City, CA) is a cylindrical device with a duckbill one-way valve placed in a nitinol wire cage, which permits expired air and secretions to escape through the center of the valve.

The Endobronchial Valve for Emphysema Palliation Trial (VENT) was the first prospective randomized trial to evaluate bronchoscopic LVR utilizing the Zephyr valve[41]. The VENT trial randomized 220 subjects to EBV placement compared to 101 subjects treated with maximal medical therapy. The primary endpoints of the study were percentage change in FEV_1 and 6-minute walk distance at 6 months. The primary safety endpoint was the Major Complication Composite (MCC), which included death, massive hemoptysis, empyema, pneumonia distal to the valves, and ventilator dependency for $\geq$ 24 hours. Investigators placed the valves unilaterally, targeting the lobe with the highest percentage of emphysema and greatest degree of heterogeneity defined as the difference in percent emphysema between ipsilateral lobes.

At 6 months, the FEV_1 increased 4.3% (34.5 ml) in the EBV group but decreased 2.5% (–25.4 ml) in the control group such that following EBV, the FEV_1 increased 6.8% (60 ml) compared to controls (p = 0.005). The 6-minute walk distance increased 2.5% (9.3 m) in the EBV group and fell 3.2% (–10.7 m) in the control group. The mean increase in the 6-minute walk test was 5.8% (19.1 m) following EBV compared to control (p = 0.04). Furthermore, there were modest differences in the quality of life, dyspnea, cycle ergometry peak workload, and supplemental oxygen use, all favoring the EBV group. The MCC rate was 1.2% in the control group and 6.1% in the EBV group (p = 0.08). Acute exacerbations of COPD requiring hospitalization occurred in 7.9% of the EBV cases compared to 1.2% of controls (p = 0.03). Heterogeneity of emphysema between lobes in treated lung and the presence of complete fissures were the only factors predictive of improvements in the primary endpoints. For heterogeneity of emphysema, those with $\geq$15% differences in emphysema were found to have greater improvements in FEV_1 and 6-minute walk distance at 6 months. EBV subjects with intact fissures had a 16.2% improvement in FEV_1 at 6 months (p < 0.001) and 17.9% at 12 months (p < 0.001), while those with incomplete fissures had changes of FEV_1 of only 2.0 and 2.8% at 6 and 12 months, respectively[41].

The VENT study was also performed in 23 European sites where 111 subjects were randomized to EBV and 60 to medical therapy[42]. Although the study was underpowered compared to the VENT study in the United States, the results were similar. At 6 months, there were modest improvements in FEV_1, quality of life, and 6-minute walk distance in the EBV group compared to the control group that were either significant or nearly significant. Once again, those with complete fissures had better results with improvements in FEV_1 (16 vs 2%, p =0.02) when treated with EBV compared to medical therapy. The 6-minute walk distance did not reach statistical

significance (11 vs 19%, p = 0.6). The median reduction in target lobe volume reduction (TLVR) relative to baseline TLVR was greater in those with complete fissures (–55%) compared to incomplete fissure (–13%) (p < 0.0001). In this series the level of emphysema heterogeneity did not preclude a decrease in $TLVR^{[42]}$.

The Lung Function Improvement after Bronchoscopic Lung Volume Reduction with Pulmonx Endobronchial Valves used in Treatment of Emphysema (LIBERATE) study is now recruiting patients to determine the efficacy of the Zephyr valve in patients who have intact fissures and $\geq$15% emphysema heterogeneity between lobes. This study is utilizing the Chartis system (Pulmonx, Inc.), which measures collateral ventilation during bronchoscopy in order to only enroll subjects with intact fissures. A balloon catheter with flow and pressure sensors is inflated in the target bronchus to occlude airflow, and if there is no collateral flow (i.e. intact fissure), then there will be a gradual decline expiratory flow[43].

Experience with the Spiration intrabronchial valve is limited compared to the Zephyr valve, but a pilot study involving 91 subjects who had bilateral valve placement has been published[44]. The study was a multicenter case prospective open-enrollment study designed to examine safety and effectiveness of the device. The primary outcome of the study was safety based on incidence of valve migration and erosion or infection. Subjects enrolled had upper lobe predominant emphysema and met NETT criteria. While there was a decrease in lobar lung volumes and the SGRQ compared to baseline, there was not an improvement in FEV_1, TLC or RV, or exercise performance as measured by 6-minute walk distances or cycle ergometry. There were no instances of valve migration or erosion in any patient, and two episodes of infection in the first 3 months of the valve procedure yielded a 2.4% rate. The most common complication was pneumothorax, which occurred in 12.1% of the subjects over the 12-month study period, and a total of 19 subjects (20.8%) withdrew from the study. The investigators concluded that the procedure has an acceptable safety profile and may improve quality of life, but further controlled studies are needed[44].

Self-activating coils for LVR

One method currently under study to avoid the problems with endobronchial valves and collateral flow is to place nitinol coils into subsegmental airways. These coils are placed straight bronchoscopically and then upon release recover to a predetermined shape. In a pilot study, lung volume reduction coils (LVRCs) (PneumRx, Inc., Mountain View, CA) were bronchoscopically placed into the most diseased regions in 11 severe emphysema patients (8 homogeneous, 3 heterogeneous)[45]. Safety was the primary endpoint; efficacy outcomes were secondary endpoints. The 11 patients underwent 21 treatments with a total placement of 101 LVRCs. A total of 33 adverse events were reported, and events possibly attributed to the procedure or device included dyspnea (10 events), cough (5 events), COPD exacerbations (3 events), and chest pain (1 event). Group mean values for FEV_1, RV, TLC, SGRQ, and 6 MWD at 1 and 3 months improved following the first procedure. The greatest relative changes were observed in 6 MWD, SGRQ, and mMRC in the patients with heterogeneous emphysema[45]. A prospective cohort pilot study in 16 subjects with severe heterogeneous emphysema who underwent 28 procedures using 260 LVRCs (median 10 per procedure) was performed with the primary efficacy endpoint being quality of life as measured by SGRQ[46]. In the 28 procedures, adverse events included pneumothorax (1), transient chest pain (4), self-limiting mild hemoptysis (12), and no life-threatening events. Six months post procedure, secondary endpoints including SGRQ (−14.9, $p < 0.005$), FEV_1 (14.9%, $p = 0.004$), FVC (13.4%, $p = 0.002$), RV (11.4%, $p < 0.001$), and 6-minute walk distance (84.4 m, $p < 0.001$) all improved compared to baseline. Additionally, more than 50% of subjects met the minimal clinically important difference for FEV_1, 6-minute walk distance, and SGRQ.

The RESET trial was a prospective, randomized multicenter trial comparing LVRCs to optimal medical therapy in 47 subjects with either heterogeneous or homogeneous emphysema[47]. The goal was to place 10 coils in the most diseased lobe of each lung in those randomized to the LVRC arm during two separate bronchoscopies separated by 1 month. The primary outcome was quality of life as measured by the SGRQ at 90 days. Secondary endpoints included change in FEV_1, TLC, RV, 6-minute walk distance, and dyspnea, as well as any procedure- or device-related adverse events at 90 days. The SGRQ declined in subjects randomized to LVRC placement (−8.11 with 95% CI −13.83 to −2.39) compared to optimal medical therapy (+0.25 with 95% CI −5.58 to +6.07, $p = 0.04$).

Additionally, there were significant improvements in RV (−0.51L vs −0.20L, $p = 0.03$), FEV_1 percent change (14.19% vs 3.57%, $p = 0.03$), and 6-minute walk distance (51.15 m vs −12.39 m, $p < 0.001$) for the LVRC subjects compared to optimal medical therapy, respectively. Two subjects had a pneumothorax in the LVRC arm that occurred within 2 hours following the procedure. During the first 30 days following treatment there were significantly more adverse events in the LVRC arm (two pneumothoraces, two AECOPDs, and two lower respiratory tract infections) compared to the optimal therapy arm (two AECOPDs, p = 0.02). Between days 31 and 90 there was not a significant difference in adverse events between the two groups ($p > 0.99$)[47]. While the use of LVRC is promising and avoids problems with collateral ventilation, additional prospective controlled trials are ongoing.

Biologic lung reduction

This approach uses a biodegradable sclerosant gel (BioLVR, Aeiris Therapeutics) to polymerize in small airways and alveolar spaces, reducing lung volumes by scarring and remodeling of targeted lung regions that occur over a period of several weeks. In an open-label multicenter phase 2 dose-ranging study, BioLVR hydrogel was instilled in four pulmonary subsegments in each upper lobe at a low dose (10 ml per site) and high dose (20 ml per site)[48] in patients with upper lobe predominant emphysema. There was a significant reduction in the RV/TLC at 6 months in the low-dose (−6.4%, $p = 0.002$) and high-dose protocol (−5.5%, $p = 0.028$). The FEV_1 improvement at 6 months was more robust in the high-dose (15.6%, $p = 0.002$) compared to the low-dose protocol (6.7%, $p = 0.021$), while both low- and high-dose protocols led to improvements in health-related quality of life scores[48]. A separate study also administered BioLVR to 25 subjects with homogeneous emphysema distribution utilizing the same protocol in the upper lobe predominant group[49]. Compared to baseline, changes at 6 months in FEV_1, FVC, RV/TLC, dyspnea, and SGRQ were better with high-dose but only met statistical significance following high-dose therapy in FEV_1 (13.8, $p = 0.007$), dyspnea (−0.8 mMRC score, $p = 0.001$), and SGRQ (−12.2, $p = 0.0001$).

Aeris Therapeutics halted plans for larger studies with BioLVR to focus efforts on a new polymeric sealant coined AeriSeal. An initial pilot study was conducted at six European centers to test the safety profile and effectiveness of the AeriSeal Emphysematous Lung Sealant System (ELS)[50]. Investigators treated 25 subjects with severe upper lobe predominant emphysema in up to six subsegments in one lung with the primary outcome being RV/TLC ratio as well as the incidence of adverse events. All subjects experienced a flu-like reaction 8–24 hours following the procedure. The most common adverse events were dyspnea ($n = 25$), fever ($n = 22$), and leukocytosis ($n = 21$). Additionally, all subjects had elevated inflammatory markers such as erythrocyte sedimentation rate and/or C-reactive protein, and there were eight treatment-related COPD exacerbations. While there were improvements in FEV_1, FVC, RV/TLC, 6-minute walk distance, SGRQ, and dyspnea scores, only the FVC met statistical significance. The change in RV/TLC at 6 months had significant correlations with FEV_1 ($r = -0.759$, $p < 0.001$), FVC ($r = -0.703$, $p < 0.001$), and SGRQ ($r = 0.481$, $p = 0.05$)[50]. Another pilot study treated 20 subjects (10 with homogeneous disease and 10 with upper lobe predominant disease) in two subsegments of each upper lobe[51]. The primary outcome of this study was reduction in lung volume as measured by CT imaging, and compared to baseline, there was a decrease of 895 ml ($p < 0.001$). At 6 months post treatment there was a significant improvement in FEV_1 (31.2%, $p = 0.02$) and in RV/TLC (-7.2%, $p = 0.027$). One subject developed tension pneumothorax following the procedure and subsequently died 9 days later after developing sepsis. Remaining procedure-related events included AECOPD (three), pneumonia (two), and upper respiratory tract infection (one).

Airway bypass tract stent placement

Airway bypass is a bronchoscopic technique designed for homogeneous emphysema in which airway passages are created to deflate trapped air using paclitaxel eluding-eluting stents to maintain patency of the bypass tracts (Broncus Technologies, Mountain View, CA). The Exhale Airway Stents for Emphysema (EASE) Trial is a randomized, sham-controlled study designed to investigate the safety and efficacy of these stents[52]. EASE enrolled 315 subjects (208 in stent arm) with severe homogeneous emphysema that were severely gas trapped. Up to six stents were placed in each patient with no more than two per lobe, and none were placed in the right middle lobe. The

investigators had a coprimary endpoint of an increase in FVC by 12% as well as a decrease in modified Medical Research Council (mMRC) dyspnea scale of 1 point. There was no difference between the sham procedure or airway bypass stenting in regards to the coprimary endpoints. Compared to baseline mMRC scores, airway bypass stenting did decrease dyspnea (-0.47 points) to a greater degree than the sham procedure (-0.22 points, $p = 0.045$), but this effect was lost at 12 months. There was no difference in lung function or lung volumes at 6 or 12 months. Possible explanations for these results included loss of stents either from expectoration or occlusion from tissue debris. The number of subjects meeting one of the predetermined safety endpoints was not different in the airway bypass stent (14.4%) or the sham (11.2%) group[52].

Bronchoscopic thermal vapor ablation (BTVA) for LVR

BTVA uses heated water vapor to produce thermal injury in airways resulting in an inflammatory response followed by fibrotic and atelectatic changes to induce volume reduction. Forty-four subjects with upper lobe predominant emphysema (FEV_1 31.4% predicted) were treated in either the left or right upper lobe at a dose of 10 cal/g of tissue with BTVA[53]. The treated lobar lung volume decreased by 715.9 ml compared to baseline ($p < 0.001$), while the FEV_1 improved 17% ($p < 0.001$) compared to baseline at 6 months. The SGRQ score decreased by 14.0 points ($p < 0.001$), and 73% of the subjects met the minimal clinically important difference of 4 points 6 months following the procedure. The 6-minute walk distance increased by 46.5 m ($p < 0.001$) at 6 months as well. There were a total of 29 serious adverse events following the procedure, with the most common being COPD exacerbation (9), pneumonia (6), respiratory tract infection (5), and hemoptysis (3)[53]. While the risk-to-benefit ratio appears to be favorable with BTVA, larger clinical trials with an appropriate control group are required.

Conclusion

LVRS is one of the few interventions for the select emphysematous patient (upper lobe predominant and low exercise) that can improve survival from a morbid and mortal disease. Just as importantly, severely emphysematous patients with upper lobe predominant disease (high or low exercise capacity) can expect improved dyspnea, exercise tolerance, and quality of life following LVRS. LVRS remains a vastly underutilized intervention, and its role in treating severely emphysematous patients appears to be undervalued. Less invasive methods of lung reduction are currently being studied, and although results are promising, it would seem unlikely that these procedures would offer a similar degree of lung volume reduction as surgical intervention. Future studies will be required to determine who should undergo LVRS vs. bronchoscopic LVR.

References

1   Kochanek KD, Xu J, Murphy SL, et al. Deaths: Preliminary data for 2009. *National Vital Statistics Reports* 2011; 59(4): 1–51.

2   Vestbo J, Hurd SS, Agusti AG, et al. Global strategy for the diagnosis, management and prevention of chronic obstructive pulmonary disease, GOLD executive summary. *Am J Respir Crit Care Med* 2012.

3   Continuous or nocturnal oxygen therapy in hypoxemic chronic obstructive lung disease: a clinical trial. nocturnal oxygen therapy trial group. *Ann Intern Med* 1980; 93(3):391–8.

4   Long term domiciliary oxygen therapy in chronic hypoxic cor pulmonale complicating chronic bronchitis and emphysema. Report of the Medical Research Council Working Party. *Lancet* 1981; 1(8222):681–6.

5   Anthonisen NR, Skeans MA, Wise RA, et al. The effects of a smoking cessation intervention on 14.5-year mortality: A randomized clinical trial. *Ann Intern Med* 2005; 142(4):233–9.

6   Naunheim KS, Wood DE, Mohsenifar Z, et al. Long-term follow-up of patients receiving lung-volume-reduction surgery versus medical therapy for severe emphysema by the national emphysema treatment trial research group. *Ann Thorac Surg* 2006; 82(2):431–43.

7   Fishman A, Martinez F, Naunheim K, et al. A randomized trial comparing lung-volume-reduction surgery with medical therapy for severe emphysema. *N Engl J Med* 2003; 348(21): 2059–73.

8   O'Donnell DE, Revill SM, Webb KA. Dynamic hyperinflation and exercise intolerance in chronic obstructive pulmonary disease. *Am J Respir Crit Care Med* 2001; 164(5):770–7.

9   Casanova C, Cote C, de Torres JP, et al. Inspiratory-to-total lung capacity ratio predicts mortality in patients with chronic obstructive pulmonary disease. *Am J Respir Crit Care Med* 2005; 171(6):591–7.

10 Washko GR, Martinez FJ, Hoffman EA, et al. Physiological and computed tomographic predictors of outcome from lung volume reduction surgery. *Am J Respir Crit Care Med* 2010; 181(5):494–500.

11 Fessler HE, Scharf SM, Ingenito EP, et al. Physiologic basis for improved pulmonary function after lung volume reduction. *Proc Am Thorac Soc* 2008; 5(4):416–20.

12 Fessler HE, Permutt S. Lung volume reduction surgery and airflow limitation. *Am J Respir Crit Care Med* 1998; 157(3 Pt 1):715–722.

13 Brantigan OC, Mueller E, Kress MB. A surgical approach to pulmonary emphysema. *Am Rev Respir Dis* 1959; 80(1, Part 2): 194–206.

14 Cooper JD, Trulock EP, Triantafillou AN, et al. Bilateral pneumectomy (volume reduction) for chronic obstructive pulmonary disease. *J Thorac Cardiovasc Surg* 1995; 109(1):106–16; discussion 116–9.

15 Cooper JD, Patterson GA, Sundaresan RS, et al. Results of 150 consecutive bilateral lung volume reduction procedures in patients with severe emphysema. *J Thorac Cardiovasc Surg* 1996; 112(5):1319–29; discussion 1329–30.

16 Criner GJ, Cordova FC, Furukawa S, et al. Prospective randomized trial comparing bilateral lung volume reduction surgery to pulmonary rehabilitation in severe chronic obstructive pulmonary disease. *Am J Respir Crit Care Med* 1999; 160(6):2018–27.

17 Geddes D, Davies M, Koyama H, et al. Effect of lung-volume-reduction surgery in patients with severe emphysema. *N Engl J Med* 2000; 343(4):239–45.

18 Weinmann GG, Chiang YP, Sheingold S. The National Emphysema Treatment Trial (NETT): a study in agency collaboration. *Proc Am Thorac Soc* 2008; 5(4):381–4.

19 Rationale and design of the national emphysema treatment trial: A prospective randomized trial of lung volume reduction surgery. the national emphysema treatment trial research group. *Chest* 1999; 116(6):1750–61.

20 Fishman A, Martinez F, Naunheim K, et al. A randomized trial comparing lung-volume-reduction surgery with medical therapy for severe emphysema. *N Engl J Med* 2003; 348(21): 2059–73.

21 National Emphysema Treatment Trial Research Group. Patients at high risk of death after lung-volume-reduction surgery. *N Engl J Med* 2001; 345(15):1075–83.

22 Naunheim KS, Wood DE, Krasna MJ, et al. Predictors of operative mortality and cardiopulmonary morbidity in the national emphysema treatment trial. *J Thorac Cardiovasc Surg* 2006; 131(1):43–53.

23 DeCamp MM, Blackstone EH, Naunheim KS, et al. Patient and surgical factors influencing air leak after lung volume reduction surgery: lessons learned from the national emphysema treatment trial. *Ann Thorac Surg* 2006; 82(1):197–206; discussion 206–7.

24 McKenna RJ,Jr, Benditt JO, DeCamp M, et al. Safety and efficacy of median sternotomy versus video-assisted thoracic surgery for lung volume reduction surgery. *J Thorac Cardiovasc Surg* 2004; 127(5):1350–60.

25 Stoller JK, Gildea TR, Ries AL, et al. National Emphysema Treatment Trial Research Group. Lung volume reduction surgery in patients with emphysema and alpha-1 antitrypsin deficiency. *Ann Thorac Surg* 2007; 83 (1):241–51.

26 Chandra D, Lipson DA, Hoffman EA, et al. Perfusion scintigraphy and patient selection for lung volume reduction surgery. *Am J Respir Crit Care Med* 2010; 182(7):937–46.

27 Washko GR, Fan VS, Ramsey SD, et al. The effect of lung volume reduction surgery on chronic obstructive pulmonary disease exacerbations. *Am J Respir Crit Care Med* 2008; 177(2):164–9.

28 Snyder ML, Goss CH, Neradilek B, et al. Changes in arterial oxygenation and self-reported oxygen use after lung volume reduction surgery. *Am J Respir Crit Care Med* 2008; 178(4): 339–45.

29 Criner GJ, Scharf SM, Falk JA, et al. Effect of lung volume reduction surgery on resting pulmonary hemodynamics in severe emphysema. *Am J Respir Crit Care Med* 2007; 176(3): 253–60.

30 Criner GJ, Belt P, Sternberg AL, et al. Effects of lung volume reduction surgery on gas exchange and breathing pattern during maximum exercise. *Chest* 2009; 135(5):1268–79.

31 Vestbo J, Prescott E, Almdal T, et al. Body mass, fat-free body mass, and prognosis in patients with chronic obstructive pulmonary disease from a random population sample: findings from the Copenhagen City Heart study. *Am J Respir Crit Care Med* 2006; 173(1):79–83.

32 Kim V, Kretschman DM, Sternberg AL, et al. National Emphysema Treatment Trial Research Group. Weight gain after lung reduction surgery is related to improved lung function and ventilatory efficiency. *Am J Respir Crit Care Med* 2012; 186 (11):1109–16.

33 Mineo TC, Pompeo E, Mineo D, et al. Resting energy expenditure and metabolic changes after lung volume reduction surgery for emphysema. *Ann Thorac Surg* 2006; 82(4):1205–11.

34 Ramsey SD, Berry K, Etzioni R, et al. Cost effectiveness of lung-volume-reduction surgery for patients with severe emphysema. *N Engl J Med* 2003; 348(21): 2092–102.

35 Ramsey SD, Shroyer AL, Sullivan SD, Wood DE. Updated evaluation of the cost-effectiveness of lung volume reduction surgery. *Chest* 2007; 131 (3):823–32.

36 Anonymous, Centers for Medicaid and Medicare Services. Part B National summary data file (previously known as BESS): Centers for Medicaid and Medicare Services. Part B National summary data file (previously known as BESS): Centers for Medicaid and Medicare Services website:

www.cms.gov/Research-Statistics-Data-and-Systems/Files-for-Order/NonIdentifiableData Files/PartBNationalSummary DataFile.html. Updated 2012. Accessed 20 September 2013.

37 Akuthota P, Litmanovich D, Zutler M, et al. An evidence-based estimate on the size of the potential patient pool for lung volume reduction surgery. *Ann Thorac Surg* 2012; 94(1):205–11.

38 Criner GJ, Sternberg AL. National Emphysema Treatment Trial Research Group. A clinician's guide to the use of lung volume reduction surgery. *Proc Am Thorac Soc* 2008; 5(4):461–7.

39 Kim V, Criner GJ, Abdallah HY, et al. Small airway morphometry and improvement in pulmonary function after lung volume reduction surgery. *Am J Respir Crit Care Med* 2005;171(1):40–7.

40 Hogg JC, Chu FS, Tan WC, et al. Survival after lung volume reduction in chronic obstructive pulmonary disease: Insights from small airway pathology. *Am J Respir Crit Care Med* 2007; 176(5):454–9.

41 Sciurba FC, Ernst A, Herth FJ, et al. A randomized study of endobronchial valves for advanced emphysema. *N Engl J Med* 2010; 363(13):1233–44.

42 Herth FJ, Noppen M, Valipour A, et al. Efficacy predictors of lung volume reduction with zephyr valves in a European cohort. *Eur Respir J* 2012; 39(6):1334–42.

43 Shah PL, Herth FJ. Current status of bronchoscopic lung volume reduction with endobronchial valves. *Thorax* 2013.

44 Sterman DH, Mehta AC, Wood DE, et al. A multicenter pilot study of a bronchial valve for the treatment of severe emphysema. *Respiration* 2010; 79(3):222–33.

45 Herth FJ, Eberhard R, Gompelmann D, et al. Bronchoscopic lung volume

reduction with a dedicated coil: a clinical pilot study. *Ther Adv Respir Dis* 2010; 4(4): 225–31.

46 Slebos DJ, Klooster K, Ernst A, et al. Bronchoscopic lung volume reduction coil treatment of patients with severe heterogeneous emphysema. *Chest* 2012; 142(3):574–82.

47 Shah PL, Zoumot Z, Singh S, et al. Endobronchial coils for the treatment of severe emphysema with hyperinflation (RESET): a randomised controlled trial. *Lancet Respiratory Medicine* 2013; 1(3):233–40.

48 Criner GJ, Pinto-Plata V, Strange C, et al. Biologic lung volume reduction in advanced upper lobe emphysema: Phase 2 results. *Am J Respir Crit Care Med* 2009; 179 (9):791–8.

49 Refaely Y, Dransfield M, Kramer MR, et al. Biologic lung volume reduction therapy for advanced homogeneous emphysema. *Eur Respir J* 2010; 36(1): 20–7.

50 Herth FJ, Gompelmann D, Stanzel F, et al. Treatment of advanced emphysema with emphysematous lung sealant (AeriSeal(R)). *Respiration* 2011; 82(1):36–45.

51 Kramer MR, Refaely Y, Maimon N, et al. Bilateral endoscopic sealant lung volume reduction therapy for advanced emphysema. *Chest* 2012; 142(5):1111–17.

52 Shah PL, Slebos DJ, Cardoso PF, et al. Bronchoscopic lung-volume reduction with exhale airway stents for emphysema (EASE trial): randomised, sham-controlled, multicentre trial. *Lancet* 2011; 378(9795):997–1005.

53 Snell G, Herth FJ, Hopkins P, et al. Bronchoscopic thermal vapour ablation therapy in the management of heterogeneous emphysema. *Eur Respir J* 2012; 39(6):1326–33.

Surgical aspects of infectious conditions of the lung

Elaine Teh and Elizabeth Belcher

Empyema

Background

Pleural empyema is defined as collection of pus in the pleural space. It was first described by an Egyptian physician in 3000 BC, but Hippocrates was more famously credited with its description. The mainstay of early treatment was open drainage; however, associated mortality was high. In 1917–1919, during the influenza epidemic, an Empyema Commission recommended closed chest tube, avoidance of early open drainage, obliteration of pleural space and nutritional support for the patient. These principles remain the basis of treatment today.

Empyema remains a common clinical problem, with an incidence of about 80,000 in the UK and United States[1]. The mortality and morbidity associated with the condition remain high[1].

Etiology

Empyema may be caused by spread of infection from organs contiguous to the pleural space, direct inoculation of the pleura due to trauma or as a result of haematogenous spread. Contiguous spread is the most common modality and accounts for over half of all cases. Most commonly it arises from the lung or structures such as mediastinum, deep cervical organs, chest wall and spine or organs below the diaphragm. The other major route is secondary to thoracic procedures such as thoracocentesis, post-operatively following thoracic or oesophageal surgery or secondary to trauma. Rarely empyema develops as a result of haematogenous spread from a distant source.

Chronic respiratory diseases, diabetes mellitus, malignancies, immunosuppression, gastro-oesophageal reflux disease and alcohol and drug addiction increase the risk of developing empyema.

The incidence of complicated parapneumonic effusion or empyema in patients requiring hospital admission for community-acquired pneumonia is over 7%. Hypoalbuminemia, hyponatremia, thrombophilia, raised C-reactive protein (CRP) and alcohol and intravenous drug abuse were independently associated with the development of complicated parapneumonic effusion or empyema. Interestingly, it appears COPD is protective against the development of empyema[2].

Over half of patients with community-acquired pneumonia develop pleural effusions; however, the majority are sterile sympathetic effusions destined to resolve. In about 30% of these patients, the condition progresses to complicated parapneumonic effusion (CPPE) or to empyema[3].

The incidence of empyema following post-traumatic haemothorax is over 25%. Risk factors for its development include rib fractures, (injury severity score) ISS > 25 and the need for additional interventions to evacuate retained haemothorax[4]. The use of prophylactic antibiotics in patients with chest trauma can decrease the incidence of post-traumatic empyema and pneumonia[5].

Pathophysiology and microbiology

When empyema develops, three stages are observed, with distinct characteristics of the pleural fluid and space (Figure 9.1).

In a normal, healthy person, pleural fluid amounts to less than 1 ml. The early simple exudative stage (Stage I) occurs within the first 2 weeks of the developing empyema. The pleural fluid is increased in quantity; however, it has normal pH, with glucose

Core Topics in Thoracic Surgery, ed. Marco Scarci, Aman Coonar, Tom Routledge and Francis Wells. Published by Cambridge University Press. © Cambridge University Press 2016

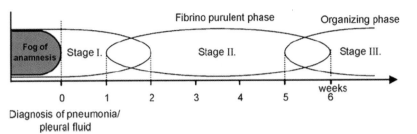

Figure 9.1 Time-scale and overlapping of stages of thoracic empyema. [Adapted from Molnar 2007.]

level equivalent to serum level, low white cell count and absence of micro-organisms. If the patient is adequately treated with antibiotics, the exudate normally will resolve spontaneously at this stage, with preservation of the thoracic dimensions. However, if there is persistent infection, it may progress to the fibrinopurulent stage (stage II) between week 1 and week 6. This stage is characterized by neutrophil phagocytosis, with inhibition of plasminogen activator and decreased tissue-type plasminogen activator leading to increased fibrin deposition, low pH, low glucose ($<$ 2.2 mmol/L) and high lactase dehydrogenase ($>$ 1000 IU/L). This is typically manifested by thick and purulent secretions with formation of septae causing loculations. The final phase, which develops from week 5 onwards, the organizing phase (stage III), is characterized by formation of a fibrous peel which leads to restriction of lung expansion.

The bacteriology of empyema has changed with the advent of antibiotic therapy. In the pre-antibiotic era, *Streptococcus* was the most common organism. Currently in community-acquired pneumonia, the majority of the infections continue to be caused by gram-positive aerobes or facultative organisms. *Streptococcus* and *Staphyloccus aureus* account for 65% of isolated organisms. Streptococcal organisms include *Streptococcus pneumoniae*, beta-haemolytic streptococci group A and *Streptococcus 'milleri'* groups. Commonly isolated gram-negative bacilli include *Escherichia coli*, *Klebsiella pneumonia*, *Haemophilus influenzae* and *Pseudomonas aeruginosa*. *Staphylococcus aureus* accounts for 50% of hospital-acquired empyema. Anaerobic organisms account for 13% of isolates. The frequency of pathogens such as anaerobic cocci, *Fusobacterium* and *Bacteroides* species is increasing in the community-acquired infection. These organisms are particularly seen in association with aspiration pneumonia and lung, dental and oropharyngeal abscess. The remainder of cases are due to mixed aerobic and anaerobic isolates (23%)[6].

In many cases no organism is ever isolated, which may relate to early speculative antibiotic use.

Diagnosis

Empyema should be suspected in patients presenting with acute respiratory illness associated with pleural effusion. Symptoms and signs include dyspnoea, cough, pleuritic chest pain, fever, tachycardia, malaise, anorexia and weight loss. Extension of a pleural infection, outside of the thoracic cage and into the neighbouring chest wall and surrounding soft tissues, is known as empyema necessitans. Empyema necessitans may be observed in patients in whom presentation is late or in association with particular organisms such as *Mycobacterium tuberculosis* and *Actinomyces* species. *Mycobacterium tuberculosis* account for approximately 70% of cases[7] and *Actinomycosis* for most of the remainder.

Investigations should include haematology, biochemistry and cultures of blood and sputum for aerobic and anaerobic bacteria. There are seven clinical variables that are found to be positively predictive of pleural infection: albumin $<$ 30 g/L, CRP $>$ 100 mg/L, platelet count $> 400 \times 10^9$/L, sodium $<$ 130 mmol/L, intravenous drug and alcohol abuse.

New biomarkers such as tumour necrosis factor alpha (TNF-α), myeloperoxidase, matrix metalloproteinase-2, interleukin 8 and CRP may have potential as future biomarkers in the diagnosis and management of empyema[3].

Imaging

Radiological investigation in empyema facilitates image-guided aspiration for diagnostic purposes, is an aid to chest drain insertion and allows assessment of loculations to guide relative merits of drain insertion versus operative intervention. Chest radiograph is the first-line imaging investigation. A lateral chest radiograph may help distinguish between free-flowing or loculated collection in the pleural space. CT, however, may be more useful in aiding the diagnosis of empyema, as well as staging the disease, as it facilitates differentiation between pleural effusion, lung abscess and consolidation. Classically, empyemas are usually posterolateral, and most extend to the diaphragm. CT also allows better visualization of septations, thickness of pleura, the presence or absence of trapped lung and associated underlying abnormalities.

Ultrasound (US) is able to differentiate between pleural effusion and consolidation, facilitates image-guided aspiration of effusion and is superior compared with CT in the assessment of loculations. US-guided aspiration will yield higher pleural aspirates and a lower risk of organ perforation compared to non-image-guided aspiration. Although US and CT have established roles in the investigation of parapneumonic effusions, neither technique reliably identifies the stage of pleural infection or predicts those patients who subsequently require surgical intervention after failed management by chest tube drainage[8].

Pleural aspiration

US-guided pleural aspiration is recommended in effusion > 10 mm in depth, especially if associated with pneumonic illness, ongoing sepsis or recent history of chest trauma or surgery. Frank pus indicates the need for formal drainage. Anaerobic pus is usually foul-smelling, whilst aerobic pus usually has little or no odour. Biochemical analysis (pH, glucose and protein concentration), microbiological culture and cytology are indicated. Pleural pH of < 7.2 is the single most powerful predictor of the need for chest tube drainage. Glucose level of fluid < 400 mg/L, LDH above 1000 IU/ml, protein level > 3 g/ml and WCC > 15,000 cells/mm[3] are also consistent with infection of the pleural space. Microbiological yield for suspected empyema is usually low. In the MIST-1 (Multicenter Intrapleural Sepsis Trial), positive pleural culture was only obtained in about 15% of patients. Polymerase chain reaction and immunological analysis may also identify the offending organisms.

Underlying causes of empyema should be sought. In patients with anaerobic empyema, examination of the oropharynx should be undertaken to exclude periodontal and oropharyngeal abscess. Bronchoscopy should be considered to exclude foreign bodies or endobronchial tumours. Bronchoscopy also facilitates

bronchoalveolar lavage, which will increase the rate of isolation of positive microbiological culture when performed in addition to pleural fluid microcopy and culture.

Management

The principles of empyema management are drainage and sterilization of the pleural space, obliteration of empyema cavity, lung expansion and nutritional support. However, individual therapy should be tailored to the cause, clinical stage, underlying lung, presence or absence of bronchopleural fistula and patient's clinical and nutritional status.

Drainage of pleural fluid

Presentation of patients in the earliest stage facilitates conservative management without empyema drainage. However, the presence of frankly purulent or turbid fluid, presence of bacteria confirmed with Gram stain, pleural pH < 7.2, poor clinical progress with signs of ongoing sepsis despite antibiotic therapy and loculated effusion are indications for closed tube drainage of empyema. The chest drain should be inserted under image guidance. There are no substantial data to recommend the optimal size of the chest drain or management of the chest drain such as regular flushing or suction. Historically, large-bore surgical chest drains were used, but currently, there is an increasing use of small intercostal chest drains, which are inserted percutaneously. Small-bore catheters (10–14F) facilitate ease of insertion, and evidence for the optimal size of chest tube is scarce[1].

Antibiotics

British Thoracic Society guidelines recommend that all patients should be treated with adequate and appropriate antibiotics, guided when available by culture based on pleural and blood culture results, and microbiological review taking into account local patterns of resistance[1]. Antibiotic therapy should cover anaerobic infections, except in patients with culture-proven *Streptococcus* infection. Penicillins, penicillins combined with β-lactamase inhibitor, metronidazole and cephalosporins penetrate the pleural space well; aminoglycosides should be avoided due to poor pleural penetration. In the absence of positive culture results, antimicrobial therapy should be directed based on local hospital policy and resistance pattern. Antimicrobial therapy may be needed for 2 to 3 weeks; however, the ultimate duration should be guided by clinical progress. Intravenous treatment is recommended initially, with change to the oral route once the patient shows improvement.

Intrapleural fibrinolytics

In an attempt to improve drainage of empyema, fibrinolytics have been utilized intrapleurally to lyse fibrinous septations. A number of case series and small trials suggested that these agents may improve outcome. However, the MIST-1, a large multicenter UK trial, showed no overall benefit in using streptokinase, when given intrapleurally. This large study enrolled 454 patients randomized in doubleblind fashion to intrapleural streptokinase twice daily for 3 days or placebo. No benefits were noted in either mortality or the need for surgical intervention at either 3 or 12 months after randomization with intrapleural streptokinase compared to placebo (31% streptokinase group versus 27% placebo group). Moreover, patients receiving streptokinase had a greater tendency to suffer serious adverse effects such as chest pain, fever, rash and allergy (7 versus 3%, RR = 2.49, 95% CI 0.98–6.36, p = 0.08)[9]. Following this study, fibrinolytics alone fell out of favour for the management of adult empyema. More recently, the MIST-2 of four study treatments – intrapleurally tissue plasminogen activator (t-PA), DNase, each agent alone and double placebo – showed intrapleural t-PA–DNase therapy improved fluid drainage in patients with pleural infection with improvement in chest radiograph. Secondary outcome measures reduced frequency of surgical referral, and the duration of hospital stay was also improved. Treatment with either agent alone was ineffective[10].

Prognosis

The prognosis is generally good in young and otherwise fit patients, especially if treatment was initiated early. There are rarely any long-term functional sequelae, although radiographically, there may be residual pleural thickening. Very rarely, a patient could develop fibrothorax with impairment of respiratory function.

Overall, however, the mortality and morbidity associated with the condition remains high, with 20% mortality if not effectively treated, as many of those affected are elderly with significant co-morbidities.

Indications for surgery

Surgery is indicated in patients with persistent sepsis and pleural effusion despite adequate therapy. Surgical options will be discussed in the next section. However, if surgery is not a feasible option due to the patient's clinical condition, re-imaging with consideration for further chest drain insertion, with or without intrapleural fibrinolytics, may be considered.

Operative approaches (Figure 9.2)

Stage I: Drainage

Antibiotic therapy and simple drainage by either aspiration or intercostal chest drain are most useful in the early stage I exudative phase of empyema. If this is used as a treatment modality in primary thoracic empyema, the success rate ranges from 67 to 74%[11–13]. The thoracic surgeon rarely meets the patient at this early stage as patients are adequately managed by respiratory physicians.

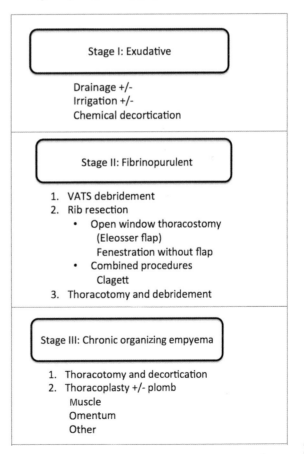

Figure 9.2 Summary of management of the three stages of empyema.

Stage II: Debridement

When the disease progresses to stage II, simple drainage alone is inadequate to resolve the infection, and debridement is then necessary to achieve local control. Surgical debridement of the pleural cavity can be carried out via open or video-assisted thoracoscopic surgery. Thoracoscopic debridement has gained popularity since the late 1990s with the general benefits associated with its minimally invasive nature compared to open, such as reduced post-operative pain and analgesic requirement, decreased air leak, decreased duration of chest tube drainage and shorter post-operative hospital stay.

In early stage empyema (stage II), two small randomized, controlled studies comparing VATS debridement with conservative drainage in patients with early/mixed-stage disease reported success rates of 83–93% in patients treated with VATS[14,15]. In other small case series, the reported conversion rates to open thoracotomy with VATS increased with increasing stage of the disease: 3–28% in early stage, 15–21% in mixed stage and 7–44% in late disease[16–26]. Between days 2 and 16 from presentation of empyema, the conversion rates to open with VATS increased from 22% to about 86%. A recent review of VATS decortication compared to open decortication in adults with primary empyema found that in stage II empyema, VATS is superior in the treatment of empyema with reduced post-operative morbidity, complications such as pain and air leak and reduced length of hospital stay[27].

The other major factor ensuring a higher success rate of treating empyema with VATS is the underlying condition of the parenchymal lung. In patients with empyema secondary to trauma, underlying normal lung will facilitate lung re-expansion with VATS drainage and debridement, hence preventing persistent space and infection in the pleural cavity.

Stage III: Decortication

Once the disease progresses to the advanced stage of organizing fibrous tissue encasing the underlying lung, decortication is usually a necessary therapeutic intervention. Decortication is defined as removal of constricting peel over the lung. It is usually indicated if the history of empyema is longer than 6 weeks, diagnostic assessment suggests progression to stage III disease and the patient is symptomatic. In these patients, lung perfusion can decrease by 20–25% in the affected lung, and decortication can improve vital capacity from 62 to 80% and forced expiratory volume in 1 second (FEV1) from 50 to 69%[28]. There is, however, controversy regarding the optimal timing of decortication. Advocates of early surgery will argue that there is less injury to the underlying lung parenchyma with early surgery as there is less significant ingrowth of fibrous tissue. However, on the other hand, late decortication after 3 months may achieve maximal functional respiratory recovery. The presence of intact visceral pleura, expandable lung and pleural space that will be completely obliterated by lung expansion are vital to the success of the therapy.

The mortality associated with decortication is high, ranging between 1.3 and 6.6%, with significant morbidity such as persistent air leak, bleeding, prolonged intubation with mechanical ventilation, persistent infection with prolonged ITU and hospital stay[11,29].

Many surgeons now advocate the use of VATS in decortication, even at the advanced stage. Many series and reviews suggests that VATS is as safe and effective in treating stage III empyema, with the added advantage of less post-operative pain, superior functional recovery of respiratory function, safer in high-risk patients and shorter hospital stay. Readers are directed to many good series and reviews of comparison between VATS and open decortication[16,17,19,30–32]. The conversion rate for patients treated with VATS decortication to open thoracotomy is between 3.5 and 41%. The main aim is to achieve sufficient decortication to allow full expansion of the underlying lung. VATS may be attempted in suitable patients; however, if this technique does not result in the desired outcome, open decortication will be required.

Management of persistent pleural space

Thoracoplasty

Thoracoplasty or collapse therapy was first introduced at the end of the nineteenth century, but due to its mutilating nature and being a poorly tolerated procedure, it rapidly lost popularity as a therapeutic option. However, with the advance in other aspects of surgery such as improvement in thoracic anaesthesia, blood transfusion and ITU support, thoracoplasty may be a good surgical option to treat a persistent pleural space in empyema in highly selected group of patients. The aim of thoracoplasty is to decrease the distance between the lung parenchyma and the chest wall. Collapsing the chest wall and filling the space with viable tissue such as omentum or viable muscle flap can achieve this. The modern indications, as described by Botianu, are

The lack of dissecting plane for decortication

Inability of the underlying to fully re-expand following decortication

Post-operative empyema, when decortication has failed or is not possible

Presence of bronchopleural fistula (BPF) – as this has to be dealt with by safe closure and suture reinforcement with a muscle flap

Presence of unresectable lesion in the lung parenchyma

Modern technique has achieved much better results due to an improved understanding and experience in raising muscle flaps and reducing the extent of chest wall mutilation by limiting the extent of rib resection. Meticulous assessment and planning pre- and peri-operatively are absolutely essential. With good planning and management, the operative mortality reported in the recent years is around 5%[33–37], with varying length of hospital stay and post-operative morbidity. Success rates of >90% have been reported when the procedure was performed in suitable patients.

Open window thoracostomy/fenestration

In debilitated patients who are unable to tolerate a major thoracic procedure as described earlier to manage a persistent pleural space, open window thoracostomy drainage is a useful option. The cavity is marsupialized via rib resection and open drainage. This long-term treatment plan involves multiple outpatient attendances for dressing changes and irrigation of the cavity. The cavity may eventually heal with time, fill with granulation tissue or require undergoing surgical closure.

Eloesser described a procedure involving a U-shaped incision through skin, subcutaneous tissue and muscle down to the ribs, creating a soft-tissue flap[38]. The exposed two or three adjacent ribs should be resected into 5-cm-long segments to fashion an approximately 5 to 7-cm opening to prevent contraction and spontaneous closure. Following drainage of empyema, the superiorly attached skin

flap is folded inward underneath the chest wall and sutured both to the parietal pleura and empyema peel, and the cavity packed.

Theron Claggett described a similar two-stage open procedure in 1963. The superficial fascia is sutured down to the periosteum of resected ribs to leave a large window for daily irrigation and delayed closure.

Simple rib resection to facilitate adequate drainage of the empyema space is another alternative in high-risk patients who are medically unfit for major surgery. It is a minor procedure, performed under general anaesthesia. A short segment of the rib over the most dependent part of empyema is resected, with the space opened and deloculated, followed by insertion of either a large-bore chest drain or multifenestrated tube into the cavity to ensure adequate drainage. Mortality of rib resection in empyema reported in various small retrospective series ranged between 5 and 14%, with a low failure rate of <10% and median hospital stay of between 11 and 21 days[11,39,40]. However, in cases of late referral to a thoracic surgical unit for management of chronic empyema, Cham and associates reported a failure rate as high as 83% in patients who initially underwent rib resection subsequently requiring decortication[41].

Post-pneumonectomy empyema

Post-pneumonectomy empyema (PPE) is a serious complication of pneumonectomy with high morbidity and mortality in excess of 10%[42]. (See also Chapter 20 on BPF.) PPE must be treated immediately. However, there are various techniques to manage PPE; it very much is dependent on the presence of bronchopleural fistula and the patient's general condition. Conservative treatment with chest tube drainage only seemed to result in a low success rate[43,44]. Surgical debridement, via either VATS or open thoracotomy, is associated with low mortality[45–48]. Even when more complex thoracoplasty was required to manage PPE, especially in the presence of BPF, the outcome reported was encouraging, with a success rate of between 81 and 100%[49–53]. A recent review by Zahid and colleagues found that open surgery is superior to minimally invasive management (which the authors have included chest tube drainage with or without chemical irrigation and video-assisted thoracoscopic debridement) in reducing empyema recurrence rate, mortality and re-intervention rate[54].

A study by Colice demonstrated the mortality associated with the natural history of the condition and inability to perform aggressive intervention[55] (Figure 9.3). Escalating mortality rate can be observed with reduction in intervention. Partly this reflects the fitness of the patients to undergo aggressive surgical intervention; it also serves to demonstrate the mortality of the condition when it is untreated or there is inability to undertake the treatment due to the patient's condition.

Empyema in children

In children, empyemas almost always occur as a complication of respiratory tract infection. The goals of

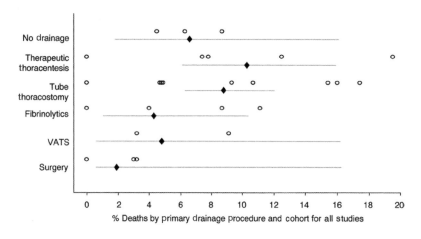

Figure 9.3 Deaths by primary drainage procedure. (Colice et al., 2000[55]).

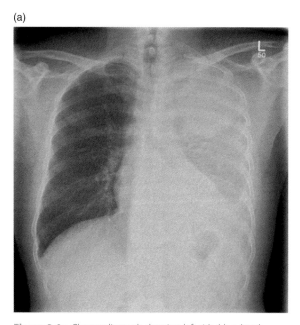

(a)

Figure 9.4a Chest radiograph showing left-sided loculated empyema.

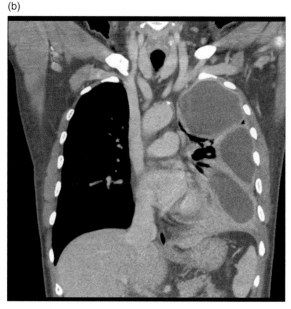

(b)

Figure 9.4b Chest CT demonstrating loculations prior to VATS drainage. No organism was isolated in this patient despite culture of pleural fluid.

(c)

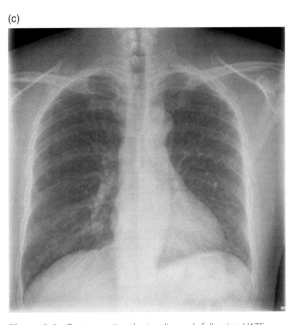

Figure 9.4c Post-operative chest radiograph following VATS and drainage of empyema.

management of empyema in children are similar to those in adults, which are to eliminate the empyema, re-expand trapped lung, restore mobility of chest wall and diaphragm, return respiratory function to normal, eliminate complications of chronicity and reduce length of hospital stay. Two randomized, controlled trials have found that there is no difference in the length of hospital stay and success rate between VATS and chest tube drainage with fibrinolytics[56,57]. However, when patients were randomized to either VATS or chest tube, with fibrinolytics as indicated, Kurt and colleagues found that patients treated with VATS had significantly shorter hospital stay[58]. A systematic review which included 3418 patients from 54 different studies concluded that VATS significantly improved mortality (0 vs 3.3%), re-intervention rate (2.5 vs 23.5%), duration of chest drains (4.4 vs 10.6 days) and length of hospital stay (10.8 vs 20 days)[59].

(b)

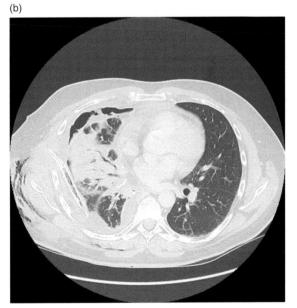

(a)

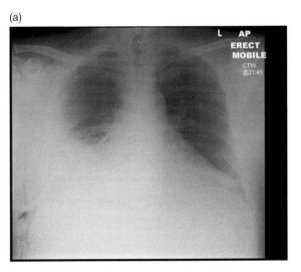

Figure 9.5a Chest radiograph demonstrating right lower zone opacification despite drain insertion. Patient presented with staphylococcal empyema following basal segmentectomy for metastastic thyroid carcinoma.

Figure 9.5b Chest CT showing incomplete drainage of pleural despite intercostal drain, consolidation of undergoing lung and surgical emphysema. Patient underwent re-thoracotomy and drainage of empyema.

93

(a)

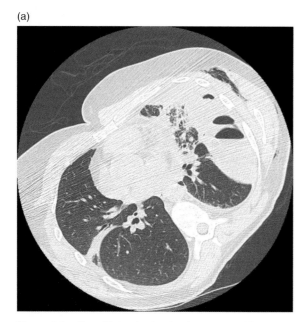

Figure 9.6a Chest CT showing loculated empyema with hydropneumothorax 6 weeks following aspiration of *Streptococcus pneumoniae* parapneumonic effusion.

(b)

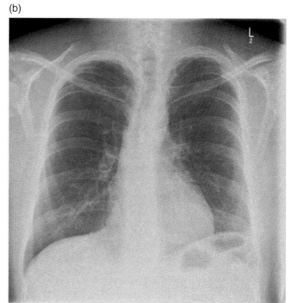

Figure 9.6b Chest radiograph of same patient 2 months following VATS and drainage of empyema.

(b)

(a)

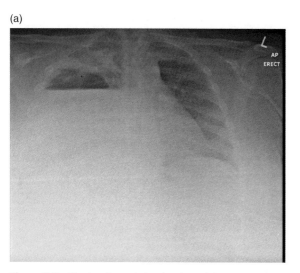

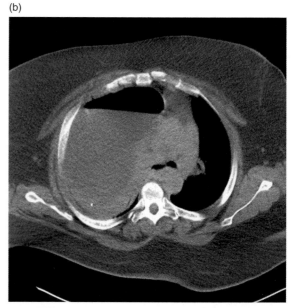

Figure 9.7a Chest radiograph showing large right hydropneumothorax secondary to ruptured pulmonary abscess. Patient presented with sepsis and multiple organ failure requiring admission to intensive care.

Figure 9.7b Chest CT demonstrating large right hydropneumothorax with contralateral mediastinal shift. Patient underwent drainage of 2.5 L of pus from pleural cavity and cavernostomy of underlying lung abscess.

(a)

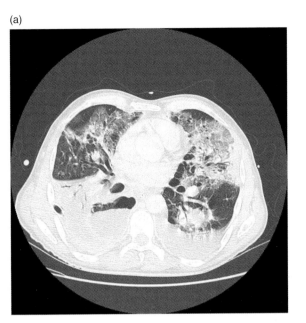

Figure 9.8a Chest CT of patient presenting with complications of right lung abscess. Abscess was associated with bronchopleural fistula, empyema and contamination of bilateral lung parenchyma. Patient developed acute respiratory distress syndrome requiring prolonged intubation and ventilation.

(b)

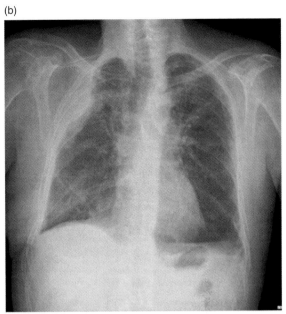

Figure 9.8b. Follow-up chest radiograph showing resolution of changes and opacification of right upper zone in area of interposition muscle flap.

(a)

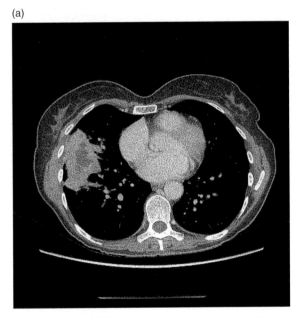

Figure 9.9a Chest CT demonstrating right lung abscess. Patient had associated poor dentition.

(b)

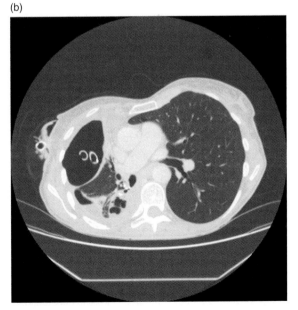

Figure 9.9b Chest CT showing lung abscess and empyema. *Klebsiella* species were cultured from pleural drain fluid.

(c)

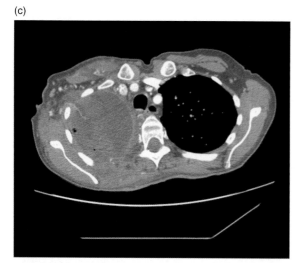

Figure 9.9c Chest CT showing pectoralis muscle flap utilized to obliterate residual pleural space following thoracotomy and drainage in same patient.

(a)

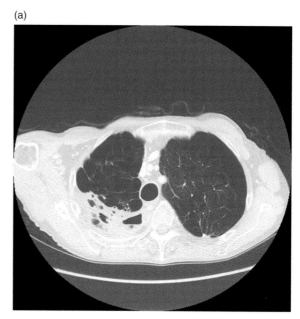

Figure 9.10a Chest CT showing pleural aspergilloma associated with emphysema.

(b)

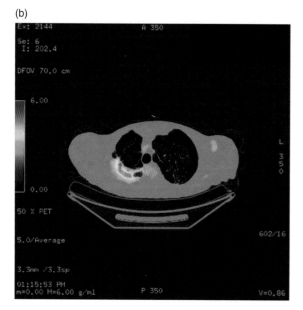

Figure 9.10b Fludeoxyglucose positron emission tomography (FDGPET) demonstrating FDG avidity of pleural aspergilloma prior to resection in a patient with significant emphysema.

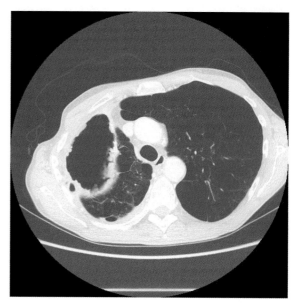

Figure 9.11 Aspergilloma cavity occurring late following earlier lung volume reduction surgery.

Landmark and important publications

Maskell NA, Davies CW, Nunn AJ, et al. First Multicenter Intrapleural Sepsis Trial (MIST1) Group. UK controlled trial of intrapleural streptokinase for pleural infection. *N Engl J Med* 2005 Mar 3; 352(9):865–74.

Rahman NM, Maskell NA, West A, et al. Intrapleural use of tissue plasminogen activator and DNase in pleural infection. *N Engl J Med*. 2011 Aug 11; 365(6):518–26.

Molnar TF. Current surgical treatment of thoracic empyema in adults. *Eur J Cardiothorac Surg* 2007 Sep; 32(3):422–30.

Lung abscess

Aetiology

Lung abscess is defined as a localized area of suppuration occurring in association with cavitation within the lung. Abscess formation may occur primarily as a consequence of initial necrotizing infection or result from secondary causes including infection of a pre-existing cavity, bronchial obstruction due to foreign body or tumour or due to septic emboli. Cavitating conditions of the lung including pulmonary infarction, sarcoid and Wegener's granulomatous; all pre-dispose to lung abscess.

The risk of developing necrotizing infection is increased in the immunocompromised patient and by factors that increase the risk of aspiration such as altered mental state particularly alcohol misuse, vocal cord paralysis, poor dental hygiene and oesphageal pathology such as diverticulae or malignancy. Poor dental hygiene is so commonly associated that suspected lung abscess in the edentulous should cause reconsideration of the diagnosis and further efforts to exclude underlying malignancy should be made.

Such pre-disposing factors are identified in the majority of patients diagnosed with lung abscess. In a series of 259 patients presenting with lung abscess, overall poor health was seen in over 97%, 82.5% had associated dental disease, 78.6% reported having lost consciousness at least once and 70.2% described alcohol misuse[60].

Pathophysiology/microbiology

The process has arbitrarily been divided into acute and chronic phases based on a 6-week time period; however, in practice, the onset is insidious, and these phases are not therefore useful in the diagnosis and management of the condition.

The classic studies of lung abscess were performed by David Smith at Duke in the 1920s[61]. He noted the similarity between bacteria in the mouth and those identified in the walls of the lung abscesses at post mortem, leading him to postulate that aspiration was the mechanism of infection, which he confirmed by an inoculation model of lung abscess.

Lord Brock later radiologically demonstrated that the segmental localization we observe in lung abscess is associated with aspiration by using iodized oil in patients in the recumbent position. In the supine position, aspiration preferentially targeted the posterior segment of the right upper lobe and the apical segment of the lower lobes[62].

Anaerobic bacteria accounted for 60–80% of cases of lung abscess, with the predominant isolates being mixed *Peptostreptococcus*, *Fusobacterium*, *Prevotella* and *Bacteroides* species[60,63]. In primary necrotizing pneumonia, *Staphylococcus aureus*, *Streptococcus pneumoniae* and gram-negative organisms especially *Klebsiella* are more commonly seen to predominate rather than mixed cultures[64]. Other culprit pathogens include *Haemophilus influenzae*, *Actinomyces* species, *Aspergillus*, *Cryptococcus*, *Histoplasma*, *Blastomyces* and *Coccidioides*.

Enatamoeba histolytica results in lung abscess following haematogenous spread and is almost always associated with empyema. It is classically associated with anchovy paste sputum due to expectoration of amoebae and liver tissue. Metronidazole is the antibiotic of choice.

Diagnosis
Clinical features

Onset of symptoms is typically insidious. Features include productive foul-smelling cough (67%), fever, malaise, weight loss (97%), chest pain (64%)

haemoptysis (15%), complicated by empyema (10%), clubbing (30%), poor dental hygiene (82%), amphoric breath sounds and cachexia[60].

Investigation

Routine haematology, biochemistry and blood cultures for aerobic and anaerobic bacteria should be obtained for these patients.

Radiological investigation facilitates diagnosis of abscess, identification of underlying causes such as proximal obstruction or pre-existing lung disease and image-guided biopsy when required to exclude tumour. Chest radiograph is the first-line imaging investigation and identifies an air-fluid level within a cavitating lesion.

CT is the most sensitive and specific imaging modality to diagnose a lung abscess. Contrast should be administered to enable identification of the abscess margins. Abscess cavities are usually rounded externally with irregular luminal surface. Classically they contain an air-fluid level with evidence of surrounding consolidation. It should be remembered that the commonest cause of a cavitating lesion is carcinoma.

Lung abscess is unilateral in 96% of cases and is more frequently observed on the right[60]. Anatomically, the apical segments of the lower lobes and posterior segments of upper lobes are preferentially involved in 85% of patients[60]. In a series of patients presenting with lung abscess, the lesion was identified in the right upper lobe in 28.4%, middle lobe 7.1%, right lower lobe 29%, left upper lobe 14.2% and left lower lobe 21.3%[64].

Management

Antibiotic therapy, nutritional support and treatment of underlying cause are the mainstay of the management of lung abscess. Most patients will respond to treatment with parenteral clindamycin within 2 weeks, although treatment should be continued for 8 weeks. This regimen is superior to penicillin in published trials as several anaerobes may produce beta-lactamase and therefore penicillin resistance[65]. The response rate to metronidazole is only 50% due to the polymicrobial nature of the abscess in most cases[66].

CT-guided percutaneous drainage has been shown to be a useful and safe procedure for the treatment of patients with lung abscesses who do not respond to medical therapy. In a study of patients with lung abscesses over a 3-year period in which antibiotic therapy failed and patients were managed with CT-guided percutaneous drainage, the abscess completely resolved in 33 of 40 patients (83%). Five (13%) patients developed pneumothorax. Seven patients (17.5%) had a residual cavity, and surgery was performed[67].

Failure of conservative therapy will occur in approximately 5–10% of patients, who will require surgical intervention[64, 68].

Complications of lung abscess and indications for surgery

Rates of surgery have decreased over time due to increasing effectiveness of antibiotic therapy. However, surgery continues to play an important role in a minority of patients. Indications for surgery are failure of medical treatment with ongoing sepsis and complications of lung abscess. Complications include massive significant haemoptysis, bronchopleural fistula and inability to exclude carcinoma. Surgery should be also considered in patients with associated empyema (see later in chapter).

Initial bronchoscopy should be undertaken if not previously performed to exclude proximal obstruction. Single lung ventilation should be instituted as early as possible in order to protect the contralateral lung from spillover contamination and certainly before establishment of lateral positioning. Consideration of repeat bronchoscopy to facilitate bronchial toilet should be given at the end of the procedure if there are concerns that contamination of the tracheobronchial tree has been significant.

Anatomical resection, usually lobectomy, is the resection of choice with early control of the bronchus to reduce contamination with drainage of empyema and obliteration of pleural space as indicated. In patients where the risk of resection is prohibitively high, surgical drainage of the abscess cavity is indicated[69]. It is critical that the nutritional support, antibiotic therapy and treatment of underlying conditions initiated during the conservative management phase should continue despite the move to a surgical approach. In the series examined by Moreira et al., surgical intervention was indicated in 52 (20.6%) of 252 patients. Procedures performed included drainage of the empyema in 24 patients (9.5%), pulmonary resection in 22 cases (8.7%) and drainage of abscess in 6 others (2.3%)[60].

Prognosis

The mortality associated with lung abscess has reduced significantly over time from rates of over 34% in the first half of the twentieth century to 5–6% today[60,70]. This is due to advances in antimicrobial therapy and improvements in health over time.

Risk factors for worse outcome have been identified in certain patients with lung abscess. Approximately 8% of lung abscesses will occur in association with empyema. In a series of 259 patients with empyema, 22 had associated lung abscess (8%). This conferred a higher requirement for intensive care admission (64 vs 40%, p = 0.032) and a higher operative mortality (23 vs 5.9%, OR = 4.69, 95% CI 1.057–14.56)[71]. Early surgical intervention should be considered in these patients.

Prognosis is poor for patients requiring ventilatory support prior to surgical intervention. In a series of 35 patients undergoing requiring surgery for lung abscess, of those ventilated pre-operatively, three died and four remain ventilator dependent longterm. In this series there were no deaths in patients not ventilated pre-operatively[72].

Harding and Hagan noted in their series of 252 patients that cavity size >6 cm prolonged symptoms for longer than 8 weeks; necrotizing pneumonia, old age, immunocompromised patients, bronchial obstruction and aerobic pathogens were independently associated with worse outcomes.

The mortality of patients undergoing surgery for lung abscess ranges from 11 to 28%[64,73].

Landmark and important publications

Moreira Jda S, Camargo Jde J, Felicetti JC, et al. Lung abscess: analysis of 252 consecutive cases diagnosed between 1968 and 2004. *J Bras Pneumol* 2006 Mar-Apr; 32(2):136–43.

Smith DT. Experimental aspiration abscess. *Surgery* 1927; 14:231–9.

Bartlett JG. Anaerobic bacterial infections of the lung. *Chest* 1987; 91:901–9.

Schweigert M, Dubecz A, Stadlhuber RJ, Stein HJ. Modern history of surgical management of lung abscess: from Harold Neuhof to current concepts. *Ann Thorac Surg* 2011 Dec; 92(6):2293–7.

Aspergillosis
Aetiology

Aspergillus species are a group of fungi, usually acquired by inhalation. They can be isolated from soil, plant debris or an indoor environment. The most common species isolated is *Aspergillus fumigatus*, although other species are also found. *Aspergillus* may cause a spectrum of pulmonary syndromes dependent on the physiological state of the host.

Pathophysiology/microbiology

Aspergillus infection results in one of three distinct patterns of disease depending on host susceptibility[74]. Allergic bronchopulmonary aspergillosis (ABPA) is an Immunoglobulin E (IgE)–mediated condition affecting patients with asthma, cystic fibrosis and bronchiectasis.

Aspergilloma consists of fungal hyphae, inflammatory cells, fibrin, mucus and tissue debris. Aspergilloma may be simple or complex. Simple aspergilloma is associated with a thin-walled cyst lined with ciliated epithelium in contrast to complex aspergilloma with thick-walled cavities and radiological evidence of surrounding disease. Aspergilloma generally develops in pre-existing lung cavities, most commonly tuberculosis. The decline in cases of tuberculosis has resulted in both a reduction in cases of aspergillosis and improvement in outcome for patients who develop and undergo treatment for aspergilloma[75,76]. Other disease processes associated with aspergilloma development include sarcoidosis, bronchiectasis, bronchial cyst, bullae, neoplasm and pulmonary infection.

Invasive aspergillosis occurs in the immuno-suppressed patient including solid organ and bone marrow transplant recipients, following radiotherapy and HIV infection.

Diagnosis

Patients with aspergilloma are usually asymptomatic. When symptoms develop, haemoptysis is the usual presentation as a consequence of invasion of local bronchial artery, secondary to endotoxins released by the fungus ball or to mechanical irritation of the fungal ball itself. Other than haemoptysis, other symptoms may include dyspnea, cough and fever.

Diagnosis is made on clinical, radiological, serological and microbiological basis. Chest radiograph and CT show one or more cavitating lesions. Lesions are commonly seen in upper lobes. Monad sign describes the air surrounding the mycetoma.

However, this sign is not specific to aspergilloma but may be present in other conditions, including malignancy and abscess. Serum immunoglobulin G (IgG) antibodies to *Aspergillus* are almost always positive, except in patients on immunosuppression therapy including steroids. Sputum culture is positive in about 50% of patients.

A diagnosis of ABPA relies on the following criteria: bronchospasm, eosinophilia, immediate skin test reactivity to *Aspergillus* antigens, precipitating (IgG) antibodies to *Aspergillus*, elevated total IgE, elevated *Aspergillus*-specific IgE, central bronchiectasis and history of pulmonary infiltrates on chest radiograph. The presence of all eight factors confers diagnostic certainty.

Galactomannan antigen is an *Aspergillus*-specific antigen that is released during the growth phase of invasive aspergillosis. Galactomannan assay is useful for the diagnosis of invasive aspergillosis with a sensitivity of 81% and specificity of 89%. The halo sign describes an area of ground-glass attenuation surrounding a pulmonary nodule. It is most commonly associated with invasive aspergillosis but may also be associated with haemorrhagic nodules, tumours, or inflammatory processes. Lung biopsy may be required to provide definitive diagnosis. The air crescent sign refers to air around the nodule and may indicate improvement.

Management

The treatment of ABPA is medical. Steroids and antifungals are first-line therapy. There is currently no consensus on the optimal management strategy for asymptomatic aspergilloma. Anti-fungal therapy remains the mainstay of treatment. A number of small studies advocate the benefits of various routes of administration including transcutaneous and inhalation. Oral itraconazole is an effective therapy due to its penetration for elective therapy; however, its role as a first-line treatment for life-threatening haemoptysis is limited owing to the significant length of time from administration to action.

Thoracic surgery has a limited role in the management of most of the clinical syndromes except for aspergilloma. Whilst surgery for aymptomatic patients is controversial, results are good for selected patients. Patient presenting with haemoptysis should receive tranexamic acid, and radiologically guided coil embolization should be considered. Where this is ineffective or unavailable, surgery is indicated.

Indications for surgery

Surgery for aspergilloma has been recognized as technically challenging with a high complication rate due to multiple adhesions, obliterated pleural space, indurated hilar structures and failure of residual lung to re-expand post-resection. Lobectomy is the operation of choice.

Surgical resection is indicated in patients with life-threatening haemoptysis, recurrent chest infection or weight loss. In the complex form, surgical intervention must be considered as a last resort. In the simple form, surgery is relatively benign and prevents disease progression. Pleural aspergillosis can occur, usually as a consequence of previous resection. Given the loss of lung parenchyma, thoracoplasty is often the only option.

Whilst surgical intervention should generally be avoided in invasive aspergillosis, it may be considered in the event of massive haemoptysis and to prevent relapse during or following antifungal therapy[77].

Operative approaches

Open anatomical lung resection is the operation of choice in low-risk patients. Loboectomy is the operation of choice; however, segmentectomy or wedge resection are alternative options. Postoperative complications are significant, including haemorrhage, residual pleural space, prolonged air leak, empyema, bronchoalveolar fistula, respiratory failure and recurrence.

Cavernostomy is an alternative procedure in older patients or in whom the risk of resection is prohibitively high[78]. This may be performed as an isolated procedure or in combination with limited thoracoplasty and latissimus dorsi myosplasty.[79]

In one medically inoperable patient, a satisfactory result is reported following bronchoscopic removal of a large intracavitary pulmonary aspergilloma[80].

Thoracoplasty is often the only surgical option for semi-invasive aspergillosis and pleural disease. In a series of 16 patients with pleural aspergillosis who underwent surgical management, all patients experienced complications including bleeding pleural space problems, respiratory failure and post-pneumonectomy empyema. Mortality associated with thoracoplasty was 15% (vs 6% for patients with all types of aspergilloma not receiving thoracoplasty). These findings lead the authors to conclude that only symptomatic pleural aspergilloma should be operated on and pleuropneumonectomy should be avoided[81].

More recently, VATS has been advocated for patients with both simple and complex aspergilloma. In a series of 20 patients undergoing a minimal access approach, early mortality was 5%, with a 5-year survival of 89%[82].

Prognosis and complications

Aspergilloma generally runs a chronic course with 10% regressing; however, 30% of patients will experience significant haemoptysis with an associated mortality rate of between 2 and 14%[83].

In a series of 64 cases of aspergilloma undergoing surgical intervention, 10-year cumulative survivals in simple and complex aspergilloma were 88.3 and 70.6%, respectively ($p = 0.042$). Certain patient factors are associated with a worse prognosis. These include older age, underlying lung disease, greater number of lesions, immunosuppression, increasing *Aspergillus*-specific IgG titers, recurrent large volume of haemoptysis, underlying sarcoid and presence of HIV[84], whilst female gender, forced expiratory volume in

1 second greater than >75% and simple aspergilloma are independent favourable prognostic factors. However, in routine use adjuvant antifungals did not significantly affect morbidity or survival in this series[85].

The surgical mortality associated with aspergilloma is high, between 7 and 23% in the published case series[81,86–88]. Improved outcomes over time have been associated with a reduction in complex cases of aspergilloma as a result of a reduction in tuberculosis. Only 17% of patients in a contemporary cohort had a history of tuberculosis compared with 57% in a former series. Reduced morbidity of surgery in terms of bleeding, pleural space issues and hospital stay have all decreased such that modern-day surgery for aspergilloma may be offered at lower risk in order to interrupt the course of the disease[75,76].

Invasive aspergillosis continues to carry a high mortality of up to 80%. Bone marrow transplant patients or those with cerebral involvement are particularly at risk [89].

Landmark and important publications

The Aspergillus website: www.aspergillus.org.uk

Belcher JR, Plummer NS. Surgery in bronchopulmonary aspergillosis. *Br J Dis Chest* 2011; 54:335–41.

Lejay A, Falcoz PE, Santelmo N, et al. Surgery for aspergilloma: time trend towards improved results? *Interact Cardiovasc Thorac Surg* 2011 Oct; 13(4):392–5.

References

1   Davies HE, Davies RJ, Davies CW. Management of pleural infection in adults: British Thoracic Society Pleural Disease Guideline 2010. *Thorax* 2010; 65(Suppl 2): ii41–53.

2   Chalmers JD, Singanayagam A, Murray MP, et al. Risk factors for complicated parapneumonic effusion and empyema on presentation to hospital with community-acquired pneumonia. *Thorax* 2009; 64:592–7.

3   Porcel JM. Pleural fluid tests to identify complicated parapneumonic effusions. *Curr Opin Pulm Med* 2010; 16:357–61.

4   DuBose J, Inaba K, Okoye O, et al. Development of posttraumatic empyema in patients with retained hemothorax: results of a prospective, observational AAST study. *J Trauma Acute Care Surg* 2012; 73:752–7.

5   Sanabria A, Valdivieso E, Gomez G, Echeverry G. Prophylactic antibiotics in chest trauma: a meta-analysis of high-quality studies. *World J Surg* 2006; 30:1843–7.

6   Park DR. The microbiology of ventilator-associated pneumonia. *Respir Care* 2005; 50:742–63; discussion 63–5.

7   Choi JA, Hong KT, Oh YW, et al. CT manifestations of late sequelae

in patients with tuberculous pleuritis. *AJR Am J Roentgenol* 2001; 176:441–5.

8   Kearney SE, Davies CW, Davies RJ, Gleeson FV. Computed tomography and ultrasound in parapneumonic effusions and empyema. *Clin Radiol* 2000; 55:542–7.

9   Maskell NA, Davies CW, Nunn AJ, et al. UK controlled trial of intrapleural streptokinase for pleural infection. *N Engl J Med* 2005; 352:865–74.

10   Rahman NM, Maskell NA, West A, et al. Intrapleural use of tissue plasminogen activator and DNase in pleural infection. *N Engl J Med* 2011; 365:518–26.

11 Thourani VH, Brady KM, Mansour KA, et al. Evaluation of treatment modalities for thoracic empyema: a cost-effectiveness analysis. *Ann Thorac Surg* 1998; 66:1121–7.

12 Athanassiadi K, Gerazounis M, Kalantzi N. Treatment of post-pneumonic empyema thoracis. *Thorac Cardiovasc Surg* 2003; 51:338–41.

13 Suchar AM, Zureikat AH, Glynn L, et al. Ready for the frontline: is early thoracoscopic decortication the new standard of care for advanced pneumonia with empyema? *Am Surg* 2006; 72:688–92; discussion 92–3.

14 Wait MA, Sharma S, Hohn J, Dal Nogare A. A randomized trial of empyema therapy. *Chest* 1997; 111:1548–51.

15 Bilgin M, Akcali Y, Oguzkaya F. Benefits of early aggressive management of empyema thoracis. *ANZ J Surg* 2006; 76:120–2.

16 Landreneau RJ, Keenan RJ, Hazelrigg SR, et al. Thoracoscopy for empyema and hemothorax. *Chest* 1996; 109:18–24.

17 Kim BY, Oh BS, Jang WC, et al. Video-assisted thoracoscopic decortication for management of postpneumonic pleural empyema. *Am J Surg* 2004; 188:321–4.

18 Solaini L, Prusciano F, Bagioni P, et al. Video-assisted thoracic surgery (VATS) of the lung: analysis of intraoperative and postoperative complications over 15 years and review of the literature. *Surg Endosc* 2008; 22:298–310.

19 Luh SP, Chou MC, Wang LS, et al. Video-assisted thoracoscopic surgery in the treatment of complicated parapneumonic effusions or empyemas: outcome of 234 patients. *Chest* 2005; 127:1427–32.

20 Angelillo-Mackinlay T, Lyons GA, Piedras MB, Angelillo-Mackinlay D. Surgical treatment of postpneumonic empyema. *World J Surg* 1999; 23:1110–3.

21 Striffeler H, Gugger M, Im Hof V, et al. Video-assisted thoracoscopic surgery for fibrinopurulent pleural empyema in 67 patients. *Ann Thorac Surg* 1998; 65:319–23.

22 Lardinois D, Gock M, Pezzetta E, et al. Delayed referral and gram-negative organisms increase the conversion thoracotomy rate in patients undergoing video-assisted thoracoscopic surgery for empyema. *Ann Thorac Surg* 2005; 79:1851–6.

23 Cassina PC, Hauser M, Hillejan L, et al. Video-assisted thoracoscopy in the treatment of pleural empyema: stage-based management and outcome. *J Thorac Cardiovasc Surg* 1999; 117:234–8.

24 Waller DA, Rengarajan A. Thoracoscopic decortication: a role for video-assisted surgery in chronic postpneumonic pleural empyema. *Ann Thorac Surg* 2001; 71:1813–6.

25 Petrakis I, Katsamouris A, Drossitis I, et al. Usefulness of thoracoscopic surgery in the diagnosis and management of thoracic diseases. *J Cardiovasc Surg (Torino)* 2000; 41:767–71.

26 Wurnig PN, Wittmer V, Pridun NS, Hollaus PH. Video-assisted thoracic surgery for pleural empyema. *Ann Thorac Surg* 2006; 81:309–13.

27 Chambers A, Routledge T, Dunning J, Scarci M. Is video-assisted thoracoscopic surgical decortication superior to open surgery in the management of adults with primary empyema? *Interact Cardiovasc Thorac Surg* 2010; 11:171–7.

28 Rzyman W, Skokowski J, Romanowicz G, et al. Decortication in chronic pleural empyema – effect on lung function. *Eur J Cardiothorac Surg* 2002; 21:502–7.

29 Mandal AK, Thadepalli H, Chettipally U. Outcome of primary empyema thoracis: therapeutic and microbiologic aspects. *Ann Thorac Surg* 1998; 66:1782–6.

30 Shahin Y, Duffy J, Beggs D, et al. Surgical management of primary empyema of the pleural cavity: outcome of 81 patients. *Interact Cardiovasc Thorac Surg* 2010; 10:565–7.

31 Solaini L, Prusciano F, Bagioni P. Video-assisted thoracic surgery in the treatment of pleural empyema. *Surg Endosc* 2007; 21:280–4.

32 Tong BC, Hanna J, Toloza EM, et al. Outcomes of video-assisted thoracoscopic decortication. *Ann Thorac Surg* 2010; 89:220–5.

33 Botianu PV, Dobrica AC, Butiurca A, Botianu AM. Complex space-filling procedures for intrathoracic infections - personal experience with 76 consecutive cases. *Eur J Cardiothorac Surg* 2010; 37:478–81.

34 Garcia-Yuste M, Ramos G, Duque JL, et al. Open-window thoracostomy and thoracomyoplasty to manage chronic pleural empyema. *Ann Thorac Surg* 1998; 65:818–22.

35 Icard P, Le Rochais JP, Rabut B, et al. Andrews thoracoplasty as a treatment of post-pneumonectomy empyema: experience in 23 cases. *Ann Thorac Surg* 1999; 68:1159–63; discussion 64.

36 Okumura Y, Takeda S, Asada H, et al. Surgical results for chronic empyema using omental pedicled flap: long-term follow-up study. *Ann Thorac Surg* 2005; 79:1857–61.

37 Regnard JF, Alifano M, Puyo P, et al. Open window thoracostomy followed by intrathoracic flap transposition in the treatment of empyema complicating pulmonary resection. *J Thorac Cardiovasc Surg* 2000; 120:270–5.

38 Eloesser L. An operation for tuberculous empyema. *Chest* 1935; 1:8–23.

39 Ferguson AD, Prescott RJ, Selkon JB, et al. The clinical course and management of thoracic empyema. *QJM* 1996; 89:285–9.

40 Galea JL, De Souza A, Beggs D, Spyt T. The surgical management of empyema thoracis. *J R Coll Surg Edinb* 1997; 42:15–8.

41 Cham CW, Haq SM, Rahamim J. Empyema thoracis: a problem with late referral? *Thorax* 1993; 48:925–7.

42 Deschamps C, Pairolero PC, Allen MS, Trastek VF. Management of postpneumonectomy empyema and bronchopleural fistula. *Chest Surg Clin N Am* 1996; 6:519–27.

43 Kacprzak G, Marciniak M, Addae-Boateng E, et al. Causes and management of postpneumonectomy empyemas: our experience. *Eur J Cardiothorac Surg* 2004; 26:498–502.

44 Massera F, Robustellini M, Pona CD, et al. Predictors of successful closure of open window thoracostomy for postpneumonectomy empyema. *Ann Thorac Surg* 2006; 82:288–92.

45 Gossot D, Stern JB, Galetta D, et al. Thoracoscopic management of postpneumonectomy empyema. *Ann Thorac Surg* 2004; 78:273–6.

46 Ng T, Ryder BA, Maziak DE, Shamji FM. Treatment of postpneumonectomy empyema with debridement followed by continuous antibiotic irrigation. *J Am Coll Surg* 2008; 206:1178–83.

47 Schneiter D, Grodzki T, Lardinois D, et al. Accelerated treatment of postpneumonectomy empyema: a binational long-term study. *J Thorac Cardiovasc Surg* 2008; 136:179–85.

48 Goldstraw P. Treatment of postpneumonectomy empyema: the case for fenestration. *Thorax* 1979; 34:740–5.

49 Jadczuk E. Postpneumonectomy empyema. *Eur J Cardiothorac Surg* 1998; 8:123–6.

50 Wong PS, Goldstraw P. Post-pneumonectomy empyema. *Eur J Cardiothorac Surg* 1994; 8:345–9; discussion 9–50.

51 Gharagozloo F, Trachiotis G, Wolfe A, et al. Pleural space irrigation and modified Clagett procedure for the treatment of early postpneumonectomy empyema. *J Thorac Cardiovasc Surg* 1998; 116:943–8.

52 Zaheer S, Allen MS, Cassivi SD, et al. Postpneumonectomy empyema: results after the Clagett procedure. *Ann Thorac Surg* 2006; 82:279–86; discussion 86–7.

53 Seify H, Mansour K, Miller J, et al. Single-stage muscle flap reconstruction of the postpneumonectomy empyema space: the Emory experience. *Plast Reconstr Surg* 2007; 120:1886–91.

54 Zahid I, Routledge T, Bille A, Scarci M. What is the best treatment of postpneumonectomy empyema? *Interact Cardiovasc Thorac Surg* 2011; 12:260–4.

55 Colice GL, Curtis A, Deslauriers J, et al. Medical and surgical treatment of parapneumonic effusions : an evidence-based guideline. *Chest* 2000; 118:1158–71.

56 Sonnappa S, Cohen G, Owens CM, et al. Comparison of urokinase and video-assisted thoracoscopic surgery for treatment of childhood empyema. *Am J Respir Crit Care Med* 2006; 174:221–7.

57 St Peter SD, Tsao K, Spilde TL, et al. Thoracoscopic decortication vs tube thoracostomy with fibrinolysis for empyema in children: a prospective, randomized trial. *J Pediatr Surg* 2009; 44:106–11; discussion 11.

58 Kurt BA, Winterhalter KM, Connors RH, et al. Therapy of parapneumonic effusions in children: video-assisted thoracoscopic surgery versus conventional thoracostomy drainage. *Pediatrics* 2006; 118: e547–53.

59 Avansino JR, Goldman B, Sawin RS, Flum DR. Primary operative versus nonoperative therapy for pediatric empyema: a meta-analysis. *Pediatrics* 2005; 115:1652–9.

60 Moreira Jda S, Camargo Jde J, Felicetti JC, et al. Lung abscess: analysis of 252 consecutive cases diagnosed between 1968 and 2004. *J Bras Pneumol* 2006; 32:136–43.

61 Smith DT. Experimental aspiration abscess. *Surgery* 1927; 14:231–9.

62 Brock RC. *The Anatomy of the Bronchial Tree*. Oxford University Press; 1946.

63 Bartlett JG. Anaerobic bacterial infections of the lung. *Chest* 1987; 91:901–9.

64 Hagan JL, Hardy JD. Lung abscess revisited: a survey of 184 cases. *Ann Surg* 1983; 197:755–62.

65 Appelbaum PC, Spangler SK, Jacobs MR. Beta-lactamase production and susceptibilities to amoxicillin, amoxicillin-clavulanate, ticarcillin, ticarcillin-clavulanate, cefoxitin, imipenem, and metronidazole of 320 *non-Bacteroides fragilis Bacteroides* isolates and 129 fusobacteria from 28 US centers. *Antimicrob Agents Chemother* 1990; 34:1546–50.

66 Perlino CA. Metronidazole vs clindamycin treatment of anerobic pulmonary infection. Failure of metronidazole therapy. *Arch Intern Med* 1981; 141:1424–7.

67 Kelogrigoris M, Tsagouli P, Stathopoulos K, et al. CT-guided percutaneous drainage of lung abscesses: review of 40 cases. *JBR-BTR* 2011; 94:191–5.

68 Erasmus JJ, McAdams HP, Rossi S, Kelley MJ. Percutaneous management of intrapulmonary air and fluid collections. *Radiol Clin North Am* 2000; 38:385–93.

103

69 Schweigert M, Dubecz A, Stadlhuber RJ, Stein HJ. Modern history of surgical management of lung abscess: from Harold Neuhof to current concepts. *Ann Thorac Surg* 2011; 92:2293–7.

70 Allen CI, Blackman JR. Treatment of lung abscess: with report of 100 consecutive cases. *Thorac Surg* 1936; 6:156

71 Huang HC, Chen HC, Fang HY, et al. Lung abscess predicts the surgical outcome in patients with pleural empyema. *J Cardiothorac Surg* 2010; 5:88.

72 Reimel BA, Krishnadasen B, Cuschieri J, et al. Surgical management of acute necrotizing lung infections. *Can Respir J* 2006; 13:369–73.

73 Delarue NC, Pearson FG, Nelems JM, Cooper JD. Lung abscess: surgical implications. *Can J Surg* 1980; 23:297–302.

74 Belcher JR, Plummer NS. Surgery in bronchopulmonary aspergillosis. *Bri J Dis Chest* 1960; 54:335–41.

75 Chatzimichalis A, Massard G, Kessler R, et al. Bronchopulmonary aspergilloma: a reappraisal. *Ann Thorac Surg* 1998; 65:927–9.

76 Lejay A, Falcoz PE, Santelmo N, et al. Surgery for aspergilloma:

time trend towards improved results? *Interact Cardiovasc Thorac Surg* 2011; 13:392–5.

77 Shah R, Vaideeswar P, Pandit SP. Pathology of pulmonary aspergillomas. *Indian J Pathol Microbiol* 2008; 51: 342–5.

78 Cesar JM, Resende JS, Amaral NF, et al. Cavernostomy x resection for pulmonary aspergilloma: a 32-year history. *J Cardiothorac Surg* 2011; 6:129.

79 Igai H, Kamiyoshihara M, Nagashima T, Ohtaki Y. Pulmonary aspergilloma treated by limited thoracoplasty with simultaneous cavernostomy and muscle transposition flap. *Ann Thorac Cardiovasc Surg* 2012; 18:472–4.

80 Stather DR, Tremblay A, MacEachern P, et al. Bronchoscopic removal of a large intracavitary pulmonary aspergilloma. *Chest* 2013; 143:238–41.

81 Massard G, Roeslin N, Wihlm JM, et al. Pleuropulmonary aspergilloma: clinical spectrum and results of surgical treatment. *Ann Thorac Surg* 1992; 54:1159–64.

82 Ichinose J, Kohno T, Fujimori S. Video-assisted thoracic surgery

for pulmonary aspergilloma. *Interact Cardiovasc Thorac Surg* 2010; 10:927–30.

83 Zmeili OS, Soubani AO. Pulmonary aspergillosis: a clinical update. *QJM* 2007; 100:317–34.

84 Sagan D, Gozdziuk K, Korobowicz E. Predictive and prognostic value of preoperative symptoms in the surgical treatment of pulmonary aspergilloma. *J Surg Res* 2010; 163:e35–43.

85 Sagan D, Gozdziuk K. Surgery for pulmonary aspergilloma in immunocompetent patients: no benefit from adjuvant antifungal pharmacotherapy. *Ann Thorac Surg* 2010; 89:1603–10.

86 Aslam PA, Eastridge CE, Hughes FA Jr. Aspergillosis of the lung – an eighteen-year experience. *Chest* 1971; 59:28–32.

87 Daly RC, Pairolero PC, Piehler JM, et al. Pulmonary aspergilloma. Results of surgical treatment. *J Thorac Cardiovasc Surg* 1986; 92:981–8.

88 Kilman JW, Ahn C, Andrews NC, Klassen K. Surgery for pulmonary aspergillosis. *J Thorac Cardiovasc Surg* 1969; 57:642–7.

89 Doffman SR, Agrawal SG, Brown JS. Invasive pulmonary aspergillosis. *Expert Rev Anti Infect Ther* 2005; 3:613–27.

Chapter 10

Treatment of haemoptysis

Odiri Eneje and Katharine Hurt

Introduction

Haemoptysis is defined as coughing up blood or bloody sputum from the airways. It is a relatively common presenting symptom in clinical practice[1]. The symptoms can range from small volume specks mixed in with sputum through to massive life-threatening haemoptysis. It can be difficult to accurately quantify the volume of haemoptysis, as this mostly relies on patients' subjective recollections, often in moments of high stress. In the clinical setting, the degree of compromise depends on the underlying cause, the patient's current health status and co-morbidities. There is no absolute volumetric definition of massive haemoptysis, with quoted volumes ranging from 100 ml to 1000 ml over 24 hours[2]. In general 200–600 ml in 24 hours appears to be an acceptable definition for massive haemoptysis[3]. A functional definition can also be useful to account for physiological effect of haemoptysis[4,5].

Massive haemoptysis is rare but a potential life-threatening emergency, which carries a mortality rate of up to 38%[6]. It is estimated that 400 ml of blood in the alveolar space is sufficient to inhibit gaseous exchange significantly[7]. In cases of massive haemoptysis, death commonly occurs as a result of asphyxiation as opposed to exsanguination[8]. The patient's current health status greatly predicts severity, morbidity and mortality. Identified independent predictors of mortality include chronic alcohol dependency, malignancy, aspergillosis, pulmonary artery involvement, infiltrates involving two quadrants or more on the admission radiograph and requirement for mechanical ventilation[9]. Haemoptysis is associated with many conditions. It warrants prompt investigation, although a cause may never be found. This so-called idiopathic or cryptogenic haemoptysis is quoted to be responsible for 3–42% of cases and carries a better prognosis[10]. Key elements of the history can often suggest an aetiology; investigations can be focused around this, and management should be directed at the underlying cause. Massive haemoptysis is a medical emergency where initial management will centre on resuscitation, especially airway protection. In this chapter, we will discuss common causes of haemoptysis. We will also discuss history and key investigatory algorithms before reviewing current medical, radiological and surgical management options.

Causes

Haemoptysis is caused by many conditions. A full list is summarized in Table 10.1. The commonest causes vary according to geography, ethnicity, socioeconomic status and age. They can be broadly divided into being associated with infection, neoplastic disease, airway disease, systemic disease, cardiovascular disease and coagulopathy. In the UK, the most common causes are bronchiectasis, lung cancer, pulmonary emboli, pulmonary tuberculosis (TB) and pneumonia. Worldwide, TB is the leading cause of haemoptysis[11,12]. As stated, no underlying aetiology is found in 3–42% of cases[12,13]. Rarer causes include endobronchial capillary haemangioma[14] and Hughes-Stovin syndrome; there are fewer than 40 cases described, and the condition is characterized by thrombophlebitis and multiple pulmonary and/or bronchial aneurysms[15].

History

Haemoptysis needs to be differentiated from haematemesis, epistaxis or bleeding from the oropharynx. This information is sometimes more difficult to elicit than one may think, and confirmation of understanding of what constitutes coughing blood needs to be

Core Topics in Thoracic Surgery, ed. Marco Scarci, Aman Coonar, Tom Routledge and Francis Wells. Published by Cambridge University Press. © Cambridge University Press 2016

Table 10.1 Causes of hemoptysis

Neoplastic	Systemic disease
Bronchogenic carcinoma	Goodpasture's syndrome
Pulmonary metastatic disease	Wegner's granulomatosis
	Microscopic polyarteritis
Kaposi's sarcoma	Behcet's disease
	Systemic lupus erythematosus
	Idiopathic pulmonary hemosiderosis

Infection	Coagulopathy
Bacterial pneumonia	Use of anticoagulants or thrombolytic agents
TB	Von Willebrand's disease
Mycetoma	Haemophilia
Respiratory viral infections	Thrombocytopenia
	Disseminated intravascular coagulation
Lung abscess	
Parasitic disease	

Airways disease	Miscellaneous
Bronchiectasis	Trauma
Bronchitis	Foreign body
Cystic fibrosis	Iatrogenic
	Pulmonary sequestration
	Endometriosis/catamenial
	Lymphangioleiomyomatosis
	Cryptogenic or idiopathic

Primary vascular disease

Pulmonary AV malformation
Pulmonary emboli
Pulmonary hypertension
Congestive cardiac failure
Mitral stenosis

[Reproduced from Hurt K, Bilton D. Haemoptysis: diagnosis and treatment. *Acute Medicine* 2012; 11(1):39–45.]

made. An assessment of volume also needs to be performed. Doing this accurately is difficult. A small volume of blood can seem large, especially when the reporter is frightened. If the patient is in hospital, ongoing measurement of volume needs to be documented. In the era of smart phones, patients often photograph initial episodes of haemoptysis, so it is worth asking about. Onset and frequency then needs to be established. In women, take note of association with menses (catamenial haemoptysis). The patient

may describe a gurgling sound, which could indicate the side from which the bleeding is coming. A clear, detailed history will help identify or exclude causes.

It is important to establish associated symptoms that may suggest a particular aetiology. For example, the presence of fevers and night sweats may suggest infection. Associated weight loss should prompt immediate exclusion of malignancy and TB. Acute breathlessness and chest pain may suggest infection or pulmonary embolism. Associated sputum production acutely may suggest pneumonia or bronchitis but chronically may suggest bronchiectasis.

A full systemic review should be performed. For example, joint pains and rashes should prompt investigation for vasculitis. A thorough past medical history needs to be made, with particular attention to childhood respiratory disease (bronchiectasis and TB reactivation). Cardiovascular disease can cause haemoptysis, so enquire about previous cardiovascular disease, paroxysmal nocturnal dyspnoea, orthopnoea and peripheral oedema.

It is important to elicit a drug history, in particular, anti-coagulation and anti-platelet therapy. Smoking and travel history may also add information to assessment of risk for lung cancer, TB and pulmonary embolism. A summary of key points of the history is made in Table 10.2.

Examination

After the history is taken, assessment of the patient's physical status is essential (In the case of massive haemoptysis, this will be performed simultaneously.) Observations should be recorded, and an assessment of physiological compromise should be made. This should involve the application of an early warning score if in hospital.

The examination may be normal. Features on general examination to ascertain are the presence or absence of cachexia, pallor, cyanosis, clubbing, lymphadenopathy, rashes, telangiectasia or ecchymoses.

Respiratory examination is mandatory. Clinical signs of deep vein thrombosis should be excluded. In addition, a cardiovascular examination should be performed to ascertain signs of heart failure, pulmonary hypertension or valvular disease.

Abdominal examination may reveal signs of hepatic failure, congestion, intra-abdominal masses or scars.

Table 10.2 Summary of key aspects of the history

History of presenting compliant

Establish true haemoptysis	Onset (acute vs chronic)
Frequency	Progression
Weight loss	Volume
Sputum production	Fevers
Rashes	Night sweats
Chest discomfort	Wheeze
Shortness of breath	Recent illness/Ill contacts
Recent travel	History of trauma
Calves tenderness	Peripheral oedema
Orthopnoea	Paroxysmal nocturnal dyspnoea
Association with menses	

Past medical history

Previous TB/TB exposure	Previous lung disease
Recent operations	History of PE/DVT
Recent bronchoscopy	Cardiovascular disease
Previous breast colon or renal cancers	Childhood illness/failure to thrive
HIV status	

Drug history

Allergies
Anticoagulation/anti-platelets

Social history

Smoking and pack year history
Alcohol intake

Family history

Congenital illness

Investigations

Most patients will have small-volume haemoptysis and can be investigated as an outpatient[16]. The National Institute for Clinical Excellence (NICE) lung cancer guidelines suggest urgent (2 week wait) referral to respiratory medicine for patients with persistent haemoptysis who are smokers or ex-smokers aged 40 years and older. They suggest an urgent chest radiograph for all patients with haemoptysis to be arranged by their general practitioner (GP)[17]. Investigations will be guided by history and examination.

Chest radiograph is an essential test, as it will rapidly identify gross pathology such as tumours and consolidation and may help localize the site of bleeding. It will fail to identify pathology in up to 46% of cases[18].

Initial blood tests should include full blood count, urea and electrolytes, liver function and clotting. Second-line tests that may offer a diagnosis are anti-neutrophil cytoplasmic antibodies or anti-nuclear antibodies if concerned about a vasculitis or autoimmune process. If vasculitis is a possibility urine analysis (protein and blood) and microscopy (for cast cells) should also be performed.

Sputum examination and culture are important to exclude bacterial infection and tuberculosis[19].

Computed tomographic (CT) scanning increases diagnostic yield, especially in distal bronchial and parenchymal abnormalities. It should be done prior to bronchoscopy as it will help locate the abnormality, improving diagnostic yield especially in cases of possible malignancy[17,20]. The choice of scan and protocol will depend on the likely underlying cause – for example, CT staging in cases of malignancy and high-resolution CT scan in cases where it is felt to be due to an interstitial process or bronchiectasis. CT may fail to identify small endobronchial lesions, early mucosal abnormalities, bronchitis, squamous metaplasia and a benign papilloma[21]. CT angiography may also be performed to assess bronchial arteries and potential bleeding source. This should be performed in patients with known bronchiectasis or cystic fibrosis when bronchial artery embolization is the treatment of choice if conservative options fail.

Fibreoptic bronchoscopy should be considered in high-risk patients if the chest X-ray and CT scan are normal and no cause has been found for the haemoptysis such as infection. Those at high risk include ongoing haemoptysis, smokers and those over the age of 40[22]. This could be diagnostic, allowing visualization of the airways and endobronchial or transbronchial biopsies to be taken. This could also be therapeutic; interventions such as cold saline, adrenaline or balloon tamponade can be performed[23].

Second-line investigations include CT pulmonary angiogram (CTPA) to rule out pulmonary embolism, echocardiography to assess for pulmonary hypertension and nasopharyngoscopy performed by an ear, nose and throat specialist may be beneficial.

Management of haemoptysis

The sequence and timing of investigations and management will depend on whether the patient is having a massive or non-massive haemoptysis. The next section

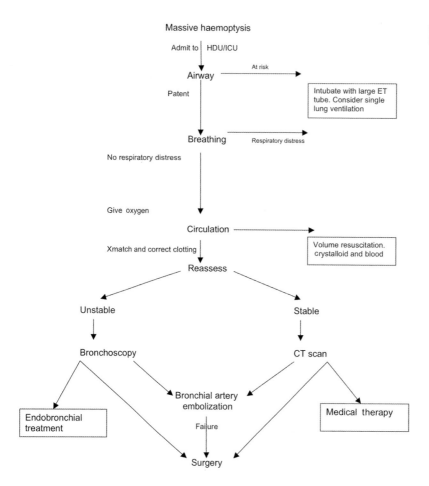

Figure 10.1 Management of massive hemoptysis.

describes an algorithm for investigation and management. This is summarized in Figure 10.1.

The mortality rate for patients with mild to moderate haemoptysis is low (2.5 and 6%, respectively)[13]. Investigations and management are similar to that of massive haemoptysis; however, conservative approaches play more of a role and surgical intervention less.

Management of massive haemoptysis

Patients should be resuscitated in accordance with the Resuscitation Council (UK) guidelines, using the ABCDE approach in assessment and management[24]. Senior doctors from intensive care and respiratory medicine should be called immediately. These patients are best managed in a high dependency or intensive care setting and nursed bleeding side down (if known)[19]. Thoracic surgery and interventional radiology need to be informed at an early stage.

The immediate priority, to prevent asphyxiation, is to protect the airway and ensure adequate oxygenation. This may require tracheal intubation, in which case a large-caliber single-lumen ET tube should be inserted. It should be large enough to allow suctioning and the introduction of a fibreoptic bronchoscope, preferably size 8 or more[25]. Once the airway is clear, if the side of haemoptysis is known, unilateral intubation can be performed, allowing protective ventilation of the collateral lung and preventing aspiration from the side actively bleeding. This can be done with a double-lumen tube; however, this requires equipment and expertise to prevent misplacement and the complications that may arise as a result[26]. An alternative to protect the left lung is, under fibreoptic bronchoscopic guidance, the left main bronchus is intubated. This is best avoided on the right, as a pitfall is the inadvertent occlusion of the right upper lobe, preventing it from participating in gaseous exchange. In this situation, an ET tube is inserted over a bronchoscope; and a Fogarty catheter of size 14F/100 cm length is passed through the vocal cords and guided via bronchoscopy in to the left main bronchus and inflated, allowing continued ventilation of the right lung and tamponade of the left[19].

Two large-bore cannulae should be inserted to allow adequate volume replacement. Samples should be sent for full blood count, urea and electrolytes, liver function tests, cross-match, clotting and inflammatory markers. Cross-match at least 6 units of blood. Coagulopathy should be corrected, which may include reversing anticoagulants[7]. Arterial blood gases are useful to look at parameters such as lactate, pH and base excess and provide an instant estimate of haemoglobin concentration. Replace volume with crystalloids and blood products, once available. Tranexamic acid can be given; however, there is little evidence to support its use. Other medical treatments that should be commenced include antibiotics for infection, antituberculous therapy in the case of TB and systemic antifungals for *Aspergillus* lung disease.

Localizing the bleeding

Once the patient has been stabilized, the next priority is to locate the bleeding point. The patient may need transfer to a specialist centre if he or she is being managed in a unit without interventional radiology or thoracic surgery. If that is the case, an expert in transfer medicine should assess the patient.

There is no consensus on the best diagnostic approach to massive haemoptysis. Broadly, though, an assessment of stability needs to be made. In the case of haemodynamic instability (where time taken for CT scanning could threaten life), patients should proceed immediately to bronchoscopy. Exceptions to this are patients with known bronchiectasis or cystic fibrosis. These patients, no matter how severe the bleeding is, should not undergo bronchoscopy at this stage.

Bronchoscopy

Urgent rigid bronchoscopy should be preformed where possible; it is preferable to fibreoptic bronchoscopy for maintaining airway patency, preserving ventilation, allowing for suctioning and therefore better visualization of the airways. Definitive procedures can also be performed. The major limitation of rigid bronchoscopy is the inability to identify more peripheral lesions or view the upper lobes easily; however, a fiberoptic bronchoscope can be introduced through

it. It is more suitable for patients with large-volume active bleeding requiring endobronchial management or in cases with bilateral lung involvement, where radiographic intervention may be limited[23]. Bronchoscopy identifies the site of bleeding in 73–93% of episodes of massive bleeding[27,28].

Therapeutic techniques include instillation of epinephrine (1:20,000) to a bleeding point; however, its effectiveness is uncertain in life-threatening haemoptysis[25]. There is limited evidence for the use of cold saline lavage, fibrinogen compounds and tranexamic acid[29–31]. Endobronchial balloon tamponade can be performed. This involves identifying the site of bleeding and wedging the bronchoscopy against it. A 4–7F Fogarty catheter is inserted through the bronchoscope and inflated. The bronchoscope can then be removed over the catheter, which is left in place for 24 hours. Complications with balloon tamponade include mucosal necrosis and obstructive pneumonia[19].

Neodymium: yttrium-aluminium-garnet (Nd:YAG) laser photocoagulation has been used with some success in the literature[32].

Stable patients

Haemodynamically stable patients with no evidence of respiratory distress should have a CT scan. CT is more effective than bronchoscopy at locating the site of bleeding and identifying the aetiology of the bleeding (60–77 vs 2.5–8%)[23]. New multi-detector CT scans allow more accurate identification of bronchial and non-bronchial systemic arteries in comparison with conventional angiography; quoted success rates are 62–100%[33]. This can be used for planning for bronchial artery embolization.

Bronchial artery embolization (BAE)

BAE (Figure 10.2) is a minimally invasive procedure that is well established in the management of massive haemoptysis. Success depends on the underlying disease, with better outcomes in TB and less favorable outcomes in lung cancer. Immediate control of haemoptysis is achieved in 73–99%, but the overall recurrence rate long term is unchanged[34].

The procedure starts with a descending thoracic aortogram to identify bronchial artery anatomy, any collaterals and bleeding site. Selective catheterizations of the arteries are then carried out. The most commonly used catheter is the cobra catheter. Alternative micro-catheters are available for cases where the bleeding vessel is small and tortuous requiring

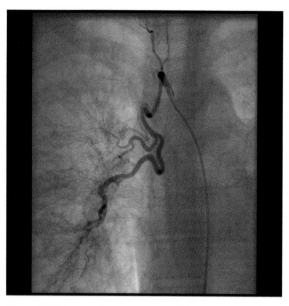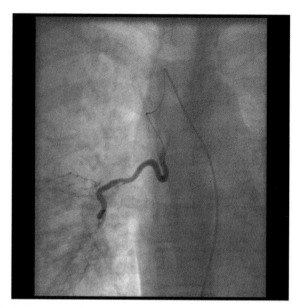

Figure 10.2 Images demonstrate bronchial arteries pre- and postembolization [Reproduced from Hurt K, Bilton D., Haemoptysis: diagnosis and treatment. *Acute Medicine* 2012; 11(1):39–45.]

super-selective catheterization in order to successfully access the bleeding vessels and avoid damage to surrounding vessels. This is important in the case of the right bronchial artery, to prevent occlusion of the anterior medullary artery and the spinal cord supply[10].

Contrast may demonstrate hypertrophic and tortuous bronchial arteries, areas of hypervascular and neovascular change as well as aneurysms. Rarely do you see extravasation of contrast medium, and this finding is reported in between 3.6 and 10.7% of cases[35,36]. The most commonly used embolic material is polyvinyl alcohol foam granules, but isobutyl-2-cyanoacrylate, Gianturco steel coils and absorbable gelatin pledgets have also been used[19]. A detailed search for ongoing bleeding vessels should be preformed, especially from the collateral blood supply. Early re-bleeding may be due to incomplete embolization or, as aforementioned, the bleeding may be coming from the pulmonary or non-bronchial arteries. Late re-bleeding is generally as a result of revascularization of collateral arteries. The re-bleed rate depends on the underlying disease[34].

Complications of bronchial artery embolization include chest pain (24–91%), dysphasia (1–18%) and spinal cord ischaemia (1.4–6.5%). Systemic embolization can lead to ischemic colitis or cortical blindness[34].

Pulmonary angiography has been advocated in patients with early recurrent haemoptysis, after bronchial artery embolization or in the presence of normal bronchial arteries. In certain conditions such as pulmonary TB, bleeding arises from the pulmonary circulation. The most common cause of bleeding from the pulmonary circulation is from a Rasmussen's aneurysm. This is a result of erosion of a peripheral pulmonary artery by chronic inflammation seen in TB. They are seen as nodules within the walls of TB cavities; reported incidence varies from 4 to11%[10].

Surgery

Until two decades ago, surgery was regarded as the treatment of choice for massive haemoptysis. Surgery has now been largely superseded by safer endovascular techniques. It does, however, remain the treatment of choice in the following clinical situations[23]:

1. AV malformations
2. Trauma
3. Pulmonary artery rupture
4. Mycetoma that has failed medical treatment
5. Failed BAE
6. Immediate life-threatening haemoptysis, where the risk of temporizing measures are considered too great

The patient's fitness for surgery should be assessed early in the admission and discussed with the thoracic team. Surgical resection will not be an option for patients with a poor performance status and poor respiratory reserve. Lung cancer that is deemed 'inoperable' due to spread is also a contraindication.

Morbidity and mortality are high following surgery, with mortality ranging between 20 and 30%[37–40].

Recent studies looking at patients with significant haemoptysis presenting to specialist centres have demonstrated surgery rates of 10–15% in patients with massive haemoptysis (who also underwent BAE). These mortality rates were lower than in some older studies quoted earlier and were around 13%[41, 42].

Management of haemoptysis in special cases

Cystic fibrosis (CF)

Haemoptysis is a common complication in CF, occurring in 9.1% of patients. Massive haemoptysis is associated with older patients with more severe disease and carries a high mortality rate. Current guidelines for treatment from the Cystic Fibrosis Foundation (CFF) are based on consensus opinion of experts[44]. There is limited evidence to support current practice. Patients should receive specialist centre treatment and should receive treatment for respiratory infection. There is a limited amount of data to support the use of tranexamic acid and terlipressin, and these are routinely used[45,46].

BAE is the treatment of choice when these measures have failed. Bronchoscopy should not be routinely performed as it may delay time to BAE. Immediate control is gained in most cases, but there are few data to support improved outcomes longer term. Surgery is a last resort in patients with CF.

There should be a lower threshold for patients with cavitatory disease. Lobectomy is the most common procedure performed. It should be considered in cases of ongoing bleeding despite BAE or recurrent severe haemoptysis that has not responded to BAE. For patients undergoing recurrent life-threatening haemoptysis, lung transplantation may play a role. This needs a full risk-benefit discussion with the CF team, transplant team and patient.

Vasculitis and alveolar haemorrhage

These patients should be managed medically (joint care with renal physicians). Therapeutic options include immunosuppression and plasma exchange. Bronchoscopy may have a role if super-added infection is suspected[47].

Conclusion

Haemoptysis is a serious symptom that needs further investigation, usually by a respiratory physician. Massive haemoptysis carries a high mortality, yet there are no agreed guidelines for treatment. Patients with massive haemoptysis should generally be managed in a high-dependency setting. Initial stabilization includes airway protection, possible single lung ventilation, volume resuscitation, isolation of the bleeding source and definitive treatment.

There are some established endobronchial techniques for control of bleeding with a limited evidence base and some newer treatments that need further trials. BAE is now a well-established treatment for massive haemoptysis and has reduced the amount of patients requiring surgery. Surgery still has a significant role to play in cases that won't settle with these measures.

References

1 Haponik EF, Fein A, Chin R. Managing life-threatening hemoptysis: has anything really changed? *Chest* 2000; 118(5): 1431–5.

2 Amirana M, Frater R, Tirschwell P, et al. An aggressive surgical approach to significant hemoptysis in patients with pulmonary tuberculosis. *Am Rev Respir Dise* 1968; 97(2): 187–92.

3 Hurt K, Bilton D. Haemoptysis: diagnosis and treatment. *Acute Medi* 2012; 11(1):39–45.

4 Hankanson E, Konstantinov IE, Fransson SG, Svedjeholm R. Management of life threatening haemoptysis. *Br J Anaesth* 2002; 88(2):291–5.

5 Ibrahim WH. Massive haemoptysis: the definition should be revised. *Eur Respir J* 2008; 32(4):1131–2.

6 Hirshberg B, Biran I, Glazer M, Kramer MR. Hemoptysis:

etiology, evaluation, and outcome in a tertiary referral hospital. *Chest* 1997; 112(2):440–4.

7 Jean-Baptiste E. Clinical assessment and management of massive hemoptysis. *Crit Care Med* 2000; 28(5):1642–7.

8 Crocco JA, Rooney JJ, Fankushen DS, et al. Massive hemoptysis. *Arch Intern Med* 1968; 121(6): 495–8.

9 Fartoukh M, Khoshnood B, Parrot A, et al. Early prediction of

in-hospital mortality of patients with hemoptysis: an approach to defining severe hemoptysis. *Respir Int Rev Thorac Dis* 2012; 83(2): 106–14.

10 Chun JY, Morgan R, Belli AM. Radiological management of hemoptysis: a comprehensive review of diagnostic imaging and bronchial arterial embolization. *Cardiovasc Intervent Radiol* 2010; 33(2):240–50.

11 Santiago S, Tobias J, Williams AJ. A reappraisal of the causes of hemoptysis. *Arch Intern Med* 1991; 151(12):2449–51.

12 Reisz G, Stevens D, Boutwell C, Nair V. The causes of hemoptysis revisited. A review of the etiologies of hemoptysis between 1986 and 1995. *Mo Med* 1997; 94:633–5.

13 Hirshberg B, Biran I, Glazer M, Kramer MR. Hemoptysis: etiology, evaluation, and outcome in a tertiary referral hospital. *Chest* 1997; 112(2):440–4.

14 Ozyilmaz E, Yunsel D, Hanta I, et al. Endobronchial capillary hemangioma: a very rare cause of massive hemoptysis. *Tuberkuloz ve toraks* 2012; 60(1):78–80. Epub 5 May 2012. Masif hemoptizinin nadir bir nedeni: Endobronsiyal kapiller hemanjiyom.

15 Khalid U, Saleem T. Hughes-Stovin syndrome. *Orphanet J Rare Dis* 2011; 6:15.

16 Bidwell JL, Pachner RW. Hemoptysis: diagnosis and management. *Am Fam Phys* 2005; 72(7):1253–60.

17 National Institute for Health and Clinical Excellence. *The Diagnosis and Treatment of Lung Cancer CG24.* London: National Institute for Health and Clinical Excellence 2005.

18 Marshall TJ, Flower CDR, Jackson JE. The role of radiology in the investigation and management of patients with haemoptysis. *Clin Radiol* 1996; 51(6):391–400.

19 Lordan JL, Gascoigne A, Corris PA. The pulmonary physician in critical care. Illustrative case 7: Assessment and management of massive haemoptysis. *Thorax* 2003; 58(9):814–9.

20 Thirumaran M, Sundar R, Sutcliffe IM, Currie DC. Is investigation of patients with haemoptysis and normal chest radiograph justified? *Thorax* 2009; 64(10):854–6.

21 Set PA, Flower CD, Smith IE, et al. Hemoptysis: comparative study of the role of CT and fiberoptic bronchoscopy. *Radiology* 1993; 189(3):677–80.

22 Poe RH, Israel RH, Marin MG, et al. Utility of fiberoptic bronchoscopy in patients with hemoptysis and a nonlocalizing chest roentgenogram. *Chest* 1988; 93(1):70–5.

23 Sakr L, Dutau H. Massive hemoptysis: an update on the role of bronchoscopy in diagnosis and management. *Respir Int Rev Thorac Dis* 2010; 80(1):38–58.

24 The Resuscitation Guidelines 2010. The Resuscitation Council (UK), 2010.

25 Dweik RA, Stoller JK. Role of bronchoscopy in massive hemoptysis. *Clin Chest Med* 1999; 20(1):89–105.

26 Klein U, Karzai W, Bloos F, et al. Role of fiberoptic bronchoscopy in conjunction with the use of double-lumen tubes for thoracic anesthesia: a prospective study. *Anesthesiology* 1998; 88(2): 346–50.

27 Revel MP, Fournier LS, Hennebicque AS, et al. Can CT replace bronchoscopy in the detection of the site and cause of bleeding in patients with large or massive hemoptysis? *Am J Roentgenol* 2002; 179(5): 1217–24.

28 Khalil A, Soussan M, Mangiapan G, et al. Utility of high-resolution chest CT scan in the emergency management. *Bri J Radiol* 2007; 80(949):21–5.

29 Conlan AA, Hurwitz SS. Management of massive haemoptysis with the rigid bronchoscope and cold saline lavage. *Thorax* 1980; 35(12): 901–4.

30 Tsukamoto T, Sasaki H, Nakamura H. Treatment of hemoptysis patients by thrombin and fibrinogen-thrombin infusion therapy using a fiberoptic bronchoscope. *Chest* 1989; 96(3): 473–6.

31 Solomonov A, Fruchter O, Zuckerman T, et al. Pulmonary hemorrhage: a novel mode of therapy. *Respir Med* 2009; 103(8):1196–200.

32 Edmondstone WM, Nanson EM, Woodcock AA, et al. Life-threatening haemoptysis controlled by laser photocoagulation. *Thorax* 1983; 38(10):788–9.

33 Yoon YC, Lee KS, Jeong YJ, et al. Hemoptysis: bronchial and nonbronchial systemic arteries at 16-detector row CT. *Radiology* 2005; 234(1):292–8.

34 Chun JY, Belli AM. Immediate and long-term outcomes of bronchial and non-bronchial systemic artery embolisation for the management of haemoptysis. *Eur Radiol* 2010; 20(3):558–65.

35 Hsiao EI, Kirsch CM, Kagawa FT, et al. Utility of fiberoptic bronchoscopy before bronchial artery embolization for massive hemoptysis. *Am J Roentgenol* 2001; 177(4):861–7.

36 Ramakantan R, Bandekar VG, Gandhi MS, et al. Massive hemoptysis due to pulmonary tuberculosis: control with bronchial artery embolization. *Radiology* 1996; 200(3):691–4.

37 Garzon AA, Cerruti M, Gourin A, et al. Pulmonary resection for massive hemoptysis. *Surgery* 1970; 67:633–8.

38 Gourin A, Garzon A. Control of hemorrhage in emergency pulmonary resection for massive hemoptysis. *Chest* 1975; 68:120–1.

39 Sehhat S, Oreizie M, Moinedine K. Massive pulmonary hemorrhage: surgical approach as choice of treatment. *Ann Thorac Surg* 1978; 25:12–15.

40 Corey R, Hla KM. Major and massive hemoptysis: reassessment of conservative management. *Am J Med Sci.* 1987; 294:301–9.

41 Ong TH, Eng P: Massive hemoptysis requiring intensive care. *Intensive Care Med.* 2003; 29:317–20.

42 Fartoukh M, Khalil A, Louis L, et al. An integrated approach to diagnosis and management of severe haemoptysis in patients admitted to the intensive care unit: a case series from a referral centre. *Respir Res* 2007; 8:11–20.

43 Flume PA, Yankaskas JR, Ebeling M, et al. Massive hemoptysis in cystic fibrosis. *Chest* 2005; 128(2):729–38.

44 Flume PA, Mogayzel PJ Jr, Robinson KA, et al. Cystic fibrosis pulmonary guidelines: pulmonary complications: hemoptysis and pneumothorax. *Am J Respir Crit Care Med* 2010; 182(3): 298–306.

45 Hurley M, Bhatt J, Smyth A. Treatment massive haemoptysis in cystic fibrosis with tranexamic acid. *J R Soc Med* 2011; 104 (Suppl 1):S49–S52.

46 Bilton D, Webb AK, Foster H, et al. Life threatening haemoptysis in cystic fibrosis: an alternative therapeutic approach. *Thorax* 1990; 45(12):975–6.

47 West S, Arulkumaran, Ind PW, Pusey CD. Diffuse alveolar haemorrhage in ANCA-associated vasculitis. *Intern Med* 2013; 52(1): 5–13.

Chapter

11

Evaluation of solitary pulmonary nodule

Dustin M. Walters and David R. Jones

Introduction

The solitary pulmonary nodule (SPN) is an increasingly common radiographic entity, often presenting a challenging scenario for clinicians and provoking significant anxiety in patients. The increasing incidence of SPNs is directly related to the widespread use of chest radiography, particularly computed tomography (CT). SPNs are found incidentally on 0.09–0.2% of chest X-rays[1,2] and 1.3% of CT scans[3]. Roughly half of smokers over the age of 50 will have pulmonary nodules detected by CT scan, although the majority of these will be smaller than 7 mm[4]. As data from the National Lung Screening Trial[5] show decreased lung cancer–specific mortality in high-risk patients screened with CT, it stands to reason that the incidence of SPNs will continue to increase in coming years. Thus it is imperative that thoracic surgeons understand the nuances of these lesions in order to direct an efficient evaluation and provide optimal management for their patients.

SPNs are defined as a single nodule, less than 3 cm in size, completely surrounded by lung parenchyma and without other associated features such as atelectasis, adenopathy, or effusions[6,7]. These nodules have a variety of benign and malignant etiologies (Table 11.1). Determining the risk of malignancy is the most critical duty of the clinician because this ultimately drives the management of these lesions. Establishing a firm diagnosis, while ideal, is not always possible without invasive approaches, which is not necessary for all SPNs.

Initial evaluation

The diagnostic evaluation begins with a thorough history and physical exam, as well as a careful review

Table 11.1 Differential diagnoses for SPNs

Malignant

> Non-small-cell lung cancer
> Small-cell lung cancer
> Carcinoid tumor
> Other primary pulmonary tumors
> Metastases (colorectal, breast, sarcoma, melanoma, renal cell, etc.)

Benign

> Infectious
>
> > Bacterial pneumonia/abscess/septic embolus
> > Fungal infections
> > Tuberculosis
> > Parasitic infection
>
> Inflammatory
>
> > Sarcoidosis
> > Wegener granulomatosis
> > Rheumatoid nodule
>
> Hamartoma
> Arteriovenous malformation

of imaging, particularly old radiographs or CT scans. The majority of SPNs are asymptomatic at diagnosis. However, the history should focus on tobacco abuse and exposures (such as asbestos, radon, etc.) and a search for symptoms such as cough, hemoptysis, chest pain, and weight loss. A history of solid organ cancer should be sought, as this increases the chance that the nodule represents a malignancy and should raise suspicion of metastatic disease. Knowing the previous source of cancer may provide some clues. For instance, the odds of metastatic pulmonary

Core Topics in Thoracic Surgery, ed. Marco Scarci, Aman Coonar, Tom Routledge and Francis Wells. Published by Cambridge University Press. © Cambridge University Press 2016

disease are higher for sarcomas and melanoma compared to colorectal adenocarcinoma and head and neck squamous cancer.

The next step involves thorough review of all imaging studies, with particular attention to the radiographic features of the nodule and a comparison to old studies. With few exceptions, lesions that have been stable for 2 or more years on imaging can be considered benign and require no additional follow-up. However, this "2-year" rule is not based on great data, and if the patient is high risk for developing a lung cancer, one may wish to follow-up for a longer period of time. If no previous imaging studies are available for comparison, radiographic features of the nodule can be used to estimate cancer risk. If the nodule has been identified on a chest X-ray or low-resolution CT scan, the next approach should be a high-resolution chest CT with fine-imaging cuts for better characterization.

When reviewing imaging studies, the growth rate and size of the nodule are particularly important. A nodule that demonstrates interval growth is significantly more likely to be malignant, whereas slower-growing or stable nodules are more likely benign. The exception is lesions with ground-glass opacities (GGOs), which may represent minimally invasive adenocarcinoma or adenocarcinoma-in-situ (formerly known as bronchioloalveolar carcinoma[8]) and may have much longer doubling times. While there is no absolute consensus, there is strong suggestion that these GGOs should be followed-up for longer than a 2-year period. In a study of 61 patients found to have small lung cancers on screening CT scans, the doubling time was found to be 813 days for true GGOs compared with 457 days for semisolid GGOs and 149 days for purely solid lesions[9]. Perhaps the most important information that can be gained from the imaging studies is the size of the nodule itself, which strongly correlates with risk of malignancy. In an analysis of several large series, the risk of malignancy was 0–1% for nodules less than 0.5 cm in size compared to 6–28% for lesions 0.5–1.0 cm in size and 64–82% for nodules greater than 2.0 cm in size[10].

The radiographic appearance of the nodule, including the shape, borders, density, and location, may provide further clues to the malignant potential. Nodules with spiculated, lobulated, or otherwise irregular borders are more commonly associated with malignancy, compared to benign lesions, which usually demonstrate smooth, rounded borders.

Malignant lesions are less likely to contain calcifications and cavitations than benign lesions, but calcifications do not exclude the possibility of malignancy, and thus the pattern of calcifications may provide more useful information. Benign calcification patterns are more commonly diffuse, centric, popcorn-shaped, or concentric, while malignant patterns are more likely to be stippled or eccentric[11]. Ground-glass or semisolid nodules are more likely to be malignant than purely solid lesions, while a nodule with fatty components is more likely to represent a benign lesion, most likely a hamartoma. Finally, location may provide some clue, as malignant lesions more commonly affect the upper and middle lobes.

Further management of pulmonary nodules

Stratification of SPNs into low, intermediate, and high risk can be performed on the basis of the clinical history and radiographic review (Table 11.2)[12]. Low-risk lesions are small (<8 mm in size), smooth-bordered lesions, occurring in younger nonsmokers

Table 11.2 Risk stratification for patients with SPNs

Risk factor	Low risk	Intermediate risk	High risk
Nodule size, in mm	<8	8–20	>20
Nodule shape	Smooth	Lobular	Spiculated
Age, in years	<45	45–60	>60
Personal history of cancer	No		Yes
Smoking history	Never	Current < 1 pack/day	Current > 1 pack/day
Smoking cessation	Quit ≥ 7 years ago	Quit < 7 years ago	Never quit
COPD	No	Yes	
Exposure to asbestos	No		Yes

(Adapted from: Ost DE, Gould MK., *J Respir Crit Care Med* 2012; 185(4):363–72.)

without a personal history of cancer and other risk factors. Intermediate-risk nodules include moderately sized (8–20 mm) or lobulated lesions, occurring in slightly older patients, current light smokers, or patients with mild risk factors. High-risk lesions are larger (>20 mm) or spiculated and occur in older patients, heavy smokers, or those with more significant risk factors. In general, low-risk nodules warrant either close monitoring with serial imaging or no further workup. Intermediate-risk nodules should prompt further testing, while high-risk nodules should be surgically resected in patients who are good operative candidates.

Low-risk nodules (<10% risk of malignancy)

In general, nodules considered to be low risk for malignancy should be observed with serial imaging. If there are previous comparable imaging studies that demonstrate long-term stability of the nodule, no further workup is indicated. However, the majority of low-risk nodules warrant follow-up with serial imaging by CT scan every 3–12 months for a period of 2 years. Numerous studies have shown low rates of malignant potential, particularly for nodules less than 5 mm in diameter[13–15]. The Fleischner Society has published consensus guidelines for follow-up and management of very small nodules (Table 11.3)

Table 11.3 Fleischner Society guidelines for follow-up of small nodules incidentally detected on CT

Nodule size, in mm	Low-risk patients*	High-risk patients#
≤4	No follow-up	CT at 12 months; if stable, no further follow-up
>4–6	CT at 12 months, if stable, no further follow-up	CT at 6–12 months; if stable, repeat at 18–24 months
>6–8	CT at 6–12 months; if stable, repeat at 18-24 months	CT at 3–6 months, 9–12 months, and 24 months
>8	CT at 3, 9, and 24 months, CT-FNA, or PET-CT	CT at 3, 9, and 24 months, CT-FNA, or PET-CT

(Adapted from: MacMahon et al., *Radiology* 2005; 237(2):395–400.)
* Minimal or no smoking history, without other risk factors.
# Significant smoking history or other risk factors.

based on patient clinical risk of cancer[16]. For these small nodules, the Fleischner Guidelines stratify higher-risk patients to include those with smoking history or other known lung cancer risk factors, while lower-risk patients have minimal or no history of smoking.

Intermediate-risk nodules (10–60% risk of malignancy)

Intermediate-risk nodules should prompt further investigation, either via CT-guided fine-needle aspiration (FNA) or core needle biopsy or via positron-emission tomographic (PET)–CT followed by CT-guided FNA, if necessary. Other potential diagnostic techniques include bronchoscopy, with or without endobronchial ultrasound (EBUS), and navigational bronchoscopy, although these techniques are less reliable in many patients.

CT-guided FNA has become routine for many pulmonary nodules, with a sensitivity and specificity of 90% and 65–94%, respectively[10]. CT-guided FNA is dependent on the experience of the interventional radiologist and may be less reliable in smaller nodules, with an overall rate of nondiagnostic biopsy ranging from 6–27% in large studies[17-19]. CT-guided FNA carries some risk, and the overall complication rate is approximately 40%. The most common complication is iatrogenic pneumothorax, which has been reported with a frequency as high as 25–43% in large studies, although the majority do not require chest tube insertion[10], with contemporary series demonstrating a 3–7% rate of chest tube insertion following CT-guided biopsy[20,21]. PET-CT has largely replaced standard PET scanning and has been shown to be a cost-effective strategy for intermediate-risk SPNs[22]. The sensitivity and specificity for determining pulmonary malignancy with PET-CT have been shown to be 87 and 83%, respectively[23]. The major limitation of PET-CT is false-negative and false-positive results, given the relative small size of some SPNs. Further, some tumor subtypes, such as adenocarcinoma in situ (formerly bronchioloalveolar carcinoma) and carcinoid tumors, have decreased fluorodeoxyglucose uptake and thus diminished diagnostic accuracy with PET-CT[8,24]. While little data exist on the subject, there is strong suggestion that small (<1.0 cm) nodules have poorer sensitivity, and the use of PET-CT for smaller lesions is not likely to provide definitive information[25,26].

Table 11.4 Diagnostic yield of electromagnetic navigation diagnostic bronchoscopy

Study	Technique	Nodule size	Number (n)	Diagnostic yield	p-Value
Gildea TR et al., 2006 [30]	ENB	0–20 mm	31	74.1%	0.422
		>20–40 mm	18	66.6%	0.378
		>40 mm	5	100%	
		0–30 mm	43	72.1%	
		>30 mm	11	81.8%	
Makris D et al., 2007 [31]	ENB	0–10 mm	4	75%	Not reported
		>10–20 mm	16	43.7%	
		>20–30 mm	7	71.4%	
		>30 mm	13	76.9%	
Lamprecht B et al., 2012 [32]	Combined FDG-PET, ENB, and ROSE	0–20 mm	45	75.6%	0.066
		>20 mm	67	89.6%	
Pearlstein DP et al., 2012[33]	ENB and ROSE	<15 mm	16	88%	0.331
		15–20 mm	14	71%	
		>20 mm	71	87%	

ENB = Electromagnetic navigation bronchoscopy, FDG-PET = fluorodeoxyglucose positron emission tomography, ROSE = rapid on-site examination of cytopathology.

False-positive results are known to occur in both inflammatory and infectious conditions.

Other techniques have been used as diagnostic adjuncts, including bronchoscopic biopsy, endobronchial ultrasound (EBUS)–FNA, and electromagnetic navigation bronchoscopy (ENB). In general, these techniques are associated with decreased sensitivity and lower diagnostic yield than both PET-CT and CT-FNA. Higher success rates are observed in more central or endobronchial lesions, nodules associated with air bronchograms, and larger nodules, and these techniques may be useful in these scenarios[27,28]. There is some evidence that combining ENB biopsy with EBUS is associated with higher diagnostic yield[29]. When using ENB, larger nodules are associated with increased diagnostic yield, although the data are somewhat limited[30-33] (Table 11.4). Currently, in the majority of cases, CT-FNA is preferred over these bronchoscopic techniques when obtaining tissue is a diagnostic priority.

High-risk nodules (>60% risk of malignancy)

Nodules that have radiographic features that are high risk for malignancy should be managed operatively with resection in patients who can tolerate surgery. Preoperative workup should consist of a thorough evaluation of fitness for surgery, including pulmonary function tests and assessment of baseline functional status. Surgery is performed via video-assisted thoracoscopic surgery (VATS) or robotic techniques whenever possible. We rarely recommend that a thoracotomy be performed. If a diagnosis has not been established, a wedge resection with adequate (R_0) margins should be performed with frozen histologic assessment. Benign lesions, typical carcinoid tumors, and metastatic lesions from other sources (i.e. sarcoma, renal cell carcinoma) require no further resection. Currently, the standard of care for non-small-cell lung cancer in patients with adequate pulmonary function tests (PFTs) is anatomic lobectomy with mediastinal lymph node sampling or dissection. It is worth noting that small lesions, particularly GGOs and semisolid nodules, may be difficult to locate by manual palpation, particularly using VATS techniques. In these patients, we have found that radiotracer-guided resection with technetium-99m microalbumin aggregate safely facilitates resection of the nodule and is cost-effective[34-36].

Conclusions

SPNs are becoming increasingly common clinical entities, and thus thoracic surgeons should be comfortable with the evaluation and management of these

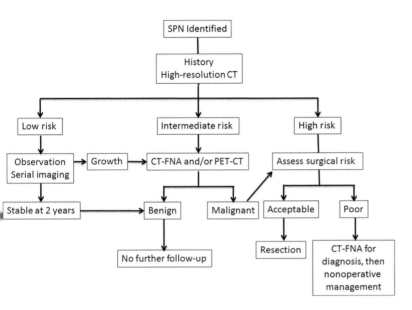

Figure 11.1 Workup algorithm for SPNs.

lesions (Figure 11.1). Patients can be risk stratified into low-, intermediate-, and high-risk groups for malignancy based on a thorough history and review of radiographic studies. High-resolution CT scan is an important component of the initial workup. In general, low-risk nodules should be followed with serial imaging, intermediate-risk nodules should trigger additional workup via CT-FNA and/or PET-CT, and high-risk nodules should be managed surgically in patients with acceptable operative risk.

References

1   Holin SM, Dwork RE, Glaser S, et al. Solitary pulmonary nodules found in a community-wide chest roentgenographic survey; a five-year follow-up study. *Am Rev Tuberc* 1959; 79(4):427–39.

2   Swensen SJ, Silverstein MD, Edell ES, et al. Solitary pulmonary nodules: clinical prediction model versus physicians. *Mayo Clin Proc* 1999; 74(4):319–29.

3   Alzahouri K, Velten M, Arveux P, et al. Management of SPN in France: pathways for definitive diagnosis of solitary pulmonary nodule: a multicentre study in 18 French districts. *BMC Cancer* 2008; 8:93.

4   Swensen SJ, Silverstein MD, Ilstrup DM, et al. The probability of malignancy in solitary pulmonary nodules: application to small radiologically indeterminate nodules. *Arch Intern Med* 1997; 157(8):849–55.

5   Aberle DR, Adams AM, Berg CD, et al. Reduced lung-cancer mortality with low-dose computed tomographic screening. *N Engl J Med* 2011; 365(5):395–409.

6   Tuddenham WJ. Glossary of terms for thoracic radiology: recommendations of the Nomenclature Committee of the Fleischner Society. *AJR Am J Roentgenol* 1984; 143(3):509–17.

7   Ost D, Fein AM, Feinsilver SH. Clinical practice: the solitary pulmonary nodule. *N Engl J Med* 2003; 348(25):2535–42.

8   Kruger S, Buck AK, Blumstein NM, et al. Use of integrated FDG PET/CT imaging in pulmonary carcinoid tumours. *J Intern Med* 2006; 260(6):545–50.

9   Hasegawa M, Sone S, Takashima S, et al. Growth rate of small lung cancers detected on mass CT screening. *Br J Radiol* 2000, 73(876):1252–9.

10   Wahidi MM, Govert JA, Goudar RK, et al. Evidence for the treatment of patients with pulmonary nodules: when is it lung cancer?: ACCP evidence-based clinical practice guidelines (2nd edition). *Chest* 2007; 132(3 Suppl): 94S–107S.

11   Webb WR: Radiologic evaluation of the solitary pulmonary nodule. *AJR Am J Roentgenol* 1990; 154(4):701–8.

12   Ost DE, Gould MK: Decision making in patients with pulmonary nodules. *Am J Respir Crit Care Med* 2012; 185(4):363–72.

13   Henschke CI, Yankelevitz DF, Naidich DP, et al. CT screening for lung cancer: suspiciousness of nodules according to size on baseline scans. *Radiology* 2004; 231(1):164–8.

14   Swensen SJ, Jett JR, Hartman TE, et al. Lung cancer screening with

CT: Mayo Clinic experience. *Radiology* 2003; 226(3):756–61.

15   Henschke CI, McCauley DI, Yankelevitz DF, et al. Early Lung Cancer Action Project: overall design and findings from baseline screening. *Lancet* 1999; 354(9173):99–105.

16   MacMahon H, Austin JH, Gamsu G, et al. Guidelines for management of small pulmonary nodules detected on CT scans: a statement from the Fleischner Society. *Radiology* 2005; 237(2):395–400.

17   vanSonnenberg E, Casola G, Ho M, et al. Difficult thoracic lesions: CT-guided biopsy experience in 150 cases. *Radiology* 1988; 167(2):457–61.

18   Yankelevitz DF, Henschke CI, Koizumi JH, et al. CT-guided transthoracic needle biopsy of small solitary pulmonary nodules. *Clin Imaging* 1997; 21(2):107–10.

19   Yamagami T, Iida S, Kato T, et al. Usefulness of new automated cutting needle for tissue-core biopsy of lung nodules under CT fluoroscopic guidance. *Chest* 2003; 124(1):147–54.

20   Poulou LS, Tsagouli P, Ziakas PD, et al. Computed tomography-guided needle aspiration and biopsy of pulmonary lesions: a single-center experience in 1000 patients. *Acta Radiol* 2013.

21   Khan KA, Zaidi S, Swan N, et al. The use of computerised tomography guided percutaneous fine needle aspiration in the evaluation of solitary pulmonary nodules. *Ir Med J* 2012; 105(2):50–2.

22   Cao JQ, Rodrigues GB, Louie AV, Zaric GS: Systematic review of the cost-effectiveness of positron-emission tomography in staging of non–small-cell lung cancer and management of solitary pulmonary nodules. *Clin Lung Cancer* 2012; 13(3):161–70.

23   Gould MK, Fletcher J, Iannettoni MD, et al. Evaluation of patients with pulmonary nodules: when is it lung cancer?: ACCP evidence-based clinical practice guidelines (2nd edition). *Chest* 2007; 132(3 Suppl):108S–30S.

24   Yap CS, Schiepers C, Fishbein MC, et al. FDG-PET imaging in lung cancer: how sensitive is it for bronchioloalveolar carcinoma? *Eur J Nucl Med Mol Imaging* 2002; 29(9):1166–73.

25   Kernstine KH, Grannis FW Jr, Rotter AJ: Is there a role for PET in the evaluation of subcentimeter pulmonary nodules? *Semin Thorac Cardiovasc Surg* 2005; 17(2):110–14.

26   Kozower BD, Meyers BF, Reed CE, et al. Does positron emission tomography prevent nontherapeutic pulmonary resections for clinical stage IA lung cancer? *Ann Thorac Surg* 2008; 85(4):1166–9; discussion 1169–70.

27   Seijo LM, de Torres JP, Lozano MD, et al. Diagnostic yield of electromagnetic navigation bronchoscopy is highly dependent on the presence of a bronchus sign on CT imaging: results from a prospective study. *Chest* 2010; 138(6):1316–21.

28   Steinfort DP, Khor YH, Manser RL, Irving LB. Radial probe endobronchial ultrasound for the diagnosis of peripheral lung cancer: systematic review and meta-analysis. *Eur Respir J* 2011, 37(4):902–10.

29   Eberhardt R, Morgan RK, Ernst A, et al. Comparison of suction catheter versus forceps biopsy for sampling of solitary pulmonary nodules guided by electromagnetic navigational bronchoscopy. *Respiration* 2010; 79(1):54–60.

30   Gildea TR, Mazzone PJ, Karnak D, et al. Electromagnetic navigation diagnostic bronchoscopy: a prospective study. *Am J Respir Crit Care Med* 2006; 174(9):982–9.

31   Makris D, Scherpereel A, Leroy S, et al. Electromagnetic navigation diagnostic bronchoscopy for small peripheral lung lesions. *Eur Respir J* 2007; 29(6):1187–92.

32   Lamprecht B, Porsch P, Wegleitner B, et al. Electromagnetic navigation bronchoscopy (ENB): increasing diagnostic yield. *Respir Med* 2012; 106(5):710–15.

33   Pearlstein DP, Quinn CC, Burtis CC, et al. Electromagnetic navigation bronchoscopy performed by thoracic surgeons: one center's early success. *Ann Thorac Surg* 2012; 93(3):944–9; discussion 949–50.

34   Grogan EL, Stukenborg GJ, Nagji AS, et al. Radiotracer-guided thoracoscopic resection is a cost-effective technique for the evaluation of subcentimeter pulmonary nodules. *Ann Thorac Surg* 2008; 86(3):934–40; discussion 934–40.

35   Grogan EL, Jones DR, Kozower BD, et al. Identification of small lung nodules: technique of radiotracer-guided thoracoscopic biopsy. *Ann Thorac Surg* 2008; 85(2):S772–7.

36   Stiles BM, Altes TA, Jones DR, et al. Clinical experience with radiotracer-guided thoracoscopic biopsy of small, indeterminate lung nodules. *Ann Thorac Surg* 2006; 82(4):1191–6; discussion 1196–7.

Chapter 12

Lung cancer staging

Bilal H. Kirmani and Aman S. Coonar

Lung cancer is the second most common cancer in the UK and a leading cause of cancer-related deaths worldwide. Prognosis and treatment options vary depending on the pathological type and the anatomical extent of the tumour. Both over-treatment of advanced disease and under-treatment of limited disease can reduce quality and length of life. Therefore, prompt and accurate staging are important to ensure delivery of appropriate therapy.

Clinical presentation

A large proportion of primary lung cancers are asymptomatic[1], and poor awareness of signs and symptoms of lung cancer in the general population[2] means that patients often present late. Clinical features identified by careful history and examination can direct tests. More recently, the increasing availability of CT screening has led to an increased detection of early cancers, and this may result in a real survival advantage by curing disease found at an early stage[3]. Alternatively, it may just represent a lead-time bias.

Staging systems

Staging helps in advising on prognosis, planning treatment and comparing data. There are two parts, the TNM (tumour, node, metastasis) and the stage groups.

Different TNM combinations have been aggregated into stage groups that differ by their prognosis. The TNM and stage groups are based on the outcomes of many pragmatically managed patients and undergo periodic review. This means there can be differences between versions, and while these may be small, users should be aware of them.

TNM status

The TNM status describes the anatomical extent of cancer based on tumour size, location and any local invasion, lymph node involvement and metastasis. Nodal involvement is described based on lymph node stations, as described by Mountain and Dresler[4].

The seventh and most recent revision of the TNM staging system for lung cancer, summarized in Table 12.1, started to be used in 2010. It is based on multicentre data from more than 80,000 patients[5]. At various stages of the diagnostic pathway, the patient's TNM status can be updated. The clinical stage (cTNM) and the pathological stage (pTNM) (post-operative) have different prognoses[6]. It is important to note that the data set employed to determine the seventh edition of the TNM classification predated the widespread use of positron-emission tomography (PET) scanning and therefore does not fully reflect the importance of that tool, which is now a standard of care for lung cancer staging in the UK and many other places.

Stage groups

The TNM classification is used to determine a prognostic stage grouping of 0, I, II, III or IV, with further subdivision of some stages into A or B, as shown in Table 12.2. Thus, patients with various combinations of tumour size and nodal involvement may have similar prognoses. The IASLC data found survival varied from 73 to 36% for completely resected stage Ia to IIb disease[5]. Treatment of stage IIIa disease is controversial and variable[7]. Some groups advocate surgery for N2 disease, some with and some without induction treatment. N2 disease is further classifiied into bulky or non-bulky. Patients with stage IIIB or IV disease are

---

Core Topics in Thoracic Surgery, ed. Marco Scarci, Aman Coonar, Tom Routledge and Francis Wells. Published by Cambridge University Press. © Cambridge University Press 2016

Table 12.1 The TNM staging system (7th edition)

Stage	Diameter	Airway	Atelectasis	Invasion	Pulmonary nodules
		Tumour extent			
T1	<2 cm	No invasion of lobar bronchus			
T2a T2b	2–3 cm 3–5 cm	Main bronchus but >2 cm to carina	Lobar	Visceral pleura	
T3a T3b	5–7 cm >7 cm	<2 cm to carina	Atelectasis to whole lung	Chest wall, diaphragm, phrenic nerve, mediastinal pleura, parietal pericardium	Nodules in same lobe
T4		Tumour in carina		Heart, great vessels, trachea, oesophagus, spine	Nodules in ipsilateral lung

Nodal involvement

N1	Ipsilateral peribronchial and/or ipsilateral hilar lymph nodes and intrapulmonary nodes
N2	Ipsilateral mediastinal and/or subcarinal nodes
N3	Contralateral mediastinal, contralateral hilar, ipsilateral or contralateral scalene or supraclavicular nodes

Metastasis

M0	No metastasis
M1a	Nodules in contralateral lung, malignant pleural or pericardial effusion
M1b	Metastases outside chest

Table 12.2 Stages I–IV

Stage	Tumour	Lymph nodes	Metastases
IA	T1a or T1b	N0	M0
IB	T2a	N0	M0
IIA	T1a or T1b or T2a	N1	M0
	T2b	N0	M0
IIB	T2b	N1	M0
	T3	N0	M0
IIIA	Any T between T1a and T2b	N2	M0
	T3	N1 or N2	M0
	T4	N0 or N1	M0
IIIB	T4	N2	M0
	Any T between T1a and T4	N3	M0
IV	Any T	Any N	M1a or M1b

usually considered incurable by surgery. However, surgery is sometimes performed as part of multi-modality treatment even in selected cases of stage IV disease[8].

The multidisciplinary team

Initial referral is usually to a chest physician, oncologist or surgeon via a fast-track clinic. After history and plain chest radiography (if not already done), contrastenhanced staging CT of chest and upper abdomen is performed and generally reviewed by the multidisciplinary team. Some units now also include the pelvis in this initial CT scan. The format and purpose of these meetings are to ensure that patients receive the most appropriate management[9]. Tests are done to determine fitness, diagnosis and stage. Practices differ between units particularly in the value put on pre-operative tissue diagnosis. Some units will rely more on a clinical-radiological diagnosis and perform intraoperative pathological confirmation, and others will prefer pre-operative tissue diagnosis assuming that it is representative of the whole specimen. If the tumour is considered suitable for surgery (all stage I, II, some

IIIa and selected higher-stage patients depending on fitness and patient preference) virtually all patients will also undergo CT-PET scan and, if still appropriate, head imaging by CT and increasingly MRI. Because of an increased availability of CT-PET and based on its efficacy, more patients are having CT-PET earlier in their pathway. This aids in targeting investigations and identifying higher-stage disease earlier.

Generally 'benefit of the doubt' is assumed, that is to say, the lowest stage is assumed for the patient, thereby allowing the most aggressive treatment. Sites suspicious for higher-stage disease are investigated with biopsies as needed.

Investigations

Diagnostic investigations are usually performed in an incremental fashion unless a single test can definitively stage the cancer (e.g. biopsy of a skin lesion, if proven to be metastatic from lung cancer would be M1b and therefore stage IV, regardless of tumour size, local involvement or regional node involvement).

Noninvasive staging

Computed tomography (CT)

CT is routinely performed for all patients. This is normally performed with intravenous contrast and includes the entire thorax and upper abdomen to incorporate the liver and adrenals. Some units also include the pelvis. CT can determine tumour size, extent and invasion; significant lymphadenopathy (>10 mm in short axis) and identify metastatic deposits. If used alone, CT has a 77% sensitivity and 55% specificity[10].

CT may not be able to discriminate between tumours close to the chest wall or mediastinum as this modality is not good at discriminating between apposition of soft tissues and invasion. Similarly, indeterminate lesions in the liver may require other evaluation such as ultrasound or MRI.

Magnetic resonance imaging (MRI)

MRI is useful in assessing for brain and hepatic metastases and has higher sensitivity than CT for the brain[11]. It also has excellent discrimination for identification of soft tissue planes and may provide an adjunct to thoracic CT where the extent of tumour invasion cannot be clearly defined[12].

Positron emission tomography (PET)

PET scanning uses intravenous glucose marked with radioactive fluorine (18-fluoro-deoxy-glucose, or ^{18}FDG). The patient is fasted and rested completely for 30 minutes in a darkened room prior to scanning to ensure that the labelled glucose is taken up by actively metabolizing cells. Rapidly dividing cells with a high mitotic index, such as those within tumours, will show as 'hotspots' of radioactivity on the PET scan. These represent positrons emitted during the radioactive decay of ^{18}FDG. Other metabolically active cells utilizing glucose also show increased activity, such as the myocardium, brain or brown fat. Renal excretion of the radioisotope may also be seen in the form of activity from the renal calyces to the bladder.

Areas of interest are compared to background radiation level measured in the caval blood pool, generating a standardized uptake value (SUV). While this can aid diagnosis, the potential for false positives and negatives must be taken into account: masses with high SUV may represent malignant tumours, inflammation or infection; those with low SUV may be tumours with low glucose uptake such as low-grade adenocarcinomas, carcinoids or other low-glucose-uptake tumours.

An SUV value > 2 is generally considered to be significant and concerning for cancer unless there is some other explanation. Deposits < 1 cm may not generate a high enough SUV to fall into this category, and this can be a cause of false negatives.

The utility of whole-body ^{18}FDG PET in the staging of lung cancer was appreciated towards the end of the data-collection period for the current TNM classification[13], which represents some limitation to that data set.

The value of PET is greater if it is performed with a CT and the images synchronized (CT-PET). This means that there is a correlation between the functional and anatomical findings. CT-PET scan is now considered a routine test in the evaluation of lung cancer, with combined PET-CT acknowledged to be significantly superior to PET and CT performed separately. CT-PET has a sensitivity of 90% and specificity of 90%[14]. The test can help to guide invasive staging and reduce the number of negative thoracotomies performed[15].

Radionuclide bone scans

Due to the age and comorbidities of the patient population presenting with lung cancer, false-positive bone scans are common, and their use should be judicious rather than universal. Bone scans tend to be performed when PET is not available.

Invasive staging

Invasive staging may be required to confirm the diagnosis of a primary tumour or for staging to identify nodal involvement or metastasis. Needle biopsies either as a fine-needle aspirate (FNA) or as a core biopsy are commonly performed. Core biopsy yields more tissue, preserves histological architecture, and is more informative than FNA.

Trans-thoracic needle biopsy

This is typically performed under CT or, if more superficial, ultrasound guidance and a biopsy taken for histological confirmation[16].

Endo-bronchial/endo-oesophageal ultrasound (EBUS/EUS)

Where CT scanning of the mediastinum identifies suspicious lymphadenopathy, invasive sampling techniques such as EBUS (for stations 2, 3, 4, 7, 10 and some 11) and EUS (for stations 7, 8, 9, left adrenal, some other abdominal sites and sometimes, with a mobile oesophagus, left sub-aortic nodes) have been demonstrated to have excellent predictive value and low morbidity compared to surgical staging of the mediastinum. These techniques use ultrasound to guide a fine needle aspiration. Sensitivity of endoscopic ultrasound-guided techniques following radiological imaging is 94%, with a 93% negative predictive value[17].

Ultrasound-guided biopsy is safer if the patient has had previous surgery, radiotherapy or inflammation to these sites.

Cervical mediastinoscopy/left anterior mediastinotomy

Surgical approaches to the mediastinum allow access to lymph node stations that have not yielded meaningful results to EBUS (2, 3, 4, 7 via mediastinoscopy) or were inaccessible (5, 6 via mediastinotomy or left VATs).

Cervical mediastinoscopy approaches the mediastinum from the neck, using an approximately 3-cm skin-crease incision, a finger's breadth above the sternal notch[18]. After dissection to the pre-tracheal plane and blunt dissection of the peri-tracheal tissues, a rigid scope is advanced to allow biopsies of lymph nodes. Particular risks include injury to the left recurrent nerve (rare) and, uncommonly, pneumothorax or significant bleeding. Thoracotomy for control of bleeding is a rare complication.

Left anterior mediastinotomy approaches the lymph nodes in the sub-aortic or aorto-pulmonary window from an approximately 5-cm incision in the left second intercostal space. Rib excision or retraction is sometimes necessary to provide adequate exposure[19]. Sometimes a biopsy is performed on the right side.

Complications after medisatinoscopy/mediastinotomy are more common following induction treatment, previous surgery or diseases such as mediastinal tuberculosis.

Scalene/supraclavicular node biopsy

Performed under ultrasound guidance, FNA or open biopsy of superficial lymph nodes can be performed.

Thoracoscopy/thoracotomy

Where other staging modalities have failed to confirm the presence of nodal involvement, video-assisted thoracoscopic surgery (VATS) or open thoracotomy can be used to sample lymph node stations or other sites. Depending on the degree of clinical suspicion and patient suitability for lung resection, this may be combined with a definitive procedure. Frozen section histological assessment is useful in determining the appropriateness of continued resection.

Stage migration

Stage migration describes the reclassification of patients from one stage to another during their care. The terms 'upstaging' and 'downstaging' may be used to describe whether the patient's stage is higher or lower than previously assessed. This may be as a result of new findings (e.g. the discovery of PET positive lymph nodes that had not appeared suspicious on CT) or the effects of treatment such as induction therapy. Planned downstaging with chemo- or radio-therapy in preparation for surgery may improve survival[20,21].

Despite the current advances in technology, the final pre-operative clinical stage (cTNM) may be revised by final pathological examination (pTNM) in up to a quarter of cases. In nearly 10%, upstaging uncovers occult N2 disease that was not identified with optimal diagnostic workup[6]. The effects of this low-volume, PET-negative micro-metastatic disease on outcome is not known, although the prognosis is likely to be better[22,23].

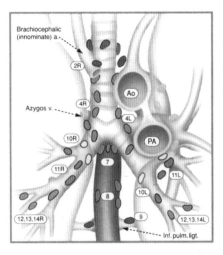

Superior mediastinal nodes

● **1** Highest mediastinal

● **2** Upper paratracheal

● **3** Pre-vascular and retrotracheal

○ **4** Lower paratracheal
(including azygos nodes)

N_2 = single digit, ipsilateral
N_3 = single digit, contralateral or supraclavicular

Aortic nodes

● **5** Subaortic (A-P window)

● **6** Para-aortic (ascending
aorta or phrenic)

Inferior mediastinal nodes

● **7** Subcarinal

● **8** Paraesophageal
(below carina)

● **9** Pulmonary ligament

N₁ Nodes

○ **10** Hilar

● **11** Interlobar

● **12** Lobar

● **13** Segmental

● **14** Subsegmental

Figure 12.1 Mountain and Dresler lymph node map[4] (used with permission).

After induction treatment patients are re-staged, and this may involve re-imaging and re-biopsy. The terminology yTNM is then sometimes used.

Key points

- Lung cancer staging is important for determining treatment and describing prognosis

- pTNM is a better guide to prognosis than cTNM.
- Lung cancer staging is usually multimodal and always multidisciplinary.
- EBUS and EUS are less-invasive effective options than mediastinoscopy and mediastinotomy.
- Stage migration is possible at any stage from diagnosis until completion of surgery.

References

1 Rostad H, Vale JR, Nesthus I. Lung cancer: symptoms, signs and diagnostic criteria. *Scand J Respir Dis* 1979; 60:184–90.

2 Simon AE, Juszczyk D, Smyth N, et al. Knowledge of lung cancer symptoms and risk factors in the UK: development of a measure and results from a population-based survey. *Thorax* 2012; 67:426–32. doi:10.1136/thoraxjnl-2011-200898.

3 International Early Lung Cancer Action Program Investigators, Henschke CI, Yankelevitz DF, et al. Survival of patients with stage I lung cancer detected on CT screening. *N Engl J Med* 2006;

355:1763–71. doi:10.1056/NEJMoa060476.

4 Mountain CF, Dresler CM. Regional lymph node classification for lung cancer staging. *Chest J* 1997; 111:1718–23. doi:10.1378/chest.111.6.1718.

5 Goldstraw P, Crowley J, Chansky K, et al. The IASLC Lung Cancer

Staging Project: proposals for the revision of the TNM stage groupings in the forthcoming (seventh) edition of the TNM classification of malignant tumours. *J Thorac Oncol Off Publ Int Assoc Study Lung Cancer* 2007; 2:706–14. doi:10.1097/JTO.0b013e31812f3c1a.

6   Kirmani BH, Rintoul RC, Win T, et al. Stage migration: results of lymph node dissection in the era of modern imaging and invasive staging for lung cancer. *Eur J Cardio-Thorac Surg Off J Eur Assoc Cardio-Thorac Surg* 2013; 43:104–9; discussion 109–110. doi:10.1093/ejcts/ezs184.

7   Robinson LA, Ruckdeschel JC, Wagner H, et al. Treatment of Non-small Cell Lung Cancer-Stage IIIA. *Chest* 2007; 132:243S–65S. doi:10.1378/chest.07–1379.

8   Sastry P, Tocock A, Coonar AS. Adrenalectomy for isolated metastasis from operable non-small-cell lung cancer. *Interact Cardiovasc Thorac Surg* 2014; 18:495–7. doi:10.1093/icvts/ivt526.

9   Coory M, Gkolia P, Yang IA, et al. Systematic review of multidisciplinary teams in the management of lung cancer. *Lung Cancer* 2008; 60:14–21. doi:10.1016/j.lungcan.2008.01.008.

10 Yasufuku K, Nakajima T, Motoori K, et al. Comparison of endobronchial ultrasound, positron emission tomography, and CT for lymph node staging of lung cancer. *Chest* 2006; 130:710–18. doi:10.1378/chest.130.3.710.

11 Yi CA, Shin KM, Lee KS, et al. Non-small cell lung cancer staging: efficacy comparison of integrated PET/CT versus 3.0-T whole-body MR imaging. *Radiology* 2008; 248:632–42. doi:10.1148/radiol.2482071822.

12 Quint LE. Staging non-small cell lung cancer. *Cancer Imaging* 2007; 7:148–59. doi:10.1102/1470–7330.2007.0026.

13 Marom EM, McAdams HP, Erasmus JJ, et al. Staging non-small cell lung cancer with whole-body PET. *Radiology* 1999; 212:803–9. doi:10.1148/radiology.212.3.r99se21803.

14 He Y-Q, Gong H-L, Deng Y-F, et al. Diagnostic efficacy of PET and PET/CT for recurrent lung cancer: a meta-analysis. *Acta Radiol Stockh Swed 1987* Published online first: 30 September 2013. doi:10.1177/0284185113498536.

15 Fischer B, Lassen U, Mortensen J, et al. Preoperative staging of lung cancer with combined PET–CT. *N Engl J Med* 2009; 361:32–9. doi:10.1056/NEJMoa0900043.

16 Coonar AS, Hughes JA, Walker S, et al. Implementation of real-time ultrasound in a thoracic surgery practice. *Ann Thorac Surg* 2009; 87:1577–81. doi:10.1016/j.athoracsur.2008.12.024.

17 Sharples LD, Jackson C, Wheaton E, et al. Clinical effectiveness and cost-effectiveness of endobronchial and endoscopic ultrasound relative to surgical staging in potentially resectable lung cancer: results from the ASTER randomised controlled trial. *Health Technol Assess Winch Engl* 2012; 16:1–75, iii–iv. doi:10.3310/hta16180.

18 Leyn PD, Lerut T. Conventional mediastinoscopy. *Multimed Man Cardio-Thorac Surg* 2005; doi:10.1510/mmcts.2004.000158.

19 Hunt I, Alwahab Y, Treasure T. Using video-assisted thorascoscopy (VATS) to aid the anterior mediastinotomy approach to mediastinal masses. *Ann R Coll Surg Engl* 2007; 89:435–6. doi:10.1308/003588407X183517d.

20 Meerbeeck JP van, Kramer GWPM, Schil PEYV, et al. Randomized controlled trial of resection versus radiotherapy after induction chemotherapy in Stage IIIA-N2 non–small-cell lung cancer. *J Natl Cancer Inst* 2007; 99:442–50. doi:10.1093/jnci/djk093.

21 DeCamp MM, Ashiku S, Thurer R. The role of surgery in N2 non-small cell lung cancer. *Clin Cancer Res* 2005; 11:5033s–7s. doi:10.1158/1078-0432.CCR-05–9013.

22 Goldstraw P, Mannam GC, Kaplan DK, et al. Surgical management of non-small-cell lung cancer with ipsilateral mediastinal node metastasis (N2 disease). *J Thorac Cardiovasc Surg* 1994; 107:19–28. doi:.

23 Andre F, Grunenwald D, Pignon JP, et al. Survival of patients with resected N2 non-small-cell lung cancer: evidence for a subclassification and implications. *J Clin Oncol Off J Am Soc Clin Oncol* 2000; 18:2981–9.

Chapter 13

Pathological considerations in lung malignancy

Doris M. Rassl

Introduction

The great majority of primary malignant lung tumours are carcinomas derived predominantly from the epithelium of bronchi, bronchioles and alveoli. These neoplasms are divided, mainly on the basis of histopathological features, into four cell types: small cell carcinoma, squamous cell carcinoma, adenocarcinoma and large cell carcinoma; the latter three cell types grouped together represent non-small cell carcinomas[1]. In recent years, it has become increasingly important to subclassify non-small cell carcinomas even in small biopsy specimens in view of therapeutic advances and the development of targeted therapies, such as tyrosine kinase inhibitors for tumours with EGFR mutations or EML4-ALK translocations, mainly seen in adenocarcinomas. Some chemotherapeutic agents, such as pemetrexed, for example, are also more efficacious in adenocarcinomas.

Small cell carcinoma is an aggressive neuroendocrine tumour, often presenting at an advanced stage. Neuroendocrine tumours of the lung are a distinct subset of tumours which share morphological, ultrastructural and immunohistochemical characteristics[2]. In addition to small cell carcinoma, the other morphologically identifiable neuroendocrine tumours of the lung are large cell neuroendocrine carcinomas and typical and atypical carcinoid tumours.

It should be noted that lung carcinomas may be mixed and composed of more than one cell type. Sarcomatoid carcinomas comprise approximately 0.3% of lung malignancies, and this group of poorly differentiated lung carcinomas expresses a spectrum of pleomorphic, sarcomatoid and sarcomatous elements[3].

Rarely, malignant salivary gland type tumours, mainly adenoid cystic carcinomas or mucoepidermoid tumours, arise from the mixed seromucous glands of the trachea and bronchi, as these are similar to the minor salivary glands and can therefore give rise to the same range of tumours.

Primary malignant neurogenic, vascular and mesenchymal tumours can also occur within the lungs and the morphological features of these types of tumours reflect those seen in extrapulmonary lesions.

Whilst the lungs are often involved in disseminated nodal lymphomas of all types, primary pulmonary lymphoma is relatively rare, accounting for less than 0.5% all of primary lung neoplasms[4].

It should also be remembered that the lungs are a very common site for metastatic disease, most commonly due to haematogenous or lymphatic spread of extrapulmonary tumours. Dissemination within pulmonary lymphatics may be widespread, producing the appearances of so-called lymphangitis carcinomatosa.

Lung cancer

Incidence and risk factors

Worldwide, lung cancer is the leading cause of cancer-related mortality, accounting for 26–29% of all cancer deaths[5]. In developed countries, geographical patterns of lung cancer incidence are a reflection of past exposure to tobacco smoking[2], the predominant aetiologic risk factor. Cigarette smoke contains over 60 chemicals that have been identified as carcinogens, the most potent of which include polycyclic aromatic hydrocarbons such as benzo(a)pyrene and nicotine-derived nitrosaminoketone (NNK).[6] For those who smoke, relative risk estimates are as high as 20–30%, depending on different aspects of tobacco smoking:

Core Topics in Thoracic Surgery, ed. Marco Scarci, Aman Coonar, Tom Routledge and Francis Wells. Published by Cambridge University Press. © Cambridge University Press 2016

average consumption, age at start, duration of smoking, time since quitting, type of tobacco product and inhalation pattern[2]. Further risk factors, in addition to smoking, include environmental and occupational factors, especially exposures to asbestos and radon and, more rarely, polycyclic aromatic hydrocarbons, chromates, crystalline silica, nickel, arsenic and chloromethyl methylether. Viruses, such as the Epstein-Barr virus (EBV) and human papilloma virus (HPV), may also play a part in the genesis of lung cancer[4,7]. Idiopathic pulmonary fibrosis is associated with a 14-fold increased incidence of lung cancer[4]. Genetic differences also influence the risk of developing lung cancer in several ways, including the enzymatic activation or elimination of carcinogens and the expression of tumour suppressor or oncogenes[4].

Clinical effects

Most lung cancers are diagnosed in view of patients presenting with symptoms, which include progressive shortness of breath, cough, chest pain, haemoptysis, hoarseness or loss of voice, paraneoplastic manifestations or evidence of intra- or extrathoracic spread via blood-borne metastases to the liver, adrenal glands, brain, kidneys and bones. Less than 15% of tumours are discovered by chance, usually during the course of radiological investigations for other reasons[4].

Paraneoplastic syndromes develop in 10–20% of lung cancer cases and are non-metastatic disorders of distant organs. Neuromuscular paraneoplastic syndromes include encephalopathies, peripheral neuropathies, myelopathies and myopathies such as dermatomyositis and polymyositis. Autoantibodies directed against a muscle cell or neuronal antigen are the cause of many carcinomatous neuromyopathies[4], including the myasthenia gravis-like Eaton-Lambert syndrome, particularly associated with small cell lung cancer.

Other paraneoplastic syndromes are due to inappropriate or ectopic hormone secretion, including the secretion of antidiuretic or adrenocorticotrophic hormone, again more commonly seen in patients with small cell carcinoma.

Tumour-related hypercalcaemia is usually due to bone metastases but may occur without metastatic disease when it is mediated by parathyroid-related hormone, most commonly seen in association with squamous cell carcinoma[4].

Prognosis

Non-small cell lung cancer (NSCLC) accounts for 80% of all lung cancer diagnoses, and as the majority of these tumours (60–80%) are diagnosed at an advanced stage, most are unresectable. In view of this, the prognosis for NSCLC remains poor, with a 5-year survival rate of ~15%[5].

Lung carcinoma is multiple (synchronous or metachronous) in about 2–5% of cases and is associated with independent cancers of the head and neck region in about 20% of cases[8].

Small cell carcinomas often present with disseminated disease; only a small percentage of limited stage tumours may be successfully resected.

Preinvasive lesions

As with other epithelial cancers, lung cancer develops over a long latent period via a series of progressive morphological changes accompanied by molecular alterations that commence in histologically normal epithelium[9]. The pathology of these pre-invasive lesions has attracted increasing interest because of the importance of early detection of lung cancer and trials of screening high-risk patients using fluorescence bronchoscopy and spiral or helical computed tomography (CT)[3]. The new 2011 IASLC/ATS/ERS classification includes adenocarcinoma in situ, in addition to atypical adenomatous hyperplasia, squamous dysplasia and carcinoma in situ (CIS), and diffuse idiopathic neuroendocrine cell hyperplasia (DIPNECH).

Squamous dysplasia and carcinoma in situ (CIS)

Bronchial carcinogenesis is believed to be a multistep process involving the transformation of the normal bronchial epithelium through a spectrum of lesions, including basal cell hyperplasia, squamous metaplasia, dysplasia and carcinoma in situ (CIS). Squamous dysplasia is graded as mild, moderate or severe depending on the degree of cytological atypia and the thickness of the abnormality within the bronchial epithelium. Full-thickness cytological atypia is seen in CIS. These morphological changes are accompanied by a series of molecular changes that accumulate as the lesions progress[3].

However, the natural history of bronchial preneoplastic lesions is based on scant data. The progression of lesions is variable, and ~50% of dysplastic lesions may regress spontaneously[9].

White light bronchoscopy is relatively insensitive for the detection of these premalignant lesions, and fluorescence bronchoscopy is much more efficient in identifying these changes.

Atypical adenomatous hyperplasia (AAH)

AAH is a bronchioloalveolar proliferation of mild to moderately atypical type II pneumocytes with associated slight fibrous thickening of alveolar septa, often encountered as an incidental finding in lung cancer resection specimens. Radiologically, these lesions represent small ground-glass opacities, which are frequently multiple. Most lesions measure less than 5 mm in diameter.

Molecular studies support the concept of AAH being a pre-malignant lesion, preceding the development of non-mucinous lepidic adenocarcinomas.

The incidence of AAH ranges from 5.7 to 21.4% depending on sampling and the criteria used for diagnosis[3].

Adenocarcinoma in situ (AIS)

In the recent IASLC/ATS/ERS adenocarcinoma classification, AIS is defined as a localized, small (≤3 cm) adenocarcinoma with growth of neoplastic cells along pre-existing alveolar structures (lepidic growth), lacking stromal, vascular or pleural invasion. AIS is subdivided into mucinous and non-mucinous variants, but the majority of cases are non-mucinous, consisting of type II pneumocytes and/or Clara cells[10].

By CT these lesions consist of a ground-glass nodule if non-mucinous and a more solid nodule if mucinous, due to the filling of alveolar spaces by mucin. If these lesions are completely resected, patients have been reported to have 100% 5-year disease-free survival; however, it is important to exclude cases with miliary spread and/or lobar consolidation, particularly for mucinous AIS.

Diffuse idiopathic neuroendocrine cell hyperplasia (DIPNECH)

This is a rare condition in which there is diffuse neuroendocrine cell hyperplasia involving the peripheral airways, which may manifest by airway obstruction due to associated bronchiolar fibrosis in approximately half of patients[3]. Other patients present with pulmonary nodules. DIPNECH is believed to represent a pre-invasive lesion for carcinoid tumours, as these tumours, often multiple, are frequently found in patients with this condition.

DIPNECH is not believed to be a precursor lesion for small cell carcinoma. No precursor lesions have been identified with certainty for the development of pulmonary small cell carcinoma.

Field effect

Exposure to carcinogens, especially tobacco smoke, results in extensive damage to the entire respiratory epithelium, and a variety of molecular lesions, often numerous, have been identified, the molecular changes preceding the onset of histologically abnormal foci. In the lungs of never smokers, the field of epithelial damage is usually more limited, being present mainly in the region surrounding a tumour. This field effect may result in the development of multiple synchronous or metachronous tumours[9].

Squamous cell carcinoma

Approximately 20–30% of all lung cancers are squamous cell carcinomas, characterized by the presence of keratinization and intercellular bridges depending on the degree of differentiation. Grading of tumours from well to moderate to poorly differentiated is of prognostic value but best limited to resection specimens as there can be substantial variation within a tumour. Historically, most squamous cell carcinomas presented as central lung tumours; however, more recently an increasing number of squamous cell carcinomas are found in the periphery.

Current squamous cell carcinoma subtypes include papillary, clear cell, small cell and basaloid variants. The papillary variant is well differentiated, and most of these lesion are endobronchial, with no or limited stromal invasion and a 5-year survival of >60%. The small cell and basaloid variants have a poor prognosis, similar to that of poorly differentiated squamous cell carcinoma.

Squamous cell carcinoma arises most often in segmental bronchi[3]. Of all bronchogenic carcinomas, squamous cell carcinoma is the one most often confined to the lung and regional lymph nodes at the time of diagnosis and therefore the most amenable to successful surgical treatment[11]. The tumours may spread along airways or form a discrete mass, sometimes with associated distal obstructive changes due to occlusion of the involved airway. Peripheral tumours often invade the pleura and chest wall.

Large squamous cell carcinomas tend to show necrosis and central cavitation.

In situ changes may be seen in the vicinity of the tumour, ranging from squamous metaplasia to dysplasia to carcinoma in situ.

Adenocarcinoma

Adenocarcinoma is the most common type of lung cancer, and there has been an increase in its incidence relative to squamous cell carcinoma. One factor may be the increasing use of filter-tipped cigarettes, which allow smaller particulate carcinogens to penetrate more deeply into the lungs. However, there is also a higher proportion of adenocarcinomas in younger patients and non-smokers[4]. Most adenocarcinomas are peripheral and arise from the terminal respiratory unit, which comprises the terminal bronchiole, the respiratory bronchioles and the alveoli and alveolar ducts. A division into central and peripheral adenocarcinomas has been suggested in view of histological heterogeneity and prognosis, and molecular studies demonstrating different mutations, such as more frequent EGFR mutations in peripheral adenocarcinomas, support the separation of adenocarcinomas into bronchial and peripheral subtypes[4,12]. Occasional peripheral adenocarcinomas may diffusely involve the pleura, mimicking mesothelioma.

Adenocarcinomas exhibit various growth patterns, including lepidic, acinar, papillary, micropapillary and solid. Tumours with a mixed subtype make up about 90% of cases, often combining an acinar and solid architecture centrally and papillary and lepidic patterns peripherally. Lung adenocarcinomas are known to be heterogeneous from various aspects: pathological, molecular, clinical, radiological and surgical, and pathological and radiological studies have demonstrated prognostic subsets of lung adenocarcinoma. In view of this, the recent 2011 IASLC/ATS/ETS lung adenocarcinoma classification has introduced several changes to the previous 2004 WHO classification[10,13]:

(1) The term 'bronchioloalveolar carcinoma' (BAC) is no longer used, and the growth pattern of BAC is referred to as lepidic pattern.
(2) The term 'adenocarcinoma in situ' (AIS) is recommended for small (≤3 cm), solitary adenocarcinomas with a pure lepidic growth pattern lacking invasion. Most AIS are non-mucinous; rarely are they mucinous.
(3) Minimally invasive adenocarcinoma (MIA) is proposed for small (≤3 cm), solitary adenocarcinomas with predominant lepidic growth and small foci of invasion measuring 0.5 cm or less. Most MIAs are non-mucinous.
(4) Invasive adenocarcinomas are classified according to the predominant subtype after comprehensive histological subtyping with semiquantative assessment of each subtype in 5% increments.

Comprehensive histological subtyping of multiple lung adenocarciomas may help to determine if tumours are metastases or separate synchronous or metachronous primaries.
(5) For non-mucinous adenocarcinomas (>3 cm) with a predominant lepidic growth pattern, the term 'lepidic predominant adenocarcinoma' is recommended.
(6) Former mucinous BACs (>3 cm) are now classified as invasive mucinous adenocarcinoma, recognizing that most of these tumours will have invasive components and a worse prognosis than non-mucinous lepidic predominant adenocarcinomas.
(7) Micropapillary adenocarcinoma is added as a major subtype due to its association with poor prognosis.
(8) Clear cell and signet ring features are considered to represent cytological changes which can be seen in various histological subtypes rather than denoting separate histological subtypes.

Studies have shown 100% 5-year disease-free survival for tumours that would be classified as AIS, and data suggest that MIAs also have 100% or near 100% disease-free survival when resected[3]. The prognostic significance of subtyping adenocarcinomas has also been demonstrated in studies of resected stage I tumours[13,14], and according to disease-free survival, three prognostic groups with low-, intermediate- and high-grade clinical behaviour were identified. The low-grade group included AIS and MIA (100% disease-free survival at 5 years), the intermediate-grade group consisted of non-mucinous lepidic predominant, acinar predominant and papillary predominant adenocarcinomas (83–90% disease-free survival at 5 years) and the high-grade tumours comprised solid predominant, micropapillary predominant and invasive mucinous and mixed mucinous tumours (67–76% disease-free survival at 5 years)[13]. Disease-free survival for patients with T1a tumours was significantly better than that for T1b tumours, and the difference was more pronounced when size of the invasive component was taken into consideration.

Lung cancer classifications have primarily addressed classification of resected tumours rather than small biopsies or cytology. However, as approximately 70% of lung cancer patients present at an advanced stage, the diagnosis in the majority of cases is based on small biopsy samples or cytology specimens[15]. Therapeutic advances – including tyrosine kinase inhibitors for tumours with EGFR mutations found mainly in adenocarcinomas, the recognition that pemetrexed is more efficacious in adenocarcinomas and NSCLC, and that there is an increased risk of haemorrhage with bevacizumab in patients with advanced squamous cell carcinoma – have highlighted the importance of subtyping non-small cell carcinomas even in small samples. To do this, light microscopy is supplemented with tinctorial stains and immunohistochemistry, and the 2011 IASLC/ATS/ERS classification includes proposed standardized criteria that apply to the pathological diagnosis in small biopsies and cytology samples.

Adenosquamous carcinoma

Adenosquamous carcinomas show both squamous and adenocarcinomatous differentiation on light microscopy, the minor component representing at least 10% of the tumour. This diagnosis can be suspected but not made on small samples and requires a resection specimen.

Large cell carcinoma

Large cell carcinomas comprise about 3% of all lung carcinomas[3], are aggressive tumours and lack differentiation on light microscopy. The diagnosis of large cell carcinoma can only be made if a resection specimen is available, as the presence of areas of squamous or adenocarcinoma differentiation cannot be excluded on biopsy or cytology specimens.

Large cell carcinomas present as large tumours, frequently with geographical areas of necrosis. The

Table 13.1 Immunophenotypic characterization of lung carcinoma

Cell type	Usual immunophenotype
Squamous cell carcinoma	CK5/6, p63, p40 +ve TTF-1, CD56 -ve, CK7+/-
Adenocarcinoma & large cell carcinoma	TTF-1 (~70%), CK7+ CK5/6, p40, CD56 -ve
Small cell carcinoma & large cell neuroendocrine carcinoma	CD56, synaptophysin, CK7 +ve TTF-1 + (70-80%)

(CK = cytokeratin, TTF-1 = thyroid transcription factor-1)
NB. Mucinous tumours show variable staining for TTF-1.

tumour cells are relatively large, possess a moderate amount of cytoplasm, vesicular nuclei with clumped nuclear chromatin and a prominent nucleolus.

Electron microscopy often reveals features of squamous or glandular differentiation, and large cell carcinoma therefore does not represent a distinct entity but a collection of poorly differentiated epithelial tumours. Some of these tumours can be classified on the basis of their immunohistochemical profile (see Table 13.1), and this is becoming increasingly important in the era of targeted drug therapy, as there is some correlation between histological type and oncogene mutation.

Five variants of large cell carcinoma are recognized in the 2004 WHO classification: basaloid, clear cell, lymphoepithelioma-like, rhabdoid and neuroendocrine.

Sarcomatoid carcinoma

Some poorly differentiated non-small cell carcinomas show areas of sarcoma or sarcoma-like (spindle and/or giant cell) differentiation. These tumours, which have undergone divergent connective tissue differentiation, are rare and account for about 1% of all lung malignancies. Histologically, five subgroups, representing a morphological continuum, are recognized, and these are pleomorphic carcinoma, spindle cell carcinoma, giant cell carcinoma, carcinosarcoma and pulmonary blastoma (see Table 13.2)[2], although 'sarcomatoid carcinoma' is the appropriate term, as there is evidence that tumours that appear to be of mixed epithelial and connective tissue phenotype, or

131

Table 13.2 Histological classification of lung cancer (modified from the 2004 WHO and 2011 IASLC/ATS/ERS classifications, based primarily on resection specimens)

Preinvasive lesions
Squamous dysplasia/carcinoma in situ (CIS)
Atypical adenomatous hyperplasia (AAH)
Adenocarcinoma in situ (AIS) (≤3 cm, formerly BAC)
    Non-mucinous
    Mucinous
    Mixed non-mucinous/mucinous
    Diffuse idiopathic pulmonary neuroendocrine
    cell hyperplasia (DIPNECH)

Squamous cell carcinoma
Variants
    Papillary
    Clear cell
    Small cell (may be discontinued)
    Basaloid

Small cell carcinoma
Combined small cell carcinoma

Adenocarcinoma
Minimally invasive adenocarcinoma (MIA)
(≤3 cm, lepidic predominant tumour with
≤5 mm invasion)
    Non-mucinous
    Mucinous
    Mixed non-mucinous/mucinous
Invasive adenocarcinoma
    Lepidic predominant (formerly non-mucinous BAC
    with >5 mm invasion)
    Acinar predominant
    Papillary predominant
    Micropapillary predominant
    Solid predominant with mucin production
    Variants of invasive adenocarcinoma
    Invasive mucinous adenocarcinoma (formerly
    mucinous BAC, >3 cm)
    Colloid
    Fetal
    Enteric

Large cell carcinoma
Large cell neuroendocrine carcinoma (LCNEC)
    Combined LCNEC
Large cell carcinoma with rhabdoid phenotype
Basaloid carcinoma
Lymphoepithelioma-like carcinoma

Adenosquamous carcinoma
Sarcomatoid carcinomas
Pleomorphic carcinoma
Spindle cell carcinoma

Giant cell carcinoma
Carcinosarcoma
Pulmonary blastoma
Other

Carcinoid tumour
Typical carcinoid
Atypical carcinoid

Carcinomas of salivary gland type
Mucoepidermoid carcinoma
Adenoid cystic carcinoma
Epimyoepithelial carcinoma

even purely sarcomatous, are epithelial and originate from the same clone[2,4].

The average age at diagnosis is 60 years, the male-to-female ratio is approximately 4 to 1 and tobacco smoking is a major aetiological factor, as for other histological types of lung cancer.

Pleomorphic carcinomas tend to be large, peripheral tumours with a tendency to invade the chest wall and a poor prognosis. Because of the histological heterogeneity of these tumours, adequate sampling of resection specimens is important, and pleomorphic carcinomas should have at least 10% of a spindle or giant cell component. In view of this, the diagnosis cannot be made based on small biopsies or cytology specimens. If the tumour has a purely spindle or giant cell morphology, the term 'spindle cell' or 'giant cell carcinoma' is used[3].

Carcinosarcomas are composed of a mixture of non-small cell carcinoma (squamous cell, adeno- or large cell carcinoma) and differentiated sarcomatous elements, such as malignant bone, cartilage or skeletal muscle. The metastases of a carcinosarcoma may consist of carcinoma or sarcoma or both.

Pulmonary blastoma is also a biphasic tumour with a glandular component that resembles well-differentiated fetal adenocarcinoma, composed of branching epithelial tubules or cords and undifferentiated stroma. Both components are malignant, and either or both may be seen in metastatic deposits. These tumours are often peripheral growths and form large, well-defined masses with foci of haemorrhage and cystic change. Pulmonary blastoma is a rare tumour, which can occur at any age, the mean age of presentation being earlier than that of carcinosarcoma, at about 40 years. It affects males three times more commonly than females[4].

Clinical outcome is stage dependent, but these tumours have a worse prognosis than conventional non-small cell carcinomas, and the 5-year survival is only about 20%, despite half the patients presenting with stage I disease[2].

The role of molecular pathology in non-small cell lung cancer

In recent years, a better understanding of mutations and rearrangements which alter the function or expression of several molecules that can either be located on the cell surface, acting as growth factor receptors, or participate in downstream intracellular pathways, leading to uncontrolled cell growth, can be used to generate prognostic information or to select patients for targeted therapies[16].

To date, effective molecularly targeted therapies have disproportionately impacted on adenocarcinomas compared to squamous cell carcinomas and on never or light smokers compared to heavy smokers. However, next-generation sequencing technologies are allowing better characterization of cancer genomes across a broad range of tumour types, and targets in squamous tumours and smokers will need to be developed to maker a greater impact on non-small cell lung cancer.

Lung cancers have a high rate of protein altering mutations, accounting for the genomic complexity of lung cancers and the comparative difficulty in effectively treating these tumours[17]. To effectively match drug therapies, it is important to distinguish 'driver' mutations, which confer growth advantage and are causally linked to cancer development, from 'passenger' mutations, which are biologically neutral[17].

These are some of the genomic changes which are currently of interest with regard to the development of targeted therapies:

EGFR

The epidermal growth factor receptor (EGFR) plays an important role in tumour development and progression through activation mechanisms including overexpression, mutation and autocrine ligand production. Derangements in the EGFR gene are associated with tumour cell proliferation, cell growth, invasion, metastatic spread, apoptosis and angiogenesis through the activation of the Ras/Raf/Mek/MAPK and PI3K/Akt/mTOR pathways.

Tumours with EGFR mutations are more frequent in East Asians (30% versus 8% in non-Asians), in women, in never smokers (66% versus 22% in ever-smokers) and in adenocarcinomas than in other types of non-small cell carcinomas[16].

Gefitinib and erlotinib are first-generation EGFR tyrosine kinase inhibitors which selectively target the intracellular tyrosine kinase domain of EGFR, blocking downstream signalling. However, patients who respond to this treatment eventually develop resistance, mostly due to the emergence of a secondary T790M mutation or amplification of mesenchymal-epithelial transition factor (c-Met)[16].

Whilst EGFR activating mutations are found in adenocarcinomas, high EGFR copy number and protein overexpression are observed more frequently in squamous cell lung cancers (82 versus 44% in adenocarcinomas)[17]. EGFR overexpression has been associated with a worse prognosis in some studies, but it has not been associated with a response to the EGFR tyrosine kinase inhibitors used clinically. One phase III study suggested that EGFR overexpression may be associated with better outcomes in the first-line chemotherapy plus cetuximab arm[18].

KRAS

Kirsten rat sarcoma viral oncogene homolog (KRAS), a member of the ras gene family, is an important downstream signalling target of EGFR and has been implicated in the development and prognosis of several cancers, including adenocarcinomas of the pancreas, colon and lung. Mutations that lead to loss of KRAS GTPase activity render the protein GT bound, resulting in sustained activation of downstream components and persistent proliferation.

Mutations in KRAS have been found in 15–30% of patients with non-small cell carcinoma[16].

KRAS mutations are most commonly detected in lung adenocarcinomas, and tumours with KRAS mutations are more frequent in Caucasian patients (20–30 versus 5% in East Asian patients) and in current or former smokers[16].

Several studies have shown that KRAS mutations correlated with poor survival in patients with non-small cell lung cancer.

Both KRAS and EGFR mutations have been described in AAH lesions, and EGFR mutations have been found in the non-neoplastic peripheral airways in the vicinity of invasive peripheral adenocarcinomas, indicating that mutations of both genes are early events that play a role in tumour initiation[19].

ALK gene rearrangements

The EML4-ALK fusion gene results from an inversion within chromosome 2p. The prevalence of EML4-ALK varies in different studies but is approximately 4% and is most commonly found in adenocarcinomas with a solid or signet ring morphology.[20] Patients with this gene rearrangement tend to be younger and are usually non-smokers or light smokers. Studies have demonstrated the therapeutic value of critozinib in patients found to be ALK-positive by fluorescence in situ hybridization (FISH).

BRAF

BRAF encodes a non-receptor serine/threonine kinase which is a member of the RAS/MAPK signalling pathway downstream of Ras protein.[16] Mutations of BRAF occur in approximately 3% of non-small cell lung cancers and are found predominantly in adeno-carcinomas (97%), with just over half being V600E mutations (57%) and the remainder non-V600E. V600E mutations appear to be more prevalent in women, in never smokers and in more aggressive tumour subtypes characterized by micropapillary features and associated with a poorer prognosis. Non-V600E mutations were found in tobacco users[21].

FGFR1

FGFR1 is a member of the FGFR family of receptor tyrosine kinases, and activation leads to downstream signalling via the PI3K/AKT and RAS/MAPK pathways, which are important for growth, migration, survival and angiogenesis in many tumours[17]. FGFR1 mutations are rare, but FGFR1 amplification was found more frequently in squamous cell carcinomas (approximately 20%) than in adenocarcinomas, and mouse models with FGFR1 amplified tumours showed tumour growth inhibition and apoptosis on inhibition of FGFR1[22]. FGFR inhibitors are in development, many of which are multitargeted tyrosine kinase inhibitors.

PIK3CA

The PIK3CA-AKT pathway is central for survival and proliferation of many cancers, and PIK3CA copy number gains have been found in about 20% of lung cancers, with a higher frequency in squamous cell carcinomas[23]. In one study, PKI3CA mutations have also been detected more often in squamous cell carcinomas than adenocarcinomas (6.5 versus 1.5%)[24].

Preclinical data suggest that cancers with activating mutations in PIK3CA are sensitive to PIK3-pathway inhibitors, and combinations of PIK3 and other cancer-related pathway inhibitors are being developed[17].

PTEN

PTEN is a tumour suppressor gene, loss of which leads to constitutive PI3K-AKT signalling. Somatic PTEN deletions and mutations and inactivation of PTEN by an epigenetic mechanism are seen in multiple cancers. Reduction or loss of PTEN has been found in up to 70% of non-small cell carcinomas (squamous and adenocarcinomas). Mutations of PTEN are more common in squamous cell carcinomas (10.2 versus 1.7% for adenocarcinomas)[25]. Cancers with PTEN loss may be more sensitive to inhibitors of the PI3K pathway[17].

EphA2

The Eph receptor family is a group of tyrosine kinases, which are important in embryonic development such as vascular development, cell migration and tissue border formation. Overexpression of EphA2 is seen in multiple tumours, including non-small cell carcinomas, and is believed to promote cell motility, invasion, metastasis and angiogenesis. EphA2 expression has been correlated with smoking and reduced survival and has been reported to be higher in metastatic lesions compared to the primary. Mutations of EphA2 have also been described, and although they are rare, they appear to be more common in squamous cell carcinomas[17].

p53/MDM2

As in other tumours, mutations in p53 are frequent in lung cancer and are seen in more than half of non-small cell carcinomas and in approximately 65% of squamous cell carcinomas[26]. The spectrum of mutations seen is affected by smoking, with frequent G→T translocations, which are linked to polycyclic aromatic hydrocarbon adducts[17].

In a number of tumours, wild-type p53 is inactivated by MDM2 overexpression or amplification. MDM2 and p53 are regulated in a negative feedback loop, where MDM2 marks p53 for degradation.

MDM2 amplification has been reported in 6–7% of non-small cell carcinomas (squamous cell and adenocarcinomas) and appears to be an exclusive event of p53 mutation. One potential treatment strategy is to try to develop small molecules that neutralize MDM2 and thereby increase p53 activity. Small molecules targeting mutant p53 are also under development[27].

DDR2

DDR2 is also a receptor tyrosine kinase involved in cell migration, proliferation and survival. Mutations have been found in lung cancer with varying frequency, with a rate of 3.8% in squamous cell carcinomas in one study[28].

Bronchopulmonary neuroendocrine tumours

Bronchopulmonary neuroendocrine tumours comprise about 20–25% of all invasive lung malignancies and represent a spectrum of tumours arising from the neuroendocrine cells of the bronchopulmonary epithelium. Although these tumours share morphological, immunohistochemical and ultrastructural features, they are classified into four subtypes: low-grade typical carcinoid tumours, intermediate-grade atypical carcinoid tumours and two high-grade malignancies: large cell neuroendocrine carcinoma and small cell carcinoma[29,30]. These exhibit different biological characteristics and data from histological and molecular studies suggests that carcinoid tumours are distinct from the more malignant large cell neuroendocrine and small cell carcinoma groups.

Large cell neuroendocrine and small cell carcinomas are strongly related to tobacco usage, whereas the link between carcinoid tumours and tobacco smoking is uncertain.[29]

Carcinoid tumours

Carcinoid tumours, typical and atypical, are well-differentiated neuroendocrine tumours which account for approximately 1–2% of all primary lung carcinomas[31]. These tumours show no sex predilection and tend to occur at a younger age than other lung cancers, with the average age at the time of diagnosis ranging from 45–55 years. Approximately 50% of patients are asymptomatic at presentation[30]. Symptoms include dyspnoea, haemoptysis, cough and post-obstructive pneumonia. The most common paraneoplastic syndromes include the carcinoid syndrome and Cushing's syndrome[30]. Classical carcinoid

syndrome with flushing and diarrhoea is rare and is generally associated with metastatic disease[32]. Approximately 5% of bronchopulmonary carcinoids may occur as a component of the multiple neuroendocrine neoplasia 1 syndrome.

Polypoid endobronchial growth is common in central carcinoids, which on bronchoscopic examination are usually red-brown masses with a smooth surface. They are often highly vascular and may bleed considerably on biopsy. Peripheral carcinoid tumours, usually within the subpleural parenchyma, occur in ~40% of cases.

Both typical and atypical carcinoid tumours are characterized histologically by an organoid growth pattern and uniform cytologic features with a moderate amount of eosinophilic cytoplasm and nuclei with finely granular chromatin. In typical carcinoid tumours nucleoli are inconspicuous, but they may be seen in atypical carcinoids, which are defined as carcinoid tumours with 2–10 mitoses per 2 mm^2 area of viable tumour or the presence of necrosis, often punctate[30]. Since necrosis and mitosis may occur only focally, small biopsies may not be representative and in such situations the lesion should be classified as carcinoid tumour until adequate material is available[29]. Carcinoid tumours stain for neuroendocrine markers such as chromogranin, synaptophysin and CD56.

Since 5–20% of typical carcinoids and 30–70% of atypical carcinoids metastasize, lymph nodes should be assessed in all cases to ensure adequate staging[29]. TNM staging is recommended for pulmonary carcinoid tumours.

Distant metastases to other organs, including adrenal glands, liver, bone and brain, are rare, and atypical carcinoids account for most cases of metastatic disease, with ~25% of patients developing distant disease even long after initial diagnosis[32].

The primary approach to treatment of pulmonary carcinoid tumours is surgical resection, as these tumours are generally resistant to radiation and various chemotherapeutic agents have yielded minimal, mostly short-lasting results[29]. Both lung conserving and radical resections have been used, and all procedures should involve lymph node dissection or sampling, as a clearly identified prognostic factor is the presence or absence of lymph node involvement[32].

Patients with typical carcinoids have an excellent prognosis, with a 5-year survival rate of 87–100% and a 10-year survival rate of 87–93%[32].

The finding of metastases should not be used as a criterion to distinguish typical from atypical carcinoid tumours, as 5–20% of typical carcinoids show lymph node involvement. Compared with typical carcinoid tumours, atypical carcinoids tend to be larger, have a higher rate of metastases and the survival is significantly reduced with 5- and 10-year survival rates of 40–59% and 31–59%, respectively, although metastatic disease has a much poorer survival rate (~25%)[3,32]. As these tumours are relatively resistant to radiation and chemotherapy, when possible, metastatic disease is best managed surgically[30].

Large cell neuroendocrine carcinoma

Some large cell carcinomas display neuroendocrine features, including neuroendocrine morphology with organoid, trabecular, pallisading or rosette-like growth patterns and positivity for at least one specific neuroendocrine marker. These tumours, termed 'large cell neuroendocrine carcinoma', represent approximately 3% of resected lung cancers, are typically found in middle-aged or elderly heavy smokers and have a poor prognosis with 5- and 10-year survival rates of 27% and 11%, respectively[3]. Surgical resection should be performed, if possible. Reports regarding their chemosensitivity are contradictory, and the clinical significance of large cell neuroendocrine carcinoma and non-small cell carcinoma with neuroendocrine differentiation has yet to be fully evaluated, but recognition of these tumours is of potential therapeutic significance[4].

Small cell carcinoma

Small cell carcinoma comprises approximately 15% of all lung cancers, and most of these tumours present as a perihilar mass, arising in major airways, typically situated in a peribronchial location with infiltration of the submucosa and peribronchial tissues. These tumours grow rapidly and metastasize early, and paraneoplastic syndromes are relatively common. Lymph node metastases are frequent, and most small cell carcinomas are unresectable at the time of presentation. At least initially these tumours are sensitive to platinum-based chemotherapy. In up to 5% of cases, small cell carcinoma may present as a solitary lesion.[3] Necrosis is often extensive, and bronchial obstruction may occur due to extrinsic compression.

Until recently, small cell carcinoma has been staged as 'limited' or 'extensive' disease, but surgery has been successful in selected early cases, especially rare peripheral lesions, and it is now recommended that the same TNM staging is applied as for other lung tumours.

With combination chemotherapy and chest radiotherapy for limited disease, the median survival is 15 months, and 5-year survival is ~10%[3].

The terms 'oat cell' and 'intermediate cell' types are no longer used, as the differences in microscopic appearance are artefactual, depending on the preservation of the tissue. The 2004 WHO classification only includes small cell and combined small cell carcinoma, the latter comprising between 3–28% of the total[4], depending on the extent of sampling, being characterized by the presence of any other type of non-small cell carcinoma in addition to small cell carcinoma.

Histologically, small cell carcinoma has a distinctive appearance, being composed of relatively small cells with scant cytoplasm and round to fusiform nuclei with finely granular chromatin and absent or inconspicuous nucleoli. Nuclear moulding and smearing of nuclear chromatin due to crush artefact is often apparent. Necrosis is usually extensive, and the mitotic rate of this type of tumour is high; hence the rapid growth rate and advanced stage at presentation.

After chemotherapy, areas of large cell, squamous cell or adenocarcinoma may be seen within any residual resected tumour in 15–45% of cases[3].

Salivary gland–type tumours

The mixed seromucous glands of the trachea and bronchi are similar to the minor salivary glands and can give rise to the same range of tumours[4]. Salivary gland-type tumours of the lung are therefore most commonly found in the proximal main airways, usually present as endoluminal lesions and rarely occur in the peripheral lung parenchyma. Salivary gland-type tumours unrelated to the bronchial tree have a possible origin from a primitive stem cell that can show variable differentiation[33]. Clinical evaluation to exclude metastasis from a salivary gland primary is essential, especially if the lung tumour is peripheral or multiple lesions are present.

The clinical presentation of these tumours depends on their location, but as most are central lesions and protrude into the airway lumen, the most common symptoms include cough, dyspnoea and haemoptysis or atelectasis and pneumonia due to proximal airway obstruction.

The two most common pulmonary salivary gland–type lung tumours are adenoid cystic carcinoma and mucoepidermoid carcinoma.

Adenoid cystic carcinoma

Adenoid cystic carcinomas of the lung account for about 0.2–0.3% of all lung cancers, and >90% arise in central rather than segmental bronchi[34,35]. These are tumours of middle age and are described as having no gender predilection, although some studies have suggested a higher incidence in females[35]. They are slow-growing, infiltrative tumours with a prolonged clinical course and are thus considered a low-grade malignancy. Adenoid cystic carcinomas form poorly defined, sessile, nodular growths which may ulcerate centrally and show a predilection for submucosal and perineural spread.

Histologically, the tumour cells form well-demarcated groups within which small cysts impart a tubular or cribriform appearance. Small, dark myoepithelial cells form the dominant cell population, amongst which are ducts lined by slightly larger cells which secrete mucin. These histological features are sufficiently distinctive to allow diagnosis, but in small biopsies it may be difficult to distinguish adenoid cystic carcinoma from adenocarcinoma, basaloid carcinoma and small cell carcinoma[4].

The first-line treatment for adenoid cystic carcinoma is surgical resection, and as these tumours often arise in the central airways, tracheobronchoplasty is also often indicated[34]. Alternative options for tumours which cannot be completely resected include stenting, local ablation and radiotherapy. Because of their tendency to exhibit submucosal and perineural extension, it is important that resection margins are checked intra-operatively by frozen section.

Although long-term survival can be expected, local recurrence is frequent, often after a number of years, and careful follow-up is recommended. Metastases are uncommon but may occur in lymph nodes, bone, liver, kidney, brain and lung[4].

The reported 5- and 10-year survival rates for adenoid cystic carcinoma are 55% and 39%, respectively[36].

Mucoepidermoid carcinoma

Mucoepidermoid carcinomas comprise 0.1–0.2% of primary lung tumours[37], occurring mostly in relatively young persons, with approximately 50% of cases presenting before the age of 30. There is a female sex predominance[4].

Mucoepidermoid carcinomas most commonly arise in the central bronchial regions and clinically may present with cough, wheezing, haemoptysis and obstructive pneumonia. Occasional lesions are peripheral.

Both low- and high-grade tumours are recognized, and the gross appearances depend on the degree of malignancy. Low-grade tumours, which comprise approximately 80%, form intraluminal smooth, partly cystic, polypoid masses compressing surrounding tissues. More aggressive tumours are less well defined, are solid and infiltrate surrounding lung[4].

Mucoepidermoid carcinoma is characterized by a mixture of mucus-producing, glandular and squamous epithelial cells, together with intermediate cells at various proportions and growth patterns, such as cystic, papillary and solid[37].

Surgical resection is the treatment of choice, with bronchoplasty for low-grade lesions. Patients with low-grade tumours have a good prognosis with a 5-year survival rate of 95%, although nodal involvement and metastases have occasionally been reported. About 25% of patients with high-grade tumours develop metastases, mainly in lymph nodes, bone or skin[4]. Effective treatment measures for high-grade mucoepidermoid carcinomas have not been established, but patients with EGFR gene mutations are reported to have responded favourably to tyrosine kinase inhibitors[37].

Primary pulmonary lymphoma

Primary pulmonary lymphoma is defined as a clonal lymphoid proliferation affecting one or both lungs, with or without mediastinal involvement, in a patient with no detectable extrapulmonary involvement at diagnosis or during the subsequent 3 months[38,39].

Although secondary involvement of the lung by malignant lymphoma is relatively frequent, with an incidence of 25–40%, primary pulmonary non-Hodgkin's lymphoma is a rare entity encompassing only 0.4% of all lymphomas[40] and 3.6% of extra-nodal lymphomas[38]. Most primary lymphomas of the lung arise from the mucosa-associated lymphoid tissue (MALT) of the airways, and it is believed that MALT is not a normal constituent of the respiratory tree but acquired in response to various antigenic stimuli such as smoking, infection or autoimmune disease[40].

Patients tend to be between 50–70 years of age, and many are asymptomatic at the time of diagnosis, with symptomatic patients presenting with cough, dyspnoea, chest pain and haemoptysis[2]. The radiological appearances of pulmonary lymphoma are non-specific and include patchy opacities with air bronchograms, solitary or multiple areas of mass-like consolidation.

Approximately 70–90% of primary pulmonary lymphomas are marginal zone B-cell lymphomas of MALT type. Most are low grade, but transformation to a higher grade occurs in a minority of cases[38]. No specific trigger has been identified so far, but MALT lymphomas have been associated with autoimmune disorders such as Sjogren's syndrome, systemic lupus erythematosus and Hashimoto's thyroiditis[39]. High-grade diffuse large B-cell lymphoma comprises about 5–20% of cases[2], most of which occur in individuals with an underlying disorder such as immunodeficiency. Patients with high-grade lymphoma are frequently symptomatic.

Bronchoscopy obtained a diagnostic yield in 30–40% of cases[41], but often a more generous VATS or open lung biopsy is required, especially since a number of non-neoplastic reactive conditions can simulate lymphoma[40]. Bronchoalveolar lavage and fine needle aspiration specimens may be diagnostic if a clonal B-cell population can be demonstrated by flow cytometry, but the specific subtype of lymphoma can rarely be determined by these techniques[2].

Low-grade marginal zone B cell lymphomas of MALT type are indolent, remain localized to the lung for a long time and have a favourable outcome, with a 5-year survival rate of >80% and a median survival time of >10 years.[39] Prognostic factors affecting survival are not well defined; the stage of the disease, extent of resection (complete versus incomplete) and presence of mediastinal lymphadenopathy do not appear to be associated with a worse prognosis[41]. Treatment options for localized disease include observation, definitive resection, chemotherapy or radiotherapy[38]. The rate of local recurrences with these tumours has been found to be as high as 50%[40].

The outcome for high-grade primary pulmonary diffuse large B-cell lymphoma is poorer, progression and relapse occurring earlier and more frequently. They are usually treated with combination chemotherapy and the overall 5-year survival ranges from 0–60%[2].

Acknowledgements

I would like to thank Dr Stephen Preston for his assistance in carrying out a literature search on carcinoid tumours.

References

1 Churgh AM, Myers JL, Tazelaar HD, Wright JL. *Thurlbeck's Pathology of the Lung* (Third Edition). New York: Thieme Medical Publishers, 2005.

2 Travis WD, Brambilla E, Muller-Hermelink HK, Harris CC. *Tumours of the Lung, Pleura, Thymus and Heart.* Lyon: IARC Press, 2004.

3 Travis WD. Pathology of lung cancer. *Clin Chest Med* 32:669–92, 2011.

4 Corrin B, Nicholson AG. *Pathology of the Lungs* (Third Edition). Churchill Livingstone, Elsevier, 2011.

5 Son JW. Year-in-review of lung cancer. *Tuberc Respir Dis (Seoul)* 73:137–142, 2012.

6 Wen J, Fu JH, Zhang W, et al. Lung carcinoma signaling pathways activated by smoking. *Chin J Cancer* 30:551–8, 2011.

7 Petersen I. The morphological and molecular diagnosis of lung cancer. *Dtsch Arztebl Int* 108:525–31, 2011.

8 Rosai J. *Rosai and Ackerman's Surgical Pathology,* Vol 1 (Tenth Edition). Elsevier, 2011.

9 Gazdar AF, Brambilla E. Preneoplasia of lung cancer. *Cancer Biomark* 9:385–96, 2010.

10 Travis WD, Brambilla E, Noguchi M, et al. International Association for the Study of Lung Cancer/American Thoracic Society/European Respiratory Society. International multidisciplinary classification of lung adenocarcinoma: executive summary. *Proc Am Thorac Soc* 8:381–5, 2011.

11 *Modern Surgical Pathology* (First Edition), 2003.

12 Yatabe Y, Kosaka T, Takahashi T, et al. EGFR mutation is specific for terminal respiratory unit type adenocarcinoma. *Am J Surg Pathol* 29:633–9, 2005.

13 Yoshizawa A, Motoi N, Riely GJ, et al. Impact of proposed IASLC/ATS/ERS classification of lung adenocarcinoma: prognostic subgroups and implications for further revision of staging based on

analysis of 514 stage I cases. *Mod Pathol* 24:653–64, 2011.

14 Kadota K, Suzuki K, Colovos C, et al. A nuclear grading system is a strong predictor of survival in epitheloid diffuse malignant pleural mesothelioma. *Mod Pathol* 25:260–71, 2012.

15 Travis WD, Rekhtman N. Pathological diagnosis and classification of lung cancer in small biopsies and cytology: strategic management of tissue for molecular testing. *Semin Respir Crit Care Med* 32:22–31, 2011.

16 Brandao GD, Brega EF, Spatz A. The role of molecular pathology in non-small-cell lung carcinoma– now and in the future. *Curr Oncol* 19:S24-32, 2012.

17 Heist RS, Sequist LV, Engelman JA. Genetic changes in squamous cell lung cancer: a review. *J Thorac Oncol* 7:924–33, 2012.

18 Pirker R, Pereira JR, von Pawel J, et al. EGFR expression as a predictor of survival for first-line chemotherapy plus cetuximab in patients with advanced non-small-cell lung cancer: analysis of data from the phase 3 FLEX study. *Lancet Oncol* 13:33–42, 2012.

19 Soh J, Toyooka S, Ichihara S, et al. Sequential molecular changes during multistage pathogenesis of small peripheral adenocarcinomas of the lung. *J Thorac Oncol* 3:340–7, 2008.

20 Rodig SJ, Mino-Kenudson M, Dacic S, et al. Unique clinicopathologic features characterize ALK-rearranged lung adenocarcinoma in the western population. *Clin Cancer Res* 15:5216–23, 2009.

21 Marchetti A, Felicioni L, Malatesta S, et al. Clinical features and outcome of patients with non-small-cell lung cancer harboring BRAF mutations. *J Clin Oncol* 29:3574–9, 2011.

22 Weiss J, Sos ML, Seidel D, et al. Frequent and focal FGFR1 amplification associates with therapeutically tractable FGFR1 dependency in squamous cell lung cancer. *Sci Transl Med* 2:62–93, 2010.

23 Yamamoto H, Shigematsu H, Nomura M, et al. PIK3CA mutations and copy number gains in human lung cancers. *Cancer Res* 68:6913–21, 2008.

24 Kawano O, Sasaki H, Endo K, et al. PIK3CA mutation status in Japanese lung cancer patients. *Lung Cancer* 54:209–15, 2006.

25 GJ, MJ K, Jeon HS, et al. PTEN mutations and relationship to EGFR, ERBB2, KRAS and TP53 mutations in non-small cell lung cancers. *Lung Cancer* 69:279–83, 2010.

26 Kishimoto Y, Murakami Y, Shiraishi M, et al. Aberrations of the p53 tumor suppressor gene in human non-small cell carcinomas of the lung. *Cancer Res* 52:4799–4804, 1992.

27 Mandinova A, Lee SW. The p53 pathway as a target in cancer therapeutics: obstacles and promise. *Sci Transl Med* 3:64–61, 2011.

28 Hammerman PS, Sos ML, Ramos AH, et al. Mutations in the DDR2 kinase gene identify a novel therapeutic target in squamous cell lung cancer. *Cancer Discov* 1:78–89, 2011.

29 Gustafsson BI, Kidd M, Chan A, et al. Bronchopulmonary neuroendocrine tumors. *Cancer* 113:5–21, 2008.

30 Travis WD. Advances in neuroendocrine lung tumors. *Ann Oncol* 21 (Suppl 7): vii, 65–71, 2010.

31 Tsuta K, Raso MG, Kalhor N, et al. Histologic features of low- and intermediate-grade neuroendocrine carcinoma

(typical and atypical carcinoid tumors) of the lung. *Lung Cancer* 71:34–41, 2011.

32 Bertino EM, Confer PD, Colonna JE, et al. Pulmonary neuroendocrine/carcinoid tumors: a review article. *Cancer* 115:4434–41, 2009.

33 Carretta A, Libretti L, Taccagni G, et al. Salivary gland-type mixed tumor (pleomorphic adenoma) of the lung. *Interact Cardiovasc Thorac Surg* 3:663–5, 2004.

34 Kitada M, Ozawa K, Sato K, et al. Adenoid cystic carcinoma of the peripheral lung: a case report. *World J Surg Oncol* 8:74, 2010.

35 Cortés-Télles A, Mendoza-Posada D. Primary adenoid cystic carcinoma of the tracheobronchial tree: a decade-long experience at a health centre in Mexico. *Lung India* 29:325–8, 2012.

36 Macarenco RS, Uphoff TS, Gilmer HF, et al. Salivary gland-type lung carcinomas: an EGFR immunohistochemical, molecular genetic, and mutational analysis study. *Mod Pathol* 21:1168–75, 2008.

37 Kitada M, Matsuda Y, Sato K, et al. Mucoepidermoid carcinoma of the lung: a case report. *J Cardiothorac Surg* 6:132, 2011.

38 Graham BB, Mathisen DJ, Mark EJ, et al. Primary pulmonary lymphoma. *Ann Thorac Surg* 80:1248–53, 2005.

39 Cadranel J, Wislez M, Antoine M. Primary pulmonary lymphoma. *Eur Respir J* 20:750–62, 2002.

40 Ferraro P, Trastek VF, Adlakha H, et al. Primary non-Hodgkin's lymphoma of the lung. *Ann Thorac Surg* 69:993–7, 2000.

41 Parissis H. Forty years literature review of primary lung lymphoma. *J Cardiothorac Surg* 6:23, 2011.

Medical treatment of lung cancer (neo and adjuvant chemoradiotherapy)

Athanasios G. Pallis and Mary E. R. O'Brien

Adjuvant chemotherapy after surgical resection

Surgery remains the only curative treatment modality for patients with stage I–IIIA non-small cell lung cancer (NSCLC). However, even after complete resection, the risk of recurrence is substantial, and 5-year overall survival (OS) is approximately 70% for patients with stage IB disease, 40–50% for stage II and less than 30% for stage IIIA patients[1]. Efforts to improve the survival of patients with operable NSCLC have examined the addition of chemotherapy (CMT) and/or radiotherapy (RT) in the post-operative setting.

In 1995, the NSCLC collaborative group reported a meta-analysis of eight trials with a total of 1394 patients treated with cisplatin-based adjuvant chemotherapy[2]. This study reported a 13% reduction in the risk of death (hazard ratio [HR] 0.87; 95% confidence interval [CI]: 0.74–1.02) corresponding to an absolute survival benefit of 3% at 2 years (95% CI 0.5% detriment to 7% benefit) and 5% (95% CI 1% detriment to 10% benefit) at 5 years in favour of chemotherapy. Despite the lack of statistical significance ($P = 0.08$), these findings encouraged the initiation of several randomized trials investigating the role of platinum-based adjuvant chemotherapy in patients with completely resected stage I, II and IIIA NSCLC (Table 14.1).

The North American Intergroup Trial INT0115 was the only trial that compared the combination of chemotherapy plus thoracic radiotherapy versus radiotherapy alone in patients with completely resected stage II or IIIA NSCLC and failed to demonstrate a benefit in favour of chemotherapy[3]. The negative results of the Adjuvant Lung Project Italy (ALPI)[4] and the Big Lung Trial (BIG)[5] further jeopardized the role of adjuvant chemotherapy in the treatment of NSCLC.

National Cancer Institute of Canada (NCIC) JBR10 trial

The National Cancer Institute of Canada (NCIC) JBR10 Trial randomly assigned 482 patients with completely resected, pathological stage IB and II (patients with T3N0 disease were excluded) to receive either post-operative adjuvant chemotherapy with cisplatin and vinorelbine or no chemotherapy[6].

At 5 years of follow-up, the 5-year survival rates were 69% for the chemotherapy arm and 54% for the control arm (HR 0.69; 95% CI 0.52–0.92; $P = 0.011$), with an absolute survival benefit of 15% for patients receiving chemotherapy[6]. An updated analysis after a median follow-up of 9.3 years continued to show a benefit in favour of adjuvant chemotherapy (HR 0.78; 95% CI 0.61 to 0.99; $P = 0.04$)[7]. Patients with stage II disease had a significant benefit in terms of 5-year OS (59 vs 44% for placebo), but in patients with stage I disease the benefit depended upon the size of tumour. For the whole group there was no benefit (5-year OS, chemotherapy vs placebo: 76 vs 69%; HR 1.03; $P = 0.79$). In patients with tumours < 4 cm, chemotherapy was associated with a *detrimental* effect (5-year OS chemotherapy vs placebo: 73 vs 79%; HR 1.73), while in those with tumours > 4 cm adjuvant treatment prolonged OS (5-year OS chemotherapy vs placebo: 79 vs 59%; HR 0.68). Compliance with chemotherapy was relatively low, with only 65% of the patients receiving three or four cycles. Neutropenia was the most common haematological toxicity, with 73% of the patients experiencing a grade III–IV neutropenia, while fatigue (15%) anorexia (10%) and vomiting (10%) were the most common grade III–IV non-haematological toxicities. Chemotherapy was not associated with an increase in secondary malignancies,

Table 14.1 Randomized phase III studies of adjuvant chemotherapy in NSCLC

Trial	No. of pts.	Disease stages included	CT regimen/ control arm	Compliance to CT (%)	Median follow-up (months)	5-Year absolute survival benefit (%)	Hazard ratio of death	p-Value
INT0115-ECOG3590[3]	488	II-IIIA	E-Cis/ Radiotherapy only (both arms received a total of 50.4 Gy radiotherapy)	69	44	−6*	0.93	0.56
ALPI Trial[4]	1209	I-IIIA	Mit-VND-Cis, for three cycles/ observation	69	64.5	1	0.96	0.589
IALT Trial[10]	1867	I-IIIA	Cis + vinka alkaloids or E/observation	74	56	4.1	0.86	<0.03
Big Lung Trial[5]	381	I-IIIA	Cis-VND, Cis-mit-If, Cis-mit-Vin or Cis-VNB/ observation	64	34.6	−2**	1.02	0.90
UFT Trial[13]	999	I	UFT for 2 years/ observation	74 (at 12 mo) 61 (at 24 mo)	72	3	—	0.047
UFT meta-analysis[14]	2003	I-III	UFT/observation	80	6.44 (years)	4.6	0.77	0.011
NCIC-JBR10 Trial[6,7]	482	IB-II	Cis-VNB/ observation	65	60	15	0.69	0.011
CALGB 9633 Trial[12]	344	IB	PCL-carboplatin/ observation	85	48	3	0.80	0.32
ANITA Trial[9]	840	IB-IIIA	Cis-VNB/ observation	56 ##	>70	8.6	0.79	0.013

* Estimated 5-year survival rates were 39% for the RT only group and 33% for the CT-RT group.
** Estimated 2-year survival rates were 60% for the observation group and 58% for the CT group.
dose density of vinorelbine

E = etoposide; Cis = cisplatin; Mit = mitomycin; PCL = paclitaxel, VND = vindesine; Vin = vinblastine; If = ifosphamide; UFT = Uracil/tegafur; VNB = vinorelbine.

but resulted in a statistically significant transient worsening of quality of life[8].

Adjuvant Navelbine International Trial Association (ANITA) trial

The Adjuvant Navelbine International Trial Association (ANITA) trial randomized 840 patients with stage IB-IIIA NSCLC to post-operative chemotherapy (4 cycles of cisplatin 100 mg/m^2 every 4 weeks and 16 cycles of vinorelbine at 30 mg/m^2 weekly) or observation only[9]. After a median follow-up of 76 months, OS was significantly longer in the chemotherapy arm (65.7 months in the chemotherapy arm vs 43.7 months in the observation arm; HR 0.80; 95% CI 0.66–0.96; p = 0.017). Overall survival at 5 years with chemotherapy improved by 8.6%, which was maintained at 7 years (8.4%). In a similar way to

141

JBR10, chemotherapy did not improve survival in stage IB disease (HR 1·10; 95% CI 0·76–1·57). Significant chemotherapy-related toxicity was reported with 84.6 and 12.5% of the patients experiencing grade 3–4 neutropenia and febrile neutropenia, respectively. It should be noted that only 50% of the patients were able to complete the planned four cycles.

International Adjuvant Lung Cancer Trial (IALT) and CALGB9633 trial

The International Adjuvant Lung Cancer Trial (IALT) was the largest adjuvant trial ($n = 1867$ patients) and included patients with stage I–IIIA disease. Patients were randomized to cisplatin-based chemotherapy or observation[10]. After a median follow-up of 56 months, the 5-year OS was significantly longer in the chemotherapy arm (5-year OS chemotherapy vs placebo 44.5 vs 40.4%; HR 0.06; $p = 0.03$), but the significant effect was no longer present after a median follow-up of 90 months (HR 0.91; $p = 0.10$)[11]. The CALGB9633 trial was the only one to use a carboplatin-based regimen and focused only on patients with stage IB disease. It failed to maintain the benefit with longer follow-up (HR 0.83; $p = 0.12$)[12]. However, exploratory analysis demonstrated a significant survival difference in favour of adjuvant chemotherapy for patients who had tumours ≥ 4 cm (HR 0.69; 95% CI 0.48–0.99; $p = 0.043$).

Uracil/tegafur (UFT)

A large phase III trial ($n = 999$) tested the role of UFT in Japanese patients with stage I adenocarcinoma and demonstrated a significant increase in the 5-year OS rate in patients with T2 tumours (85 vs 74% for the UFT and observation groups, respectively; HR 0.48; 95% CI 0.29–0.81; $p = 0.005$), while for patients with T1 disease no significant difference was observed[13]. A subsequent meta-analysis with 2,000 patients further confirmed the role of UFT in the adjuvant setting[14]. It should be noted that UFT has not been tested in Caucasians in the adjuvant setting, and the drug is not registered in the European Union for this indication.

Targeted agents

Goss et al. evaluated the role of gefitinib in 503 stage IB-IIIA NSCLC, patients not selected by EGFR status. Patients were randomized to gefitinib 250 mg or placebo daily for 2 years. After a median follow-up of 4.7 years, median disease-free survival (DFS) was 4.2 years for gefitinib versus not yet reached (NYR) for placebo (HR 1.22; 95% CI 0.93–1.61, $p = 0.15$ and median OS) 5.1 years vs NYR (HR 1.24; 95% CI 0.94–1.64, $p = 0.14$). In multivariate analysis, tumour size > 4 cm was predictive of poor DFS ($p < 0.0001$) and never smoking for better OS with gefitinib ($p = 0.02$). EGFR copy whether low/high polysomy or amplification was neither prognostic ($p = 0.77$) nor predictive of OS benefit from gefitinib[15]. A trial of erlotinib after surgery (with or without adjuvant chemotherapy) in patients who have epidermal growth factor receptor (EGFR)–positive tumours (RADIANT) is currently ongoing (NCT00373425). Adjuvant chemotherapy with or without bevacizumab as adjuvant therapy for NSCLC patients with completely resected stage IB (≥ 4 cm)–IIIA is being tested in an ongoing ECOG (E1505) trial (NCT00324805). Melanoma associated antigen (MAGE)–A3 is a tumour-specific antigen that is expressed in a large variety of cancers, including NSCLC. Vaccination with the MAGE-A3 antigen in patients with early-stage NSCLC has shown encouraging results in the context of phase II trials[16]. The vaccine reduced the risk of relapse after surgery, and its role is currently under investigation in a phase III trial (MAGRITTE trial; NCT00480025).

Meta-analyses

The survival benefit observed with adjuvant chemotherapy was confirmed by a meta-analysis of five randomized trials[4–6,9,10] with 4584 patients registered in the LACE (lung adjuvant cisplatin evaluation) database[17]. This meta-analysis demonstrated a 5.4% increase in 5-year survival in favour of adjuvant chemotherapy compared to observation (HR 0.89; 95% CI 0.82–0.96). The survival benefit varied according to stage and was most pronounced for patients with stage II and IIIA disease. The improvement in survival in patients with stage IB disease did not reach statistical significance, and patients with stage IA disease appeared to do worse with adjuvant chemotherapy. All five trials included in the LACE meta-analysis used cisplatin-based chemotherapy, and all trials except the JBR10 allowed the use of post-operative radiotherapy at the discretion of the treating physician. A more recent meta-analysis by Arriagada et al. demonstrated a similar benefit (HR 0.86, 95% CI 0.81–0.92, $p < 0.0001$), with an

Table 14.2 Meta-analyses evaluating the role of adjuvant chemotherapy

Study	Intervention	No. of studies/pts.	HR (95% CI)	p-Value
Hotta et al.[19]	Adjuvant CMT	13/5360	0.87 (0.80–0.94)	0.001
	Adjuvant C	8/3786	0.89 (0.81–0.98)	0.012
Sedrakyan et al.[20]	Adjuvant CMT	19/7200	0.87 (0.81–0.93)	< 0.0001
	Adjuvant C	12/4912	0.89 (0.82–0.96)	0.004
Berghmans et al.[21]	Adjuvant CMT	17/7644	0.84 (0.78–0.89)	NR
	Adjuvant C	16/NR	0.86 (0.80–0.92)	NR
Bria et al.[22]	Adjuvant P	12/7334		
LACE[17]	Adjuvant C	5/4584	0.89 (0.82–0.96)	0.005
NSCLC CG[18]	Adjuvant C	30/8147	0.86 (0.81–0.93)	< 0.001
	Adjuvant C +PORT	12/2763	0.90 (0.82–0.98)	0.02

CMT: chemotherapy; P: platinum based; C: cisplatin based; NR: not reported; CG: Collaborative Group; PORT: post-operative radiotherapy.

absolute increase in survival of 4% (95% CI 3–6) at 5 years (from 60 to 64%)[18]. This meta-analysis did not show significant differences in the effect of platinum chemotherapy by stage. Also, no platinum-based regimen emerged as 'goldstandard'. Numerous other meta-analyses have reported HR in the same range[19–22] (Table 14.2).

Is there an optimal regimen for adjuvant chemotherapy?

All the aforementioned trials utilized a cisplatin-based regimen in the adjuvant treatment, while in the CALGB9633 the carboplatin/paclitaxel doublet was used[12]. In the LACE meta-analysis, the effect of cisplatin plus vinorelbine was marginally better than the effect of other drug combinations[17]. However, it should be noted that these trials used relatively older drugs (etoposide, ifosfamide, vinca alkaloids) in combination with cisplatin, and no trial utilized a third-generation agent (docetaxel, gemcitabine, pemetrexed). This meta-analysis also demonstrated that patients who received a total dose of cisplatin >300 mg/m^2 had a trend towards better OS and disease-free survival compared to patients who received ≤300 mg/m^2. The total dose of cisplatin varied according to the second drug used in each regimen. In the cisplatin/vinorelbine group, 86% of the patients were able to receive >300 mg/m^2, while this percentage was 54% in the cisplatin/other drug group. Therefore, it can be questioned whether the benefit observed with the cisplatin/vinorelbine regimen is due to higher efficacy of this combination

or to the fact that higher dose of cisplatin could be achieved with this doublet[17]. Finally, patients who were treated with a triplet received significantly (p < 0.001) less cisplatin compared to patients who were treated with a doublet[17].

According to these observations, the approach of many scientific societies is to recommend the use of any cisplatin-based doublet[23–25].

Stage I treatment

With the exception of the IALT study[4], none of the studies described earlier included patients with stage IA disease. Furthermore, in the LACE meta-analysis, patients with stage IA disease (n = 347) appeared to do worse with adjuvant chemotherapy, although the number was too small to allow valid conclusions[17]. Therefore, adjuvant chemotherapy is not recommended for patients with stage IA disease[23–25].

The management of patients with stage IB disease is more controversial. CALGB9633[12], the only study that enrolled only patients with stage IB disease, failed to demonstrate a benefit. Similarly, subgroup analysis of the IALT[10], the JBR10 and the ANITA[9] studies demonstrated no benefit for these patients. Finally, in the LACE meta-analysis, there was only a trend towards an OS benefit in favour of adjuvant chemotherapy in patients with stage IB disease (HR 0.93; 95% CI 0.78–1.10)[17].

On the contrary, the more recent meta-analysis from the NSCLC Collaborative Group demonstrated an identical 5-year OS benefit in patients with stage IB, II and III disease (5% in all groups)[18]. Also, the

CALGB9633 trial[12] and the JBR10 demonstrated a benefit in patients with tumours larger than 4 cm. However, these analyses were not pre-planned or adequately powered, and therefore, their results cannot be considered conclusive.

Currently, adjuvant chemotherapy is not considered as standard of care for patients with stage IB disease[23–25]. Further, prospective trials are needed in order to clearly address this issue. However, a prospective phase III trial especially for patients with stage III disease is unlikely given the large number of patients required.

Treatment of elderly patients

Despite the increasing incidence of NSCLC in elderly populations, this patient group is often under-represented in clinical trials, and therefore, it is difficult to reach evidence-based recommendations for this population[26]. Unfortunately, in the adjuvant setting, only retrospective data exist for elderly patients.

Patient data included in the LACE meta-analysis[17] were categorized into three age groups (<65 [$n = 3,269$, 71%], 65–69 [$n = 901$, 20%] and ≥ 70 [$n = 414$, 9%]). The analysis of these data according to age demonstrated that although patients ≥ 70 years received lower total doses of cisplatin ($p < 0.0001$) and fewer cycles of chemotherapy ($p < 0.0001$), there was no difference in terms of OS between age groups, and elderly patients had a similar survival benefit from adjuvant chemotherapy with their younger counterparts[27]. Furthermore, toxicity rates were similar across all age groups evaluated. As expected, a higher number of elderly patients died from non-cancer-related causes ($p < 0.0001$)[27]. The more recent meta-analysis from the NSCLC Collaborative Group also did not observe any differential effect of chemotherapy according to age[18].

In a retrospective age-specific subgroup analysis of the JBR10 study, outcomes in elderly patients (age ≥ 65) and matched younger patients (age < 65) were compared[6]. Despite older patients receiving fewer doses of chemotherapy and lower mean dose-intensities, OS was significantly prolonged with chemotherapy (HR 0.61; 95% CI 0.38–0.98; $p = 0.04$)[28]. The survival benefit in the elderly group was similar to that demonstrated in younger patients with no significant differences in toxicities, hospitalization or treatment-related death. A recently published observational study based on data from the Surveillance, Epidemiology, and End Results (SEER) Registry also demonstrated that platinum-based adjuvant chemotherapy administered to elderly patients was associated with a significant OS benefit, although with higher toxicity[29].

According to these results, it can be argued that adjuvant chemotherapy should not be refused to elderly patients solely on the basis of age, and treatment decisions should take into account the estimated absolute benefit, life expectancy, treatment tolerance, presence of co-morbidities and patient preferences.[30]. However, it should also be noted that these results are based on retrospective analyses that are likely to suffer from selection bias in favour of treatment and their extrapolation to the general older population should be made with caution.

Molecular prognostic and predictive markers

Translational research projects were initiated in connection with the aforementioned studies in an attempt to characterize 'high-risk' patients who are likely to benefit from adjuvant chemotherapy while sparing the toxicity of unneeded treatment for 'low-risk' patients.

Excision repair cross-complementation group 1 (ERCC1) is a key enzyme participating in the nucleotide excision repair (NER) DNA repair pathway[31]. An immunohistochemical (IHC) analysis to determine the expression of ERCC1 was performed in operative specimens of patients participating in the IALT. A total of 761 tumours were tested, and ERCC1 expression was positive in 335 (44%) and negative in 426 (56%). Absence of ERCC1 expression was associated with a significant benefit from cisplatin-based adjuvant chemotherapy (HR 0.65; 95% CI 0.50–0.86; $p = 0.002$; test for interaction, $p = 0.009$). Patients with ERCC1-positive tumours had no benefit from adjuvant chemotherapy (HR 1.14; 95% CI 0.84–1.55; $p = 0.40$). ERCC1 expression had also a prognostic value. Among patients in the observation arm, ERCC1 expression was associated with longer OS (HR 0.66; 95% CI 0.49–0.90; $p = 0.009$)[32]. Similarly, low expression of MutS homologue 2 (MSH2), another key enzyme of the mismatch DNA repair pathway, had a borderline positive predictive role (low MSH2 expression HR 0.76; $p = 0.3$ vs high MSH2 expression HR 1.12; $p = 0.48$; p-value for interaction = 0.06)[33]. High expression had a positive prognostic role in patients in the no treatment arm (HR 0.66; $p = 0.01$).

Tumour samples from patients participating in the JBR10 trial were used to develop an mRNA-based 15-gene signature[34]. This gene signature could separate patients in the observation arm into high- and low-risk subgroups with significantly different OS (HR 15.02; 95% CI 5.12–44.04; $p < 0.001$). The prognostic value was further validated in four separate data sets and on the original data set by the use of reverse transcription polymerase chain reaction (RT-PCR). The signature also had a positive predictive value. Patients in the high-risk group benefitted from the adjuvant treatment (HR 0.33; 95% CI 0.17–0.63; $p = 0.0005$), but it was not beneficial and potentially even detrimental to low-risk patients (HR 3.67; 95% CI 1.22–1.06; $p = 0.021$).

Adjuvant radiotherapy after surgical resection

Because few and underpowered studies had evaluated the role of post-operative radiotherapy (PORT), a meta-analysis was performed in the late 1990s[35]. The last update of this meta-analysis included information from 11 trials and 2,128 patients[36]. The results of the updated analysis continued to demonstrate that PORT was associated with a detrimental effect on OS, with an 18% relative increase in the risk of death, which was more pronounced for patients with lower nodal status. Similar detriments were observed for local recurrence-free survival, distant recurrence-free survival and overall recurrence-free survival. A significant interaction with stage and nodal status was observed. Stage III and N2 patients had no detrimental effect (but no benefit as well), while in patients with earlier-stage disease, PORT was associated with shorter survival. However, the PORT meta-analysis has been criticized for its long enrolment period and use of different types of machines, techniques and doses that are abandoned in the current modern radiotherapy. For patients with N2 positive disease, a retrospective analysis demonstrated higher survival for those who had received PORT[9]. The role of PORT in patients with N2 disease is evaluated by the ongoing LUNGART study (NCT00410683). This trial randomizes NSCLC patients with pathologically confirmed mediastinal node disease to post-operative conformal RT (45 Gy) or observation. This trial is a cooperation between

Cancer Research UK (CRUK), the European Organisation for Research and Treatment of Cancer (EORTC), the Institut de Cancerologie Gustave Roussy (IGR), the National Institute for Health Research Cancer Research Network (NCRN), and the Christie NHS Foundation Trust.

On the basis of these results, routine PORT is not recommended for patients with completely resected stage I–IIIA NSCLC[23,24,37].

Neoadjuvant treatment

Induction (neoadjuvant) chemotherapy before surgery

Pre-operative chemotherapy has been evaluated as an alternative to adjuvant chemotherapy. Pre-operative chemotherapy presents several theoretical advantages including reduction of tumour volume that could enhance radical resections and local control, evaluation of response to chemotherapy, early eradication of micrometastatic disease, and higher patient compliance compared to post-operative chemotherapy.

In the early 1990s, two small, randomized phase III trials evaluated the role of neoadjuvant chemotherapy in patients with stage IIIA (mainly N2 disease)[38,39]. Both studies were prematurely terminated on the basis of interim analyses showing significant benefit in favour of the neoadjuvant arm.

In a multicentre phase III study conducted by the French Thoracic Cooperative Group, 355 patients with clinical IB–IIIA disease were randomly assigned to receive two cycles of induction chemotherapy (cisplatin/ifosfamide/mitomycin triplet) followed by surgery and two post-operative cycles versus surgery alone[40]. Patients with pT3 or pN2 received post-operative radiation. Median survival favoured the chemotherapy arm, but the difference failed to reach statistical significance (37 months for the chemotherapy arm vs 26 months for the surgery alone arm, $p = 0.15$). At an updated analysis after 14 years of follow-up, the 10-year recurrence-free survival rate was significantly higher in the chemotherapy arm (55 vs 38%; HR 0.78; 95% CI 0.62–0.98). A trend towards higher OS rate at 10 years was observed in the neoadjuvant arm, but the difference was not statistically significant (29 vs 21%; $p = 0.12$) [41,42].

The European multicentre LU22 trial randomly assigned 519 patients with clinical stage I—III to three

Table 14.3 Randomized phase III trials of neoadjuvant chemotherapy in NSCLC

Study	No. of pts.	Stage	Regimen	OS	p-Value
IFCT[40]	355	IB–IIIA	3 cy CIM→surgery vs surgery	10-year OS rate 29 vs 21%	0.12
MRC LU22[43]	519	I–III	3 cy platinum-based→surgery vs surgery	55 vs 54 months	NS
SWOG 9900[44]	354	IB–IIIA	3 cy carbo/PCL→surgery vs surgery	62 vs 41 months	0.11
NATCH[45]	624	IA–IIIA (T3N1)	3 cy carbo/PCL→surgery vs surgery	5-year OS rate: 47 vs 44%	NS
Scagliotti et al.[42]	270	IB–IIIA	3 cy C/GMB→surgery vs surgery	7.8 vs 4.8 years	0.04

C: cyclophosphamide, C: cisplatin, I: ifosphamide, M: mytomycin,, PCL=paclitaxel, Carbo=carboplatin, GMB :gemcitabine, NS: non significant; HR: Hazard ratio, cy: cycles

cycles of platinum-based treatment followed by surgery or immediate surgery. Overall, 75% of patients completed all three planned cycles of chemotherapy, but there was no evidence of a benefit in terms of overall survival (HR 1.02; 95% CI 0.80–1.31; $p = 0.86$). The results of this trial were criticized because of the high percentage of patients with stage I disease included[43].

The Southwest Oncology Group (SWOG) 9900 trial evaluated the role of carboplatin/paclitaxel doublet as neoadjuvant treatment in patients with stage IB–IIIA NSCLC. A total of 354 patients were enrolled, but the trial was prematurely terminated when positive results were obtained in the large phase III adjuvant trials[44]. The median OS was 41 months in the surgery-only arm and 62 months in the pre-operative chemotherapy arm (HR 0.79; 95% CI 0.60–1.06; $p = 0.11$). The median progression-free survival (PFS) was 20 months for surgery alone and 33 months for pre-operative chemotherapy (HR 0.80; 95% CI 0.61–1.04; $p = 0.10$).

Neoadjuvant and adjuvant chemotherapy were compared to surgery alone in the three-arm NATCH trial by Felip et al.[45]. In this trial, 624 patients with stage IA (tumour size > 2 cm), IB, II, or T3N1 were randomly assigned to surgery alone, three cycles of pre-operative paclitaxel/carboplatin followed by surgery, or surgery followed by three cycles of the same chemotherapy regimen. Although compliance with chemotherapy was better in the neoadjuvant

arm (90 vs 61% of patients receiving three cycles), no significant differences were observed in terms of 5-year disease-free survival rate (34, 38 and 37% for surgery, neoadjuvant and adjuvant arms, respectively) or 5-year OS rate (44, 47 and 46% for surgery, neoadjuvant and adjuvant arms, respectively).

Finally, another recent European phase III trial by Scagliotti et al. evaluated the role of another active doublet (cisplatin/gemcitabine) in patients with stage IB–IIIA disease. This trial was also prematurely terminated after the documentation of positive results from adjuvant trials, after only 270 patients of the 712 originally planned were enrolled[42].

The results of these trials (Table 14.3) do not support the use of neoadjuvant chemotherapy rather than immediate surgery followed by adjuvant chemotherapy[46]. Further investigation is required to select the ideal regimen in terms of efficacy and safety and to identify subgroups of patients and/or predictive factors associated with greater benefit.

Induction chemoradiotherapy

To improve resection rates, local control and pathological response, induction approaches that combined radiotherapy and chemotherapy were evaluated in the context of phase II trials[47–49]. A German phase III trial evaluated the role of neoadjuvant chemoradiotherapy in patients with IIIA–IIIB

NSCLC and invasive mediastinal assessment[50]. Patients were randomized to receive either three cycles of cisplatin/etoposide doublet, followed by twice-daily radiation with concurrent carboplatin and vindesine, and then surgical resection; or three cycles of cisplatin and etoposide, followed by surgery, and then further radiotherapy. The primary endpoint was median PFS. A total of 558 patients were enrolled. There was no difference in PFS between treatment groups – either in eligible patients (median PFS 9.5 vs 10.0 months; 5-year PFS 16 vs 14%; HR 0.99; 95% CI 0.81–1.19; p = 0.87). In patients receiving a pneumonectomy, treatmentrelated mortality increased in the experimental group compared with the control group (7/50 [14%] vs 3/54 [6%]).

Conclusions

The results of several large phase III trials have demonstrated that adjuvant chemotherapy with cisplatin-based doublets offers a significant OS prolongation. These results have been further confirmed in meta-analyses. The benefit is most evident in patients with disease stage II–IIIA, while for patients with stage IB disease the results are controversial. There is no clear 'goldstandard' doublet. Adjuvant chemotherapy should be offered also to carefully selected elderly patients. There is no strong data to support routine use of neoadjuvant chemotherapy rather than immediate surgery followed by adjuvant chemotherapy. Post-operative radiotherapy was associated with poorer outcomes, and its role remains controversial. Use is not recommended outside a clinical trial.

References

1 Groome PA, Bolejack V, Crowley JJ, et al. The IASLC Lung Cancer Staging Project: validation of the proposals for revision of the T, N, and M descriptors and consequent stage groupings in the forthcoming (seventh) edition of the TNM classification of malignant tumours. *J Thorac Oncol* 2007; 2:694–705.

2 Chemotherapy in non-small cell lung cancer: a meta-analysis using updated data on individual patients from 52 randomised clinical trials. Non-small Cell Lung Cancer Collaborative Group. *BMJ* 1995; 311:899–909.

3 Keller SM, Adak S, Wagner H, et al. A randomized trial of postoperative adjuvant therapy in patients with completely resected stage II or IIIA non-small-cell lung cancer. Eastern Cooperative Oncology Group. *N Engl J Med* 2000; 343:1217–22.

4 Scagliotti GV, Fossati R, Torri V, et al. Randomized study of adjuvant chemotherapy for completely resected stage I, II, or IIIA non-small-cell Lung cancer. *J Natl Cancer Inst* 2003; 95:1453–61.

5 Waller D, Peake MD, Stephens RJ, et al. Chemotherapy for patients with non-small cell lung cancer: the surgical setting of the Big Lung Trial. *Eur J Cardiothorac Surg* 2004; 26:173–82.

6 Winton T, Livingston R, Johnson D, et al. Vinorelbine plus cisplatin vs. observation in resected non-small-cell lung cancer. *N Engl J Med* 2005; 352:2589–97.

7 Butts CA, Ding K, Seymour L, et al. Randomized phase III trial of vinorelbine plus cisplatin compared with observation in completely resected stage IB and II non-small-cell lung cancer: updated survival analysis of JBR-10. *J Clin Oncol* 2010; 28:29–34.

8 Bezjak A, Lee CW, Ding K, et al. Quality-of-life outcomes for adjuvant chemotherapy in early-stage non-small-cell lung cancer: results from a randomized trial, JBR.10. *J Clin Oncol* 2008; 26:5052–9.

9 Douillard JY, Rosell R, De LM, et al. Adjuvant vinorelbine plus cisplatin versus observation in patients with completely resected stage IB-IIIA non-small-cell lung cancer (Adjuvant Navelbine International Trialist Association [ANITA]): a randomised controlled trial. *Lancet Oncol* 2006; 7:719–27.

10 Arriagada R, Bergman B, Dunant A, et al. Cisplatin-based adjuvant chemotherapy in patients with completely resected non-small-cell lung cancer. *N Engl J Med* 2004; 350:351–60.

11 Arriagada R, Dunant A, Pignon JP, et al. Long-term results of the international adjuvant lung cancer trial evaluating adjuvant cisplatin-based chemotherapy in resected lung cancer. *J Clin Oncol* 2010; 28:35–42.

12 Strauss GM, Herndon JE, Maddaus MA, et al. Adjuvant paclitaxel plus carboplatin compared with observation in stage IB non-small-cell lung cancer: CALGB 9633 with the Cancer and Leukemia Group B, Radiation Therapy Oncology Group and North Central Cancer Treatment Group Study Groups. *J Clin Oncol* 2008; 26:5043–51.

13 Kato H, Ichinose Y, Ohta M, et al. A randomized trial of adjuvant chemotherapy with uracil-tegafur for adenocarcinoma of the lung. *N Engl J Med* 2004; 350: 1713–21.

14 Hamada C, Tanaka F, Ohta M, et al. Meta-analysis of postoperative adjuvant chemotherapy with tegafur-uracil

in non-small-cell lung cancer. *J Clin Oncol* 2005; 23:4999–5006.

15 Goss G, Lorimer I, Tsao MS, et al. A phase III randomized, double-blind, placebo-controlled trial of the epidermal growth factor receptor inhibitor gefitinb in completely resected stage IB-IIIA non-small cell lung cancer (NSCLC): NCIC CTG BR.19. *J Clin Oncol* 2010; 28:abstr LBA7005.

16 Sienel W, Varwerk C, Linder A, et al. Melanoma associated antigen (MAGE)–A3 expression in stages I and II non-small cell lung cancer: results of a multi-center study. *Eur J Cardiothorac Surg* 2004; 25:131–4.

17 Pignon JP, Tribodet H, Scagliotti GV, et al. Lung Adjuvant Cisplatin Evaluation: a pooled Analysis by the LACE Collaborative Group. *J Clin Oncol* 2008; 26:3552–9.

18 Arriagada R, Auperin A, Burdett S, et al. Adjuvant chemotherapy, with or without postoperative radiotherapy, in operable non-small-cell lung cancer: two meta-analyses of individual patient data. *Lancet* 2010; 375:1267–77.

19 Hotta K, Matsuo K, Ueoka H, et al. Role of adjuvant chemotherapy in patients with resected non-small-cell lung cancer: reappraisal with a meta-analysis of randomized controlled trials. *J Clin Oncol* 2004; 22:3860–7.

20 Sedrakyan A, Van Der Meulen J, O'Byrne K, et al. Postoperative chemotherapy for non-small cell lung cancer: a systematic review and meta-analysis. *J Thorac Cardiovasc Surg* 2004; 128:414–9.

21 Berghmans T, Paesmans M, Meert AP, et al. Survival improvement in resectable non-small cell lung cancer with (neo)adjuvant chemotherapy: results of a meta-analysis of the literature. *Lung Cancer* 2005; 49:13–23.

22 Bria E, Gralla RJ, Raftopoulos H, et al. Magnitude of benefit of adjuvant chemotherapy for non-small cell lung cancer: meta-analysis of randomized clinical trials. *Lung Cancer* 2009; 63:50–7.

23 Scott WJ, Howington J, Feigenberg S, et al. Treatment of non-small cell lung cancer stage I and stage II: ACCP evidence-based clinical practice guidelines (2nd edition). *Chest* 2007; 132:234S–42S.

24 Pisters KM, Evans WK, Azzoli CG, et al. Cancer Care Ontario and American Society of Clinical Oncology adjuvant chemotherapy and adjuvant radiation therapy for stages I–IIIA resectable non small-cell lung cancer guideline. *J Clin Oncol* 2007; 25:5506–18.

25 Crino L, Weder W, VanMeerbeeck JP, et al. Early stage and locally advanced (non-metastatic) non-small-cell lung cancer: ESMO clinical practice guidelines for diagnosis, treatment and follow-up. *Ann Oncol* 2010; 21:103–15.

26 Pallis AG, Scarci M. Are we treating enough elderly patients with early stage non-small cell lung cancer? *Lung Cancer* 2011; 74:149–54.

27 Fruh M, Rolland E, Pignon JP, et al. Pooled analysis of the effect of age on adjuvant cisplatin-based chemotherapy for completely resected non-small-cell lung cancer. *J Clin Oncol* 2008; 26:3573–81.

28 Pepe C, Hasan B, Winton TL, et al. Adjuvant vinorelbine and cisplatin in elderly patients: National Cancer Institute of Canada and Intergroup Study JBR.10. *J Clin Oncol* 2007; 25:1553–61.

29 Wisnivesky JP, Smith CB, Packer S, et al. Survival and risk of adverse events in older patients receiving postoperative adjuvant chemotherapy for resected stages II–IIIA lung cancer: observational

cohort study. *BMJ* 2011; 343: d4013.

30 Pallis AG, Gridelli C, van Meerbeeck JP, et al. EORTC Elderly Task Force and Lung Cancer Group and International Society for Geriatric Oncology (SIOG) experts' opinion for the treatment of non-small-cell lung cancer in an elderly population. *Ann Oncol* 2010; 21:692–706.

31 Pallis AG, Karamouzis MV. DNA repair pathways and their implication in cancer treatment. *Cancer Metastasis Rev* 2010; 29:677–85.

32 Olaussen KA, Dunant A, Fouret P, et al. DNA repair by ERCC1 in non-small-cell lung cancer and cisplatin-based adjuvant chemotherapy. *N Engl J Med* 2006; 355:983–91.

33 Kamal NS, Soria JC, Mendiboure J, et al. MutS homologue 2 and the long-term benefit of adjuvant chemotherapy in lung cancer. *Clin Cancer Rese* 2010; 16:1206–15.

34 Zhu CQ, Ding K, Strumpf D, et al. Prognostic and predictive gene signature for adjuvant chemotherapy in resected non-small-cell lung cancer. *J Clin Oncol* 2010; 28:4417–24.

35 Postoperative radiotherapy in non-small-cell lung cancer: systematic review and meta-analysis of individual patient data from nine randomised controlled trials. PORT Meta-analysis Trialists Group. *Lancet* 1998; 352:257–63.

36 Burdett S, Stewart L. Postoperative radiotherapy in non-small-cell lung cancer: update of an individual patient data meta-analysis. *Lung Cancer* 2005; 47:81–3.

37 Okawara G, Ung YC, Markman BR, et al. Postoperative radiotherapy in stage II or IIIA completely resected non-small cell lung cancer: a systematic review and practice guideline. *Lung Cancer* 2004; 44:1–11.

38 Rosell R, Gomez-Codina J, Camps C, et al. A randomized trial comparing preoperative chemotherapy plus surgery with surgery alone in patients with non-small-cell lung cancer. *N Engl J Med* 1994; 330:153–8.

39 Roth JA, Fossella F, Komaki R, et al. A randomized trial comparing perioperative chemotherapy and surgery with surgery alone in resectable stage IIIA non-small-cell lung cancer. *J Natl Cancer Inst* 1994; 86:673–80.

40 Depierre A, Milleron B, Moro-Sibilot D, et al. Preoperative chemotherapy followed by surgery compared with primary surgery in resectable stage I (except T1N0), II, and IIIa non-small-cell lung cancer. *J Clin Oncol* 2002; 20:247–53.

41 Westeel V, Milleron B, Quoix E, et al. Long-term results of the French randomized trial comparing neoadjuvant chemotherapy followed by surgery versus surgery alone in resectable non-small cell lung cancer. *J Clin Oncol* 2010; 28:abstr 7003.

42 Scagliotti GV, Pastorino U, Vansteenkiste JF, et al. Randomized phase III study of surgery alone or surgery plus preoperative cisplatin and gemcitabine in stages IB to IIIA non-small-cell lung cancer. *J Clin Oncol* 2012; 30:172–8.

43 Gilligan D, Nicolson M, Smith I, et al. Preoperative chemotherapy in patients with resectable non-small cell lung cancer: results of the MRC LU22/NVALT 2/EORTC 08012 multicentre randomised trial and update of systematic review. *Lancet* 2007; 369:1929–37.

44 Pisters KM, Vallieres E, Crowley JJ, et al. Surgery with or without preoperative paclitaxel and carboplatin in early-stage non-small-cell lung cancer: Southwest Oncology Group Trial S9900, an intergroup, randomized, phase III trial. *J Clin Oncol* 2010; 28:1843–9.

45 Felip E, Rosell R, Maestre JA, et al. Preoperative chemotherapy plus surgery versus surgery plus adjuvant chemotherapy versus surgery alone in early-stage non-small-cell lung cancer. *J Clin Oncol* 2010; 28:3138–45.

46 Bradbury PA, Shepherd FA. Chemotherapy and surgery for operable NSCLC. *Lancet* 2007; 369:1903–4.

47 Albain KS, Rusch VW, Crowley JJ, et al. Concurrent cisplatin/etoposide plus chest radiotherapy followed by surgery for stages IIIA (N2) and IIIB non-small-cell lung cancer: mature results of Southwest Oncology Group phase II study 8805. *J Clin Oncol* 1995; 13:1880–92.

48 Choi NC, Carey RW, Daly W, et al. Potential impact on survival of improved tumor downstaging and resection rate by preoperative twice-daily radiation and concurrent chemotherapy in stage IIIA non-small-cell lung cancer. *J Clin Oncol* 1997; 15:712–22.

49 Eberhardt W, Wilke H, Stamatis G, et al. Preoperative chemotherapy followed by concurrent chemoradiation therapy based on hyperfractionated accelerated radiotherapy and definitive surgery in locally advanced non-small-cell lung cancer: mature results of a phase II trial. *J Clin Oncol* 1998; 16:622–34.

50 Thomas M, Rube C, Hoffknecht P, et al. Effect of preoperative chemoradiation in addition to preoperative chemotherapy: a randomised trial in stage III non-small-cell lung cancer. *Lancet Oncol* 2008; 9:636–48.

Chapter 15

Superior vena cava obstruction

Etiology, clinical presentation and principles of treatment

Federico Venuta, Marco Anile, Miriam Patella and Erino A. Rendina

Superior vena cava (SVC) syndrome: definition

The symptoms resulting from compression or obstruction of the SVC system at any level, from the left and right brachiocephalic veins to the right atrium.

Historical notes

The SVC syndrome was first described in 1757 by William Hunter in a patient with a saccular aneurysm of the ascending aorta. At autopsy, "the superior vena cava and innominate vein were both so much compressed by the dilated artery as hardly to have anything left in the natural capacity and appearance"[1]. Almost two hundred years later, Stokes, in 1837, described SVC syndrome related to a malignant tumor arising in the right lung; he observed that the underlying clinical findings were the result of the neoplastic compression on the vein and the progressive development of collateral circulation[2]. Rosenblatt published in the early 1960s a review on lung cancer in the nineteenth century[3] reporting several cases of SVC syndrome secondary to bronchogenic carcinoma.

Before the mid-twentieth century, only about one-third of the cases of SVC syndrome were related to malignant tumors; in fact, most were due to infections (syphilis causing aortic aneurysms or tuberculosis) or fibrotic mediastinitis[4]. This etiological distribution remained stable up to 30–40 years ago, when 40% of the cases were still related to these diseases[5]. From that time, improvement in treatment of granulomatous and infectious diseases and their prevention favored changes in the etiological distribution; nowadays, malignancy, in particular,

lung cancer, has far overcome benign disorders as the primary cause of the syndrome.

This etiological shift from benign to malignant disorders consequently required a change in the therapeutic approach; surgical resection of the vessel en bloc with the tumor and subsequent reconstruction progressively became a viable therapeutic option. The first SVC bypass graft with an autologous superficial femoral vein was described in 1951 by Klassen and colleagues[6]. However, complete sleeve resection and subsequent reconstruction of the SVC uniformly failed until the successful reconstruction by a spiral vein graft was described[7]. Notwithstanding the progressive improvement of long-term patency rates, the complexity of this surgical technique prevented widespread acceptance. In 1987, Dartevelle and associates described the use of polytetrafluoroethylene (PTFE) grafts with proven patency in patients with neoplastic involvement of the SVC[8]. Nowadays, excellent patency rates are achieved both with synthetic materials and with autologous and heterologous pericardium.

The potential role of stenting in patients with inoperable SVC obstruction, although it allows immediate symptoms relief, is still to be clearly defined since long-term patency remains to be assessed[9].

Etiology

SVC obstruction occurs is as many as 15 000 patients a year in the United States[10]; approximately 73 to 97% of the cases are secondary to malignancy[11–16]; bronchogenic carcinoma is certainly the most frequent cause, accounting for 65 to 80% of the cases. Approximately 3% of the patients with lung cancer develop SVC involvement[16–20]; 10% of the patients with right-sided tumors show it. SVC involvement occurs either by

Core Topics in Thoracic Surgery, ed. Marco Scarci, Aman Coonar, Tom Routledge and Francis Wells. Published by Cambridge University Press. © Cambridge University Press 2016

primary tumor invasion or compression or by enlarged peritracheal lymph nodes. The tumor may grow beyond the wall of the vessel into the lumen and favor thrombosis with progressive complete closure of the vein, branch vessels and collaterals. In most patients with this presentation of lung cancer, histology shows small cell carcinoma (SCC)[5]; this is probably due to the fact that this tumor (although it accounts for only 25% of all cases of bronchogenic carcinoma) often arises in the central or perihilar areas of the lung and gives extremely early lymphatic metastases at the omolateral (N2) or contralateral (N3) mediastinal stations.

Other causes of neoplastic involvement of the SVC are related to mediastinal tumors (20% of cases), particularly stage III thymoma and thymic carcinoma, germ cell tumors, and lymphoma (almost invariably non-Hodgkin); in children, T-cell leukemia and lymphoma are the most frequent causes of malignant SVC obstruction. Metastatic lesions (particularly breast cancer) are responsible for 5% of malignant SVC obstructions; primary vascular tumors are rarely observed[21].

The increased use of indwelling central venous catheters, cardiac pacemakers and defibrillator leads resulted in a higher incidence of benign SVC obstruction. Also postirradiation vascular fibrosis has been described[22].

Among the infectious etiologies, the most frequent is fibrosing mediastinitis due to tuberculosis, syphilis, histoplasmosis, actinomycosis, aspergillosis, blastomycosis, filariasis, and direct spread of nocardiosis.

Other, rarer causes of SVC obstruction are sarcoidosis, sclerosing colangytis, goiter, aortic aneurisms, fibrosing mediastinitis, Hughes-Stovin or Behcet's syndrome, and idiopathic fibrosing mediastinitis.

Anatomy

The confluence of the left and right innominate veins at the level of the cartilaginous portion of the first right rib gives rise to the SVC (Figure 15.1). The left brachiocephalic vein is much longer than the right one and crosses the anterosuperior mediastinum from left to right posteriorly to the thymus or its remnants. The SVC has a diameter of 2 cm and an average length of 7 cm; it descends toward the right atrium laterally to the ascending aorta and medially to the right mediastinal pleura and lung. Other anatomical structures adjacent to the SVC are the right

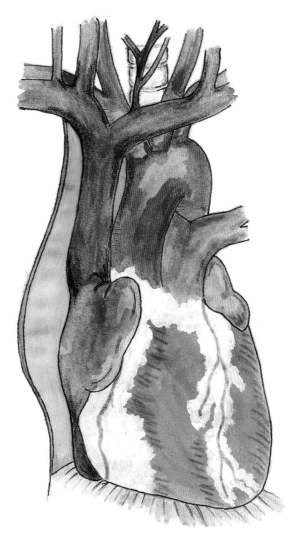

Figure 15.1 Anatomy of the superior vena cava and brachiocephalic veins.

paratracheal lymphatic chain, the right pulmonary artery, crossing the vessel posteriorly, the upper right pulmonary vein, the phrenic nerve, and the thymus or its remnants with mediastinal fat.

The junction between the SVC and the right atrium lies within the pericardium that surrounds the anterolateral surface of the vessel for about 2 cm. At the level of the anterolateral aspect of the junction with the atrium is located the sinus node.

Anatomy of the collateral SVC routes:

A) <u>Azygous venous system</u>: it drains directly into the extrapericardial posterior aspect of the SVC immediately above the level where the right pulmonary artery crosses the vein posteriorly.

151

B) Internal thoracic venous system: through this system blood converges into the inferior vena cava (IVC) from the internal thoracic vein through the epigastric veins and the external and common iliac veins.

C) Vertebral venous system: The blood flows into the IVC through the brachiocephalic veins and the intercostal, lumbar, and sacral veins.

D) External thoracic venous system: this is the superficial collateral system connecting the subclavian and axillary veins to the femoral veins through the lateral thoracic, thoracoepigastric, and superficial epigastric veins.

Clinical presentation

Obstruction of the SVC due to compression, invasion, constriction, or thrombosis shows a different pattern of clinical presentation based on its acuity and degree. The SVC drains blood from the head, neck, and upper extremities. If the SVC obstruction progresses slowly, adequate collateral drainage develops, and patients potentially show no or mild symptoms. On the other hand, if vascular obstruction develops acutely, patients are obviously more symptomatic since the collateral circulation has no time to develop and compensate. In this case the signs and symptoms might be dramatic. The eyes are usually affected first, and patients complain of tearing and swelling of eyelids. They also refer to headache, dizziness, tinnitus, and a bursting sensation in the head exacerbated when bending forward. The face, neck, and arms become red and edematous; the superficial veins of the chest may be distended if they are part of the collateral circulation. These symptoms are greatly increased when also the azygous vein is obstructed. Some patients may find some symptomatic relief in the upright position; for this reason, they sleep in a chair to avoid dyspnea. The venous hypertension might cause life-threatening complications such as cerebral edema, thrombosis, and hemorrhage or laryngeal and/or glossal edema.

Since most of the SVC obstructions are caused by bronchogenic carcinoma or mediastinal neoplasms, patients might show also symptoms related to the tumor, including paraneoplastic syndromes.

Pathophysiology

The SVC is located in an anatomic compartment that has limited distensibility; due to the thin walls and inner low pressure it is easily obstructed by compression, invasion, and constriction; also, thrombosis due to hypercoagulation, intimal damage, and/or stasis may be involved. Severe obstruction dramatically increases the endovascular pressure up to 400–500 cmH_2O. As aforementioned, in case of acute SVC obstruction, the collateral systems do not have time to accommodate the increased blood flow. On the other hand, in case of slow progression of obstruction, palliation from collateral circulation is more pronounced. The site of obstruction is extremely important: when the azygous vein orifice is not involved, the collateral pathways are more efficient since this system easily accommodates the shunted blood with acceptable flow due to its caliber and distensibility. On the other hand, when the azygous system can't compensate due to the location of the tumor, the blood flow runs through the other venous systems that are less efficient for the smaller caliber and major length of the pathway; for these reasons, in these situations, signs and symptoms are more pronounced.

Diagnosis

SVC syndrome is a clinical diagnosis; radiologic confirmation is usually not strictly necessary, although it might be helpful. However, it is crucial to diagnose the underlying disease since treatment is different according to its nature.

Routine radiologic studies include chest X-ray, computed tomography (CT), and magnetic resonance imaging (MRI). Also Doppler studies[23] and digital subtraction angiography have been employed[24].

SVC syndrome is rarely a true emergency[25]; for this reason, any treatment should be delayed until a precise histologic diagnosis is obtained. However, if urgent symptomatic treatment is deemed necessary, the diagnosis can be delayed until at least endovascular treatment is performed, especially in case of inoperable tumors.

The approach to obtain tissue for diagnosis depends on tumor location, clinical status of the patient, and available expertise. According to these key points, bronchoscopy, needle biopsy, endoscopic ultrasound (EUS) or endobronchial ultrasound (EBUS)[26], mediastinoscopy[27], anterior mediastinotomy, median sternotomy, video-assisted thoracoscopy (VATS), and even thoracotomy might be indicated.

Treatment

Management depends on etiology and severity of symptoms. It should take into account several key points. Measures such as head elevation, fluid restriction, administration of diuretics, and supplemental oxygen are useful until the diagnosis is obtained and treatment can be planned.

According to the clinical presentation and to histologic diagnosis, pharmacologic treatment, radiation therapy (with or without concomitant chemotherapy), and invasive procedures including endovascular stent deployment and surgical resection and reconstruction should be considered.

Patients affected by catheter-related SVC thrombosis should receive anticoagulant treatment and may require catheter removal. Heparin administration favors clot lysis; as an alternative, thrombolytic agents can be given through the catheter itself, especially if it is centered in the thrombus. This therapy is extremely successful when started within 48 hours of the onset of thrombosis; its efficacy strongly decreases after a longer period of time. Urokinase is usually more successful than streptokinase[28]. In patients with extensive malignancy, this treatment should be evaluated more carefully.

In patients with SVC syndrome related to inoperable tumors, radiotherapy is an effective treatment modality, and it is usually the initial choice once the diagnosis is available. Many fractional dose schemes have been proposed; however, despite the various dosing regimens described, most patients receive a total of 20 to 30 Gy[29,30].

Percutaneous delivery of metallic stents has become a viable option to treat patients with SVC obstruction not suitable for surgical resection. Several endovascular stents are available basically in two designs: self-expanding and expandable[31,32]; however, the Wallstent (Boston Scientific, Natick, MA) is certainly the most commonly used[33]. Stents are usually employed in association with adjuvant therapies: intravenous heparin is administered before and after placement[34]; thrombolysis is performed if clots occlude the lumen of the vessel.

Surgery is overall rarely indicated; however, it plays clearly an important role in patients with resectable lung cancer or mediastinal tumors without distant or lymphatic spread. Notwithstanding that, resection and reconstruction of the SVC are still considered major technical and anesthesiological challenges, clear benefits have been reported with adequate patients selection, planning of the surgical strategy, and prevention of complications[35–37].

Median sternotomy is the optimal approach for anterior mediastinal tumors, while right thoracotomy in the fourth or fifth intercostal space should be employed for upper lobe tumors invading the SVC. These approaches allow optimal exposure and access to the lung, SVC and azygous vein, trachea, pulmonary hilum, and right atrium; the left brachiocephalic vein is obviously more visible through median sternotomy. Cardiopulmonary bypass (CPBP) and shunts are easily instituted through both approaches when required.

Intraoperative management is extremely important and should be planned in advance. Partial caval clamping (tangential) or clamping of a vessel with a long history of occlusion and presence of a viable collateral circulation is usually well tolerated. In these situations, the duration of clamping is not a major issue. On the other hand, complete clamping of an unobstructed vessel causes an important hemodynamic derangement with consequent venous pressure increase, decrease in arterial pressure, and reduced brain arteriovenous gradient. This might cause brain edema, hemorrhage, or transient dysfunction. The hemodynamic imbalance is reduced by an aggressive intraoperative management; fluid implementation by macromolecules, blood, and plasma is recommended and should be obtained through a femoral vein access; diuretics should be administered to reduce brain edema; anticoagulation therapy is mandatory during and immediately after the operation. Intravascular or extravascular shunts might be useful when a prolonged complete clamping time is required; CPBP is rarely required.

If the SVC is involved for less than 30% of its circumference, partial resection is usually feasible, and reconstruction can be performed either by direct suture of the tangential resection or by interposition of a patch (Figure 15.2); in this case, autologous material (either pericardial or venous) can be successfully employed. When a more extended involvement of the vessel is present, complete resection en bloc with the primary tumor and prosthetic reconstruction are required. Reconstruction can be accomplished by SVC replacement if the confluence of the brachiocephalic veins is disease-free (Figure 15.3). To avoid kinking of the prosthesis, whatever material is used, the length of the conduit should be adapted to keep it

153

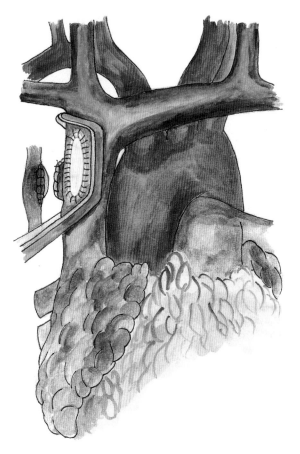

Figure 15.2 Patch reconstruction of the superior vena cava.

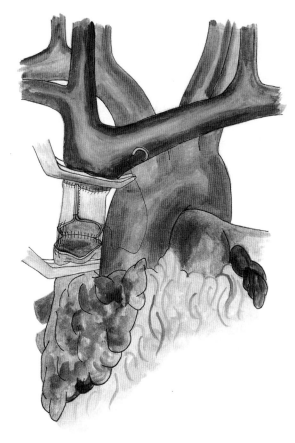

Figure 15.3 Superior vena cava reconstruction with a bovine pericardium conduit.

under moderate tension; this is particularly important when the operation is carried out through a median sternotomy, since approximation of the bone edges may cause kinking of the conduit. If the confluence of the innominate veins is involved by the tumor, the reconstruction is usually performed connecting only the two veins to the inferior SVC stump or to the right atrium, closing the contralateral vessel (Figure 15.4). Revascularization of both innominate veins connected independently to the right atrium is usually not performed for the risk of thrombosis, unless the collateral circulation in the neck is completely absent (previous neck surgery or radiotherapy). However, complete resections of the SVC and both brachiocephalic veins with a reconstruction achieved by a Y-shaped synthetic conduit have been reported[38].

Both biologic (autologous and heterologous) and synthetic materials are nowadays available for

vascular reconstructions. Biologic materials include autologous or bovine pericardium, azygous vein, and saphenous vein; they clearly show improved biocompatibility, decreased risk of infectious complications and thrombosis, and lower costs. Autologous pericardium has been used especially for patch reconstruction. It shows several advantages: it has adequate thickness and resistance; it is cost-free and available on both sides of the chest; it also offers a larger amount of tissue when compared with venous patches. An original method of fixation of autologous pericardium with glutaraldeyde[39] has been described to further improve the technical features of this material; with this technique, the fixed leaflet becomes stiffer with a reduced tendency to shrink or curl, and it is easier to tailor and suture.

Bovine pericardium is certainly the most used heterologous biologic material. It shows stiff edges and a limited tendency to retract; it is more frequently

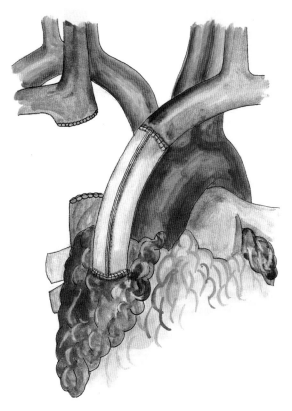

Figure 15.4 Revascularization between the left brachiocephalic vein and the right atrium with a conduit of bovine pericardium.

used for complete SVC replacement because autologous pericardium is not sufficient to create a long conduit. In our experience, the use of this material does not require long-term anticoagulation. An original technique has been described to construct a pericardial conduit suitable for SVC reconstruction[40]: the leaflet is trimmed in length and closed in a tubular shape with a mechanical GIA 75 stapler. This technique is easy and fast; it is precise and allows more regular shape of the graft, facilitating the anastomosis with the vascular stumps.

Reinforced PTFE is the option of choice among synthetic materials; it shows the highest patency rate in the long run when compared to other synthetic conduits, and shortly after the operation, it shows autologous reepithelization.

Postoperative complications of these procedures include problems at the graft anastomosis, graft thrombosis, and infection.

Results

Untreated malignant SVC obstructions usually show a very poor prognosis. The median overall survival at 1 year is 35% for non-small cell lung cancer (NSCLC) and 18% for small cell lung cancer (SCLC)[47]. In patients with operable NSCLC, overall 5-year survival is 15–30%[42–46]; the prognosis is usually better for patients with SVC involvement due to the primary tumor and not to enlarged mediastinal lymph nodes with extracapsular invasion. In 1998, the Marie Lonnelongue Hospital Group in Paris reported a 17-year experience on 89 patients with primary mediastinal tumors resected en bloc with adjacent structures (47 thymic tumors)[41]. In this series, 40% of the patients underwent resection of great vessels including SVC in 21 cases and innominate vein in 13. In 79% of the patients, the resection margins were tumor free. Overall 5-year survival was 63%; it was 69% for patients with thymoma, 42% for those with thymic carcinoma, 48% for those with germ cell tumors, and 83% for those with lymphoma. The recurrence rate was significantly higher in patients with thymic carcinoma.

Conclusion

For malignant etiologies there is rarely a role for surgical intervention with the exception of a limited number of patients with non-N2–3 NSCLC invading the SVC or mediastinal tumors, particularly thymoma. PTFE and autologous or bovine pericardium are the most frequently used replacement materials.

The currently available expandable stents provide appropriate and immediate symptomatic relief; in these cases, chemoradiotherapy is usually administered after stent deployment.

In case of SVC obstruction of benign etiologies, most commonly mediastinal fibrosis, surgical reconstruction should be performed only in patients without adequate collateral circulation.

References

1 Hunter W. History of aneurysms of the aorta with some remarks on aneurysms in general. *Medical Observations and Inquiries (London)* 1757; 1:323.

2 Stokes W. *Treatise on the Diagnosis and Treatment of Diseases of the Chest.* Dublin: Hodges and Smith, 1837: 370.

3 Rosenblatt MB. Lung cancer in the 19th century. *Bull His Med* 1964; 38:395–425.

4   Mcintyre FT, Sykes EM. Obstruction of the superior vena cava: review of the literature and report of two personal cases. *Ann Intern Med* 1949; 30:925–60.

5   Markman M. Diagnosis and management of superior vena cava syndrome. *Cleve Clin J Med* 1999; 66:59–61.

6   Klassen KP; Andrews NC, Curtis GH. Diagnosis and treatment of superior vena cava obstruction. *Arch Surg* 1951; 63:311–25.

7   Doty DB. Bypass of superior vena cava: six years experience with spiral vein graft for obstruction of superior vena cava due to benign and malignant disease. *J Thorac Cardiovasc Surg* 1982; 83:326–38.

8   Dartevelle P, Chapelier A, Navajos M, et al. Replacement of the superior vena cava with polytetrafluoroethylene grafts combined with resection of mediastinal-pulmonary malignant tumors: report of thirteen cases. *J Thorac Cardiovasc Surg* 1987; 93:361–3.

9   Sheikh MA, Fernandez BB Jr, Gray BM, et al. Endovascular stenting of nonmalignant superior vena cava syndrome. *Cathet Cardiovasc Interv* 2005; 65:405–11.

10 Wudel LJ Jr, Nesbitt JC. Superior vena cava syndrome. *Curr Treat Opt Oncol* 2001; 2:77–91.

11 Fincher RM. Superior vena cava syndrome: experience in a teaching hospital. *South Med J* 1987; 80:1243–5.

12 Parish JM, Marschke RF, Diners DE, et al. Etiologic considerations in superior vena cava syndrome. *Mayo Clin Proc* 1981; 56:407–13.

13 Banker VP, Maddison FE. Superior vena cava syndrome secondary to aortic disease: report of two cases and review of the literature. *Dis Chest* 1967; 51:656–62.

14 Kamyia K, Nahata Y, Naiki K, et al. Superior vena cava syndrome. *Vasc Dis* 1967; 4:59–65.

15 Ahmann FR. A reassessment of the clinical implications of the superior vena cava syndrome. *J Clin Oncol* 1984; 2:961–9.

16 Lockridge SK, Knobbe WP, Doty DB. Obstruction of the superior vena cava. *Surgery*; 1979; 85:14–24.

17 Perez CA, Presant CA, Van Amburg AL. Management of superior vena cava syndrome. *Semin Oncol* 1978; 5:123–34.

18 Salsali M, Clifton EE. Superior vena cava obstruction with carcinoma of the lung. *Surg Gynecol Obstet* 1965; 121:783–6.

19 Escalante CP. Causes and management of superior vena cava syndrome. *Oncology* 1993; 7:61–xx.

20 Nogeire C, Mincer F, Botsetin C. Long survival in patients with bronchogenic carcinoma complicated by superior vena cava obstruction. *Chest* 1979; 75:325–9.

21 Tuncer ON, Erbesan O, Golbasi I. Primary intravascular synovial sarcoma: case report. *Heart Surg Forum* 2012; 15:E297–9.

22 Castongue M, Rodrigues G, Vincent M, et al. Chemoradiation induced superior vena cava syndrome: a case report. *Can Respir J* 2008; 15:444–6.

23 Gooding GA, Hightower DR, Moore EH, Burke MW. Obstruction of the superior vena cava or subclavian veins: sonographic diagnosis. *Radiology* 1986; 159:663–5.

24 Sharma RP, Keller CE, Shetty PC, Burke MW. Superior vena cava obstruction evaluation with digital subtraction angiography. *Radiology* 1986; 160:845.

25 Samphao S, Eremin JM, Eremin O. Oncological emergencies: clinical importance and principles of management. *Eur J Cancer Care (Engl)* 2010; 19:707–13.

26 Wong MK, Tam TC, Lam DC, et al. EBUS–TBNA in patients presented with superior vena cava syndrome. *Lung Cancer* 2012; 77:277– 80.

27 Pop D, Venissac N, Nadeemy AS, et al. Video assisted mediastinoscopy in superior vena cava obstruction: to fear or not to fear? *J Thorac Oncol* 2012; 7:386–9.

28 Gray B, Olin JW, Graor RA, et al. Safety and efficacy of thrombolytic therapy for superior vana cava syndrome. *Chest* 1991; 99:54–9.

29 Armstrong BA, Perez CA, Simpson JR, Hederman MA. Role of irradiation in the management of superior vena cava syndrome. *Int J Radiat Oncol Biol Phys* 1987; 13:531–9.

30 Rodrigues CI, Njo KH, Karim AB. Hyperfractionated radiation therapy in the treatment of superior vena cava syndrome. *Lung Cancer* 1993; 10:221–8.

31 Crowe MTI, Davies CH, Gaines PA. Percutaneous management of superior vena cava occlusions. *Cardiovasc Intervent Radiol* 1995; 18:367–72.

32 Rosenblum J, Leef J, Messersmith R, et al. Intravascular stents in the management of acute superior vena cava obstruction of benign etiology. *J Parenteral Enteral Nutr* 1994; 18:362–6.

33 Lanciego C, Pangue C, Chacon JI, et al. Endovascular stenting as the first step in the overall management of malignant superior vena cava syndrome. *Am J Roetgenol* 2009; 193:549–58.

34 Hochrein J, Bashore TM, O'Laughlin MP, Harrison JK. Percutaneous stenting of the superior vena cava syndrome: a case report and review of the literature. *Am J Med* 1998; 104:78–84.

35 D'Andrilli A, Venuta F, Rendina EA. Surgical approaches for invasive tumors of the anterior mediastinum. *Thorac Surg Clin* 2010; 20:265–84.

36 Grunenwald DH. Resection of lung carcinomas invading the mediastinum, including the superior vena cava. *Thorac Surg Clin* 2004; 14:255–63.

37 Macchiarini P. Superior vena cava obstruction. In: Patterson JA et al. *Pearson's Thoracic & Esophageal Surgery*. Churchill Livingstone, 2008: 1684–6.

38 Chen KN, Xu SF, Gu ZD, et al. Surgical treatment of complex malignant anterior mediastinal tumors invading the superior vena cava. *World J Surg* 2006; 30:162–70.

39 D'Andrilli A, Ibrahim M, Venuta F, et al. Glutaraldeyde preserved autologous pericardium for patch reconstruction of the pulmonary artery and superior vena cava. *Ann Thorac Surg* 2005; 80:357–8.

40 D'Andrilli A, Ciccone AM, Ibrahim M, et al. A new technique for prosthetic reconstruction of the superior vena cava. *J Thorac Cardiovasc Surg* 2006; 132:192–4.

41 Engelmeers A, Goor C, Meerbeck J, et al. Palliative effectiveness of radiation therapy in the treatment of superior vena cava syndrome. *Bull Cancer Radiother* 1996; 83:153–7.

42 Spaggiari L, Thomas P, Magdelenait P. Superior vena cava resection with prosthetic replacement for non small cell lung cancer: long term results of a multicentric study. *Eur J Cardiothoracic Surg* 2002; 21:1080–6.

43 Suzuki K, Asamura H, Watanabe S, Tsuchiya R. Combined resection of superior vena cava for lung carcinoma: prognostic significance of patterns of superior vena cava invasion. *Ann Thorac Surg* 2004; 78:1184–9.

44 Thomas P, Magnan PE, Moulin G, et al. Extended operation for lung cancer invading the superior vena cava. *Eur J Cardiothoracic Surg* 1994; 8:177–82.

45 Spaggiari L, Pastorino U, Combined sleeve and superior vena cava resections for non small cell lung cancer. *Ann Thorac Surg* 2000; 70:1172–5.

46 Lanuti M, De Delva PE, Gaissert HA, et al. Review of superior vena cava resection in the management of benign disease and pulmonary or mediastinal malignancies. *Ann Thorac Surg* 2009; 88:392–7.

47 Bacha EA, Chapelier AR, Macchiarini P, et al. Surgery for invasive mediastinal tumors. *Ann Thorac Surg* 1998; 66:234–9.

Chapter 16

Robotics in thoracic surgery

Marlies Keijzers, Peyman Sardari Nia and Jos G. Maessen

Life is pretty simple: You do some stuff. Most fails. Some works. You do more of what works. If it works big, others quickly copy it. Then you do something else. The trick is the doing something else.
– Leonardo da Vinci

Introduction

Minimally invasive thoracic surgery has been a hot topic in the past decades. With the development of robotic surgery, thoracic surgeons entered a newer and more exciting field. Much progress in minimally invasive surgery has been made, and robotic surgery is accepted as a potential diagnostic and treatment modality for thoracic diseases. In this chapter, we provide a comprehensive review of the history and the current data in robotic thoracic surgery.

History of minimally invasive thoracic surgery

The first thoracoscopic procedure was described 100 years ago. In 1910, Jacobaeus examined the pleural cavity with a cytoscope and was the first to perform a thoracoscopic procedure[1]. In the late 1980s, minimally invasive surgical techniques were developed, and after the success of laparoscopic surgery, video-assisted thoracic surgery (VATS) was established in the 1990s.

The first prospective randomized studies did not meet the high expectations and showed no significant benefit for the VATS approach compared with thoracotomy[2,3]. More recent studies, however, show advantages such as reduced blood loss, less pain, lower inflammatory responses and an earlier return to work. Today, VATS plays a role in the diagnostic and therapeutic procedures for benign and malignant tumours arising from the lung or adjacent organs[4,5]. Although these studies show favourable results, there are still important limitations. The lack of three-dimensional vision, loss of wrist articulation and natural hand-eye coordination can reduce surgical precision[6].

Robotic surgical systems in the medical industry were developed to overcome these limitations. The first robotic system used for surgical procedures was the Puma 560. Kwoh et al. used the robot in 1985 to perform neurosurgical biopsies, and in 1988, Davies et al. performed a transurethral prostatectomy with the Puma 560[7]. Robotic systems developed later, originated from telepresence machines that were developed for NASA.

The rationale of developing a robotic system was to use it in the US Army in war areas by 'bringing the surgeon to the wounded soldier through telepresence'. This has been successfully tested in animal models, but it has not yet been utilized in the US Army for care of wounded soldiers in the battlefield. The researchers and surgeons of the US Army formed a research group for commercial purposes and introduced robotic surgery into civilian society[8].

The da Vinci Surgical System developed by the Stanford Research Institute was FDA approved in 2000 for general laparoscopic surgery, and in the next year it was approved for thoracic surgery. The robotic surgical approach is nowadays applied for thymectomies, lobectomies and esophagectomies. The da Vinci Surgical System is the most widely used robotic surgical system.

Core Topics in Thoracic Surgery, ed. Marco Scarci, Aman Coonar, Tom Routledge and Francis Wells. Published by Cambridge University Press. © Cambridge University Press 2016

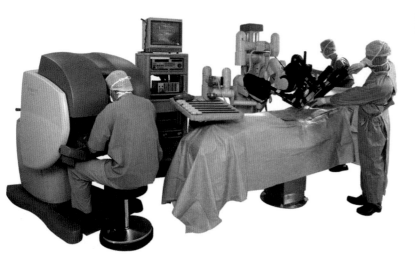

Figure 16.1 The da Vinci Surgical System set-up.

The da Vinci Surgical System

The da Vinci Surgical System was developed by Intuitive Surgical. Intuitive Surgical was created in 1995 by Frederic Moll MD Robert Younge and John Freud MD, and is based on technology developed by the Stanford Research Institute. The da Vinci Surgical System consists of an ergonomically designed master console for the surgeon, a bedside chassis with three to five interactive robotic arms, high-performance vision system and Endowrist instruments (Figure 16.1). The console contains high-definition three-dimensional optics and foot pedals to control tools. The surgeon can place fingers in the master controls, which are located below the display, with the hands and wrists in an ergonomic position.

The instruments are cable driven with 7 degrees of freedom and 360 degrees of rotation of the tip of the instruments (Figure 16.2). The three-dimensional image is displayed above the hands of the surgeon, giving the surgeon the perception of being in the surgical field.

Advantages

Compared with conventional thoracoscopic surgery, the da Vinci Surgical System has advantages (Table 16.1). One important benefit is the three-dimensional vision; the depth perception gives an improvement in the view over the cameras used in thoracoscopic surgery. The three-dimensional image is displayed above the surgeon's hands, resulting in better hand-eye coordination and eliminating the fulcrum effect, making manipulation of the instruments much easier. The instruments also offer superior manoeuvrability with

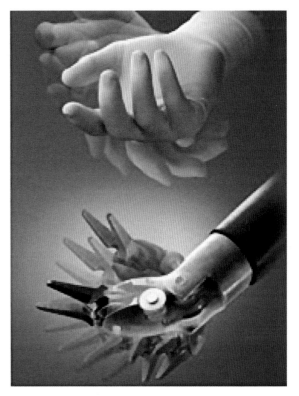

Figure 16.2 The superior manoeuvrability of the instruments.

7 degrees of freedom, 360 degrees of rotation of the tip of the instruments and elimination of physiologic tremors.

Disadvantages

Robotic surgery has a lot of advantages compared with thoracoscopic and conventional surgery, but it

159

Table 16.1 Advantages and disadvantages of robotic-assisted surgery

Advantages	Disadvantages
3-Dimensional vision	Expensive
Superior manoeuvrability	High start-up cost
No physiological tremors	Instrumental failure
No fulcrum effect	No touch sensation

has also some disadvantages. In thoracoscopic surgery, there is reduction in touch sensation; in robotic surgery, however, there is an absence of touch sensation. Robotic surgery is also very expensive; there are high start-up costs and costs in training of the staff. Another disadvantage is the possibility of failure of the instruments of the da Vinci Surgical System. A survey of the MAUDE database showed that failures occurred in a number of robotic instruments in a short period, although some failures may go unreported[9].

Thoracic applications of robotic surgery
Lung cancer

Lung cancer is the main cancer worldwide whether considered in terms of incidence or mortality. More patients die of lung cancer than breast, colon and prostate cancer together[10]. Only patients with early stage lung cancer qualify for surgical resection. With the development of new screening tools like low-dose computed tomography (LDCT), it is possible that more early-stage lung cancers suitable for surgical resection will be diagnosed in the future.

VATS lobectomy was first described in the early 1990s, and ever since, multiple studies have been published. However, only three of these published studies are randomized, controlled trials comparing VATS lobectomy to thoracotomy. There is also a great variability in the techniques described so far. The variability exists in the surgical approach for the lobectomy itself, size of the utility incision thoracotomy, number of incisions and the use of rib spreading. Despite this variability, the studies published to date have shown that VATS lobectomy is safe and effective. It is a feasible technique for early-stage lung cancer and provides at least the same oncological results. In addition to this, it has been shown that VATS lobectomy is associated with lower rates of post-operative complications and shorter duration of hospitalization.

Despite these advantages, VATS lobectomy is not very widely used by thoracic surgeons. According to the Society for Thoracic Surgeons (STS) Database (voluntary database), in 2006, around 32% of lobectomies were performed through VATS[11]. The authors showed that the percentage of lobectomies performed by VATS in the STS Database has been increasing: 21.6% in 2004 and 28.6% in 2005. In the Nationwide Inpatient Sample Database (nonvoluntary database in US), however, this number is as low as 6%[12], indicating the overall application of VATS lobectomies may be lower in nonacademic, smaller hospitals. The low application of VATS approach might be due to the limitations of VATS; it only has two-dimensional vision, hand-eye coordination is difficult, manoeuvrability is restricted and there is a steep learning curve. Robotic surgery might overcome these limitations. The use of robotic surgery for lobectomy is still in its infancy, so the literature is sparse. There are no published randomized, controlled trials comparing robotic lobectomy with VATS lobectomy.

Melfi et al. were in 2002 the first to report a series of robotic lobectomies, and they showed that it is safe and feasible[13]. Ever since, multiple series have been reported showing that robotic lobectomy is safe, feasible and has the same oncological results (Table 16.2). The early experiences with robotic lobectomy regarding chest tube drainage, morbidity, mortality, conversion rate and reasons for conversion are comparable with VATS[14–16].

The largest published series of robotic lobectomies is a multi-centre study by Park et al. The authors reported robotic lobectomies in 325 consecutive patients for early-stage non-small cell lung cancer (NSCLC) at three institutions[17]. The authors showed that robotic lobectomy for NSCLC was feasible and safe. The overall and stage-specific survival of robotic lobectomies for early-stage NSCLC was comparable with the reported series of (VATS) lobectomies in the literature[17,18]. With respect to the higher costs of robotic surgery related to purchase and maintenance of the technology, Park et al. reported that robotic surgery is more expensive than VATS but less expensive than open thoracotomy. This was mainly because of the longer hospitalization in patients who underwent open thoracotomy[19].

Table 16.2 Review of the published studies on robotic lobectomies

Authors	No. of patients	30 days mortality, %	Follow-up, mos.	OC, %	OT, minutes	LOS, days
Melfi et al. 2004[21]	23	4.3	—	8.7	192 †	5.0 †
Park et al. 2006[14]	34	0	—	12	218 *	4.5 *
Melfi et al. 2008[22]	107	0.9	—	9.4	220 *	5 †
Charagozloo et al. 2009[23]	100	3.0	32 *	0	216 †	4.0 *
Veronesi et al. 2010[24]	54	0	—	13	236 *	5.0 *
Augustin et al. 2011[25]	26	3.8	27 *	19	228 *	11.0 *
Dylewski et al. 2011[26]	154/200	3.0 ¶	—	1.5	90 *	3.0 *
Cerfolio et al. 2011[27]	104/168	0	—	7.7	132 *	2.0 *
Jang et al. 2011[28]	40	0	—	0	240 *	6.0 *
Veronesi et al. 2011[16]	91	0	24	11	239 *	5.0 *
Park et al. 2012[17]	325	0.3	27	8.0	206 *	5.0 *
Meyer et al. 2012[20]	185	1.6	—	1.6	211 †	4.0 *

¶, 60-day mortality rate; OC, open conversion; OT, operative time; LOS, length of hospital stay;
*, Median value,
† Mean value

Meyer et al. showed in a recent paper that the learning curve for robotic lobectomies in surgeons experienced with VATS was 18 ± 3 cases based on operative time, mortality and the surgeon's comfort[20].

An evaluation of the available literature shows that robotic surgery for lobectomies is comparable with the results in VATS lobectomies. However, additional research by prospective, randomized, controlled trials comparing VATS and robotic lobectomies is warranted to discern the differences between these two techniques.

Mediastinal surgery

Anterior mediastinum

In the anterior mediastinum, the most frequently found mediastinal mass is a thymoma. Thymomas and thymic carcinomas are rare tumours. Thymomas are frequently observed in patients with myasthenia gravis (MG). Up to 45% of the patients with a thymoma have MG, and in 10% of patients with MG, a thymoma is present[29]. The neurologist Oppenheim was the first who described the association between MG and the thymus[30]. The thymus gland plays a role in the complex pathogenesis of MG[31].

Therefore, thymectomy has been accepted as a standard treatment of MG for patients[32].

Myasthenia gravis (MG)

In 1936, Alfred Blalock was the first who performed a successful thymectomy by a median sternotomy in a patient with a mediastinal mass and MG[33]. Later, thymectomy by partial sternotomy, a transcervical approach, extended transcervical thymectomy, video-assisted thoracoscopic extended thymectomy and the transcervical subxyphoid-videothoracoscopic maximal thymectomy have been described[34,35]. Thymectomy has been reported as a possible treatment for nonthymomatous MG. Series comparing VATS with sternotomy in nonthymomatous MG have showed that in VATS thymectomy there is reduced operative blood loss, a shorter hospitalization and an equivalent MG remission rate[36]. Because of the heterogeneity in the surgical techniques described as VATS thymectomy, the evaluation and comparison of the studies are difficult.

On account of the lack of visualization, the unilateral procedure underwent several modifications; a bilateral approach, an addition cervical incision and an addition subxiphoid incision have been described.

Table 16.3 Review of the published studies on robotic thymectomy for thymomas

Authors	No. of patients	Masaoka stage I/II/III/IV	TS, cm	Follow-up, mos.	RR, %	OC, %	OT, minutes	LOS, days
Mussi et al. 2012[44]	13	7/6/0/0	3.3 [†]	14.5 [*]	0	7.7	139 [†]	4.0 [†]
Marulli et al. 2012[45]	79	30/49/0/0	3.7 [†]	51.7 [†]	1.3	1.3	165 [†]	4.4 [†]
Keijzers et al. 2014[46]	37	20/13/3/1	5.1 [†]	41 [†]	2.7	10.4	149 [†]	3.0 [*]

TS, tumor size; RR, recurrence rate; OC, open conversion; OT, operative time; LOS, length of hospital stay.
[*], Median value,
[†] Mean value

Proponents of the robotic approach argue that it facilitates a total extended resection for MG by a minimal invasive approach more accurately than thoracoscopic surgery. In 2004, Bodner et al. were the first to report a series of 10 robotic thymectomies with an operative morbidity and mortality of 0% and a hospitalization of less than 3 days. Multiple small series have been reported ever since and have shown that robotic thymectomy for non-thymomatous MG is feasible, safe and can produce high cumulative complete remission rates[37-39].

Rückert et al. showed in a retrospective cohort with 79 thoracoscopic and 74 robotic thymectomies that the cumulative complete remission rate of MG is higher in the robotic group. After a follow-up of 42 months, the cumulative complete remission rate was 20.3% in the thoracoscopic group and 39.25% in the robotic group. It is postulated that the superior outcome of robotic thymectomy is due to a more complete mediastinal resection because of superior three-dimensional vision and an enlargement of the operation field by insufflation with CO_2[40].

Thymomas

Minimally invasive surgery for a thymoma remains controversial. Despite advantages of less blood loss and shorter hospitalization, VATS thymectomy for thymomas is not widely used. A complete surgical resection with the resection margins free of tumour is the most important factor for the curative treatment of thymomas[41]. It is controversial whether with VATS this can be accomplished. Recurrences after resections of a thymoma, possible rupture of the capsule and seeding of the tumour during endoscopic manipulations are associated with the minimally invasive approach. Long-term oncological results are not available yet, and the prolonged learning curve is a secondary reason for the reserved attitude. In the literature, it is only recommended in highly selected patients with an early-stage thymoma[42]. A median sternotomy is the standard approach for advanced stage thymomas.

A thymectomy for a thymoma by a robotic approach might overcome the limitations of thoracoscopic thymectomy because of the three-dimensional vision and the manoeuvrability of the instruments. There are only a few studies published regarding the outcome of robotic thymectomies in patients with a thymoma (Table 16.3). Marulli et al. reported a multicentre European study of 79 early-stage thymomas resected by robotic surgery. The authors indicated that robotic thymectomy is safe for early-stage thymomas with a low complication rate, shorter hospitalization and acceptable oncological outcome. There were no vascular injuries, no nerve injuries and no peri-operative mortality. However, these results should be interpreted with caution as the median follow-up was only 40 months[43].

Keijzers et al. showed that robotic thymectomy is a safe and feasible approach for early- and late-stage thymomas. Tumour invasion in the lung, pericardium and phrenic nerve could be successfully handled with the robotic system; only invasion in major vessels was a bridge too far. Conversion to an open procedure was performed when the surgeon suspected the invasion of a major vessel. There were no conversions for surgical complications[46].

A summary of the available literature shows that robotic thymectomy is feasible in patients with MG.

In patients with an early-stage thymoma, a robotic thymectomy is also feasible; however, with a median follow-up around 40 to 50 months, a longer follow-up is indicated to evaluate the oncological outcome.

Esophageal surgery

Robotic Heller myotomy

Achalasia (Greek term that means 'does not relax') is an esophageal condition characterized by failure of the lower esophageal sphincter (LES) and a loss of peristalsis in the distal esophagus. The etiology is unknown, but different autoimmune and infectious etiologies are mentioned in the literature as possible causes. The aim of the treatment of achalasia is decreasing the pressure in the LES so that passage of nutrition is no longer difficult. Surgery by a Heller myotomy has the best long-term outcome; in 1913, Ernst Heller was the first to describe a myotomy through a thoracotomy. Over the past 20 years, minimally invasive Heller myotomy has been shown to be feasible[47]. A study of Shaligram et al. showed that robotic and laparoscopic surgery is superior to the open Heller procedures; the hospitalization is shorter, there are less post-operative complications and less need for re-admissions[48]. A robotic Heller myotomy seems similar in safety and efficacy to a pure laparoscopic approach.

Robotic esophagectomy

An esophagectomy can be performed for benign and malignant diseases. It is a complex procedure associated with significant mortality and morbidity. The 5-year overall survival rate varies between 19 and 46.5% with early-stage detection of esophagus cancer and good follow-up[49,50]. The benefits of minimally invasive esophagectomy have been described in benign diseases such as achalasia, and it is nowadays also applied in malignant esophageal diseases.

Minimally invasive surgery for esophageal oncology remains controversial. Even in experienced surgeons, dissection of the hiatus and the mediastinum can be difficult and time-consuming. With the introduction of robotic surgery, surgeons hoped to overcome these problems with the three-dimensional vision and the superior manoeuvrability of the instruments.

In 2004, Kernstine and colleagues were the first to describe a robotic esophagectomy in a 59-year-old man with an ulcerated esophageal adenocarcinoma.

And since then, many case series have been published. The described techniques differ; transthoracic and transhiatal approaches combined with different degrees of robotic assistance and a laparoscopic approach for the abdominal section of the esophagectomy have been published. The best way to perform a robotic esophagectomy remains debatable.

The largest case series of 40 robotic trans-hiatal esophagectomies showed benefits in a selected patient population with mediastinal dissection, minimal blood loss and minimal post-operative morbidity[51]. Weksler et al. compared 11 robotic esophagectomies with 26 thoracoscopic esophagectomies. The authors showed no significant differences in operative time, blood loss, number of resected lymph nodes, post-operative complications, days of mechanical ventilation and length of intensive care unit stay[52].

Robotic esophagectomy in malignant diseases is feasible, and the results are comparable with thoracoscopic esophagectomies. However, there are no published prospective, randomized, controlled studies to monitor a better long-term survival of robotic esophagectomy compared with conventional open esophagectomy. The first randomized, controlled trial comparing robot-assisted minimally invasive thoraco-laparoscopic esophagectomy with open trans-thoracic esophagectomy started in January 2012 in the Netherlands. The follow-up will be 5 years, and the short-term results will be published after discharge of the last randomized patient[53].

Conclusions

The high-definition three-dimensional optics and the superior manoeuvrability of the instruments with 7 degrees of freedom and 360 degrees of rotation are the most favorable advantages of robotic surgery. These advantages overcome the weaknesses of thoracoscopic surgery and make it possible to perform complex procedures in small operation fields more accurately. The learning curve is significantly shorter than that of the straight thoracoscopic approach. The indications in the thoracic field include esophageal diseases, early-stage lung cancer, mediastinal tumours and thymic diseases. Although the evidence is insufficient, many published series show benefits in robotic surgery for early-stage lung cancer, myasthenia gravis and thymomas. With the increased application and the promising results, it is possible that robotic surgery will markedly change thoracic surgery in the future.

References

1 Al-Mufarrej F, Margolis M, Tempesta B, et al. From Jacobeaus to the da Vinci: thoracoscopic applications of the robot. *Surgi Laparosc Endosc Percutan Tech* 2010 Feb; 20(1):1–9. PubMed PMID: 20173612. Epub 2010/02/23.eng.

2 Giudicelli R, Thomas P, Lonjon T, et al. Video-assisted minithoracotomy versus muscle-sparing thoracotomy for performing lobectomy. *Ann Thorac Surg* 1994 Sep; 58(3):712–7; discussion 7–8. PubMed PMID: 7944693. Epub 1994/09/01.eng.

3 Kirby TJ, Mack MJ, Landreneau RJ, Rice TW. Lobectomy–video-assisted thoracic surgery versus muscle-sparing thoracotomy: a randomized trial. *J Thorac Cardiovasc Surg* 1995 May; 109(5):997–1001; discussion 2. PubMed PMID: 7739262. Epub 1995/05/01.eng.

4 McKenna RJ Jr, Houck W, Fuller CB. Video-assisted thoracic surgery lobectomy: experience with 1,100 cases. *Ann Thorac Surg* 2006 Feb; 81(2):421–5; discussion 5–6. PubMed PMID: 16427825. Epub 2006/01/24.eng.

5 Jurado J, Javidfar J, Newmark A, et al. Minimally invasive thymectomy and open thymectomy: outcome analysis of 263 patients. *Ann Thorac Surg* 2012 Sep; 94(3):974–81; discussion 81-2. PubMed PMID: 22748641. Epub 2012/07/04.eng.

6 Diodato MD Jr, Damiano RJ Jr. Robotic cardiac surgery: overview. *Surg Clin North Am* 2003 Dec; 83(6):1351–67, ix. PubMed PMID: 14712871. Epub 2004/01/10.eng.

7 Lanfranco AR, Castellanos AE, Desai JP, Meyers WC. Robotic surgery: a current perspective. *Ann Surg* 2004 Jan; 239(1):14–21. PubMed PMID: 14685095. Pubmed Central PMCID: 1356187. Epub 2003/12/20.eng.

8 Satava RM. Surgical robotics: the early chronicles: a personal historical perspective. *Surg Laparosc, Endosc Percutan Tech.* 2002 Feb; 12(1):6–16. PubMed PMID: 12008765. Epub 2002/05/15.eng.

9 Friedman DC, Lendvay TS, Hannaford B. Instrument failures for the da Vinci Surgical System: a Food and Drug Administration MAUDE Database Study. *Surg Endosc* 2012 Dec 14. PubMed PMID: 23242487.

10 Siegel R, Naishadham D, Jemal A. Cancer statistics, 2012. *CA* 2012 Jan–Feb; 62(1):10–29. PubMed PMID: 22237781. Epub 2012/01/13.eng.

11 Boffa DJ, Allen MS, Grab JD, et al. Data from the Society of Thoracic Surgeons General Thoracic Surgery Database: the surgical management of primary lung tumors. *J Thorac Cardiovasc Surg* 2008 Feb; 135(2):247–54. PubMed PMID: 18242243. Epub 2008/02/05.eng.

12 Gopaldas RR, Bakaeen FG, Dao TK, et al. Video-assisted thoracoscopic versus open thoracotomy lobectomy in a cohort of 13,619 patients. *Ann Thorac Surg* 2010 May; 89(5):1563–70. PubMed PMID: 20417778. Epub 2010/04/27.eng.

13 Melfi FM, Menconi GF, Mariani AM, Angeletti CA. Early experience with robotic technology for thoracoscopic surgery. *Euro jo Cardio-thorac Surg* 2002 May; 21(5):864–8. PubMed PMID: 12062276. Epub 2002/06/14.eng.

14 Park BJ, Flores RM, Rusch VW. Robotic assistance for video-assisted thoracic surgical lobectomy: technique and initial results. *J Thorac Cardiovasc Surg* 2006 Jan; 131(1):54–9. PubMed PMID: 16399294.

15 Louie BE, Farivar AS, Aye RW, Vallieres E. Early experience with robotic lung resection results in similar operative outcomes and morbidity when compared with matched video-assisted thoracoscopic surgery cases. *Ann Thorac Surg* 2012 May; 93(5):1598–604; discussion 604–5. PubMed PMID: 22440364. Epub 2012/03/24.eng.

16 Veronesi G, Agoglia BG, Melfi F, et al. Experience with robotic lobectomy for lung cancer. *Innovations (Phila)* 2011 Nov; 6(6):355–60. PubMed PMID: 22436769.

17 Park BJ, Melfi F, Mussi A, et al. Robotic lobectomy for non-small cell lung cancer (NSCLC): long-term oncologic results. *J Thorac Cardiovasc Surg* 2012 Feb; 143(2):383–9. PubMed PMID: 22104677.

18 Flores RM, Park BJ, Dycoco J, et al. Lobectomy by video-assisted thoracic surgery (VATS) versus thoracotomy for lung cancer. *J Thorac Cardiovasc Surg* 2009 Jul; 138(1):11–8. PubMed PMID: 19577048.

19 Park BJ, Flores RM. Cost comparison of robotic, video-assisted thoracic surgery and thoracotomy approaches to pulmonary lobectomy. *Thorac Surg Clin.* 2008 Aug; 18(3):297–300, vii. PubMed PMID: 18831506. Epub 2008/10/04.eng.

20 Meyer M, Gharagozloo F, Tempesta B, et al. The learning curve of robotic lobectomy. *Int J Med Robotics Comput Assist Surg* 2012 Dec; 8(4):448–52. PubMed PMID: 22991294.

21 Melfi F, Ambrogi MC, Lucchi M, Mussi A. Video robotic lobectomy. Available from: http://mmcts.oxfordjournals.org/content/2005/0628/mmcts.2004.000448.full.pdf+html.

22 Melfi FM, Mussi A. Robotically assisted lobectomy: learning curve and complications. *Thorac Surg Clin* 2008 Aug; 18(3):289–95, vi-vii. PubMed PMID: 18831505.

23 Gharagozloo F, Margolis M, Tempesta B, et al. Robot-assisted lobectomy for early-stage lung cancer: report of 100 consecutive cases. *Ann Thorac Surg* 2009 Aug; 88(2):380–4. PubMed PMID: 19632377.

24 Veronesi G, Galetta D, Maisonneuve P, et al. Four-arm robotic lobectomy for the treatment of early-stage lung cancer. *J Thorac Cardiovasc Surg* 2010 Jul; 140(1):19–25. PubMed PMID: 20038475.

25 Augustin F, Bodner J, Wykypiel H, et al. Initial experience with robotic lung lobectomy: report of two different approaches. *Surg Endosc* 2011 Jan; 25(1):108–13. PubMed PMID: 20559664.

26 Dylewski MR, Ohaeto AC, Pereira JF. Pulmonary resection using a total endoscopic robotic video-assisted approach. *Semin Thorac Cardiovasc Surg* 2011 Spring; 23(1):36–42. PubMed PMID: 21807297.

27 Cerfolio RJ, Bryant AS, Skylizard L, Minnich DJ. Initial consecutive experience of completely portal robotic pulmonary resection with 4 arms. *J Thorac Cardiovasc Surg* 2011 Oct; 142(4):740–6. PubMed PMID: 21840547.

28 Jang HJ, Lee HS, Park SY, Zo JI. Comparison of the early robot-assisted lobectomy experience to video-assisted thoracic surgery lobectomy for lung cancer: a single-institution case series matching study. *Innovations (Phila)* 2011 Sep; 6(5): 305–10. PubMed PMID: 22436706.

29 Papatestas AE, Genkins G, Kornfeld P, et al. Effects of thymectomy in myasthenia gravis. *Ann Surg* 1987 Jul; 206(1):79–88. PubMed PMID: 3606235. Pubmed Central PMCID: 1492935. Epub 1987/07/01.eng.

30 Keesey JC. A history of treatments for myasthenia gravis. *Semin Neurol* 2004 Mar; 24(1):5–16.

PubMed PMID: 15229787. Epub 2004/07/02.eng.

31 R. Hohnfeld, Wekerle H. Reflections on the "intrathymic pathogenesis" of myasthenia gravis. *J Neuroimmunol* 2008; 201–2(0):21–7. English.

32 Diaz-Manera J, Rojas-Garcia R, Illa I. Treatment strategies for myasthenia gravis. *Expert Opin Pharmacother* 2009 Jun; 10(8): 1329–42. PubMed PMID: 19445561. Epub 2009/05/19.eng.

33 Blalock A, Mason MF, Morgan HJ, Riven SS. Myasthenia gravis and tumors of the thymic region: report of a case in which the tumor was removed. *Ann Surg* 1939 Oct; 110(4):544–61. PubMed PMID: 17857470. Pubmed Central PMCID: 1391425. Epub 1939/10/01.eng.

34 Granone P, Margaritora S, Cesario A, Galetta D. Thymectomy in myasthenia gravis via video-assisted infra-mammary cosmetic incision. *Eur Jo Cardio-thorac Surg* 1999 Jun;15(6): 861–3. PubMed PMID: 10431871. Epub 1999/08/04.eng.

35 Zielinski M, Kuzdzal J, Szlubowski A, Soja J. Transcervical-subxiphoid-videothoracoscopic 'maximal' thymectomy–operative technique and early results. *Ann Thorac Surg.* 2004 Aug; 78(2): 404–9; discussion 9–10. PubMed PMID: 15276485. Epub 2004/07/ 28.eng.

36 Zahid I, Sharif S, Routledge T, Scarci M. Video-assisted thoracoscopic surgery or transsternal thymectomy in the treatment of myasthenia gravis? *Interact Cardiovasc Thorac Surg* 2011 Jan; 12(1):40–6. PubMed PMID: 20943831.

37 Freeman RK, Ascioti AJ, Van Woerkom JM, et al. Long-term follow-up after robotic thymectomy for nonthymomatous myasthenia gravis. *Ann Thorac Surg* 2011 Sep;

92(3):1018–22; discussion 22–3. PubMed PMID: 21871293.

38 Rea F, Marulli G, Bortolotti L, et al. Experience with the 'da Vinci' robotic system for thymectomy in patients with myasthenia gravis: report of 33 cases. *Ann Thorac Surg* 2006 Feb; 81(2):455–9. PubMed PMID: 16427830.

39 Cakar F, Werner P, Augustin F, et al. A comparison of outcomes after robotic open extended thymectomy for myasthenia gravis. *Euro J Cardio-thorac Surg* 2007 Mar; 31(3):501–4; discussion 4–5. PubMed PMID: 17224274.

40 Ruckert JC, Swierzy M, Ismail M. Comparison of robotic and nonrobotic thoracoscopic thymectomy: a cohort study. *J Thorac Cardiovasc Surg* 2011 Mar; 141(3):673–7. PubMed PMID: 21335125.

41 Wilkins KB, Sheikh E, Green R, et al. Clinical and pathologic predictors of survival in patients with thymoma. *Ann Surg* 1999 Oct; 230(4):562–72; discussion 72–4. PubMed PMID: 10522726. Pubmed Central PMCID: 1420905.

42 Odaka M, Akiba T, Yabe M, et al. Unilateral thoracoscopic subtotal thymectomy for the treatment of stage I and II thymoma. *Eur J Cardio-thora sur* 2010 Apr; 37(4):824–6. PubMed PMID: 19913436.

43 Marulli G, Rea F, Melfi F, et al. Robot-aided thoracoscopic thymectomy for early-stage thymoma: a multicenter European study. *J Thorac Cardiovasc Surg* 2012 Nov; 144(5):1125–32. PubMed PMID: 22944082.

44 Mussi A, Fanucchi O, Davini F, et al. Robotic extended thymectomy for early-stage thymomas. *Euro J Cardio-thorac Surg* 2012 Apr; 41(4):e43–6; discussion e7. PubMed PMID: 22368189.

45 Marulli G, Rea F, Melfi F, et al. Robot-aided thoracoscopic thymectomy for early-stage thymoma: a multicenter European study. *J Thorac Cardiovasc Surg* 2012 Nov; 144(5):1125–30. PubMed PMID: 22944082.

46 Keijzers M, Dingemans AM, Blaauwgeers H, et al. Eight years' experience with robotic thymectomy for thymomas. *Surg Endosc* 2014 Apr; 28(4):1202–8.

47 Schuchert MJ, Luketich JD, Landreneau RJ, et al. Minimally invasive esophagomyotomy in 200 consecutive patients: factors influencing postoperative outcomes. *Ann Thorac Surg* 2008 May; 85(5):1729–34. PubMed PMID: 18442574.

48 Shaligram A, Unnirevi J, Simorov A, et al. How does the robot affect outcomes? A retrospective review of open, laparoscopic, and robotic Heller myotomy for achalasia. *Surg Endosc* 2012 Apr; 26(4): 1047–50. PubMed PMID: 22038167.

49 Portale G, Hagen JA, Peters JH, et al. Modern 5-year survival of resectable esophageal adenocarcinoma: single institution experience with 263 patients. *J Am Coll Surg* 2006 Apr; 202(4):588–96; discussion 96–8. PubMed PMID: 16571425.

50 Kim T, Grobmyer SR, Smith R, et al. Esophageal cancer–the five year survivors. *J Surg Oncol* 2011 Feb; 103(2):179–83. PubMed PMID: 21259254.

51 Dunn DH, Johnson EM, Morphew JA, et al. Robot-assisted transhiatal esophagectomy: a 3-year single-center experience. *Dis Esophagus* 2012 Mar 6. PubMed PMID: 22394116.

52 Weksler B, Sharma P, Moudgill N, et al. Robot-assisted minimally invasive esophagectomy is equivalent to thoracoscopic minimally invasive esophagectomy. *Dis Esophagus* 2012 Jul; 25(5):403–9. PubMed PMID: 21899652.

53 van der Sluis PC, Ruurda JP, van der Horst S, et al. Robot-assisted minimally invasive thoraco-laparoscopic esophagectomy versus open transthoracic esophagectomy for resectable esophageal cancer, a randomized controlled trial (ROBOT trial). *Trials* 2012 Nov 30; 13(1):230. PubMed PMID: 23199187.

Pulmonary metastasectomy

Michel Gonzalez, Jean Yannis Perentes and Thorsten Krueger

Introduction

Pulmonary metastasectomy refers to the surgical excision of metastasis to the lung originating from an extrathoracic location. Pulmonary metastases can potentially develop in any malignant tumor with a prevalence of 30% in patients diagnosed with cancer[1-3]. The pathophysiology of pulmonary metastases is thought to result from the dissemination of tumor cells from the primary tumor site to the blood circulation. These cells are stopped in the pulmonary capillary bed, and if they have the capacity, develop new tumor entities called *metastasis*. Histologic studies have demonstrated that 84% of pulmonary metastases receive their blood supply from the pulmonary arteries, while 16% receive it exclusively from bronchial arteries[1]. The probability of a new lung lesion being a metastasis is directly related to the original primary tumor. In situations of sarcoma or melanoma primary tumors, the likelihood of a new lung nodule being metastasis is approximately 80%[1-3]. If the primary tumor is urothelial or colorectal, the likelihood of a new lung nodule being metastatic is 50%. Interestingly, in situations of head and neck cancer, a new pulmonary nodule is twice as likely to be a primary tumor rather than a metastasis[4]. The latter is mostly explained by the exposure to tobacco. For these reasons, the histologic analysis of pulmonary nodules should be performed preoperatively or intraoperatively to determine the surgical strategy of resection. Fineneedle aspiration biopsy can sometimes be a good alternative; however, this approach does not always yield enough material to differentiate primary lung cancer from lung metastasis of colorectal or breast cancer.

Rationale for curative pulmonary metastasectomy

The management of the majority of patients who develop lung metastases is generally palliative including chemotherapy due to the metastatic invasion of other organs. The resection of pulmonary metastases is sometimes indicated for palliation in situations of pain due to chest wall invasion, massive hemoptysis or retention pneumonia due to centrally located metastases. However, more important, a substantial group of patients with pulmonary metastases may benefit from resection of lung metastases with curative intent. Although there are no prospectively randomized studies comparing pulmonary metastasectomy with chemotherapy or observation, surgical resection of pulmonary metastases is widely performed in carefully selected patients[5]. Several retrospective studies have suggested an increased survival for patients who underwent complete resection of lung metastases in comparison to historical results of patients who did not benefit from lung metastasectomy[6-8]. The largest multicenter study based on the International Registry of Lung Metastases reviewed retrospectively 5,206 patients from 18 centers (US, Canada, and Europe)[9]. Overall operative mortality was only 1.3%, demonstrating that pulmonary metastasectomy is safe. Complete resection was achieved in 88% of patients and was demonstrated to be an important prognostic factor of survival: overall 5-year survival of 36% for patients with complete resection compared to 13% with incomplete resection. These results suggest that pulmonary metastasectomy can offer a survival advantage when complete resection was achievable. Moreover,

Table 17.1 Five-year survival after pulmonary metastasectomy according to histologic type

Primary tumor	5-year survival
Colorectal carcinoma	24–68%
Soft tissue sarcoma	21–52%
Osteosarcoma	7–65%
Renal cell carcinoma	42–74%
Non-seminomatous germ-cell tumor	79–94%
Melanoma	21–35%
Uterine carcinoma	50%
Mammary carcinoma	36–51%

Table 17.2 Indication for a pulmonary metastasectomy

1. The primary site of cancer is controlled or controllable.

2. Absence of other extrathoracic metastases (with exception for metastases that are potentially resectable).

3. Resection of pulmonary metastases must be complete.

4. Sufficient pulmonary reserves to tolerate pulmonary resection.

5. No valid alternative therapy.

other prognostic survival factors were identified in this study: (a) a tumor-recurrence-free interval of >36 months, (b) single pulmonary metastasis, and (c) the histologic type of the primary tumor (Table 17.1)[9]. Over the past two decades, several studies have been published supporting the role of pulmonary metastasectomy in different tumors types[6–8]. Nonetheless, it is currently not possible to identify patients who may benefit mostly from this surgical strategy. Several prognostic factors have been described and should be considered in a multidisciplinary discussion before pulmonary metastasectomy including the histology of the primary tumor, the disease-free interval, the presence of other extrathoracic metastases, the number of lung metastases, the tumor doubling time, the lymph node invasion, as well as the surgical approach. The improvement of surgical techniques (video-assisted thoracoscopic surgery), radiologic images (chest CT scan with thin slices), current use of PET-CT, and advances with new chemotherapeutic agents allow increasing surgical resection of pulmonary metastases in properly selected patients. The established criteria for lung metastasectomy are (Table 17.2)[10,11] (1) the primary site of cancer is controlled or controllable with no evidence of active disease; (2) the absence of extrathoracic metastatic disease; however, involvement of other extrathoracic sites may not be a contraindication to the resection of the pulmonary disease if all metastatic sites can be resected completely before the lung resection; (3) resection of lung metastases must be complete; (4) the patient has sufficient pulmonary and cardiovascular reserves to tolerate pulmonary resection; and (5) there is no valid alternative therapy.

Preoperative evaluation
Control of the primary tumor
Surgical resection of lung metastases may be considered only if the site of the primary disease is controlled or controllable. Unresectable primary tumor is an absolute contraindication to lung metastasectomy. Staging of the primary site depends on the underlying tumor and the disease-free interval. Local tumor recurrence must always be ruled out by specific exams performed generally within 6 weeks before planning pulmonary metastasectomy. Radiologic investigations should include MRI or CT scan of the primary tumor region. A recent colonoscopy will be indicated in case of primary colorectal tumor. If the tumor and pulmonary metastases are synchronous, sequential resection is a reasonable approach if complete resection can be achieved at the two sites[10].

Exclusion of extrathoracic metastases
Staging for extrathoracic metastatic disease should be performed before the pulmonary resection, depending on the primary tumor. Abdominal CT scan is generally performed to exclude hepatic metastases or peritoneal carcinomatosis. PET scan is currently performed to assess the extrathoracic metastatic disease in patients with sarcoma, epithelial tumors (breast, colon, lung), and melanomas, offering a better sensitivity than the CT scan alone[12–14]. However, PET scan is not recommended for the detection of additional pulmonary metastases not seen on CT due to the low sensitivity for the detection of pulmonary nodules smaller than 10 mm in diameter[15]. The PET scan may be useful to determine hilar or mediastinal lymph node involvement. Lymph node invasion, which is found in approximately 15–20% of lung

metastases, represents a factor of poor prognosis[16]. If the PET scan is positive for mediastinal lymph node involvement, some authors recommend preoperative mediastinal staging with endoscopic bronchial ultrasonography (EBUS) or mediastinoscopy to histologically assess the mediastinum and potentially exclude patients from subsequent pulmonary metastasectomy[16]. In the case of neurologic symptoms, and in some tumor types with cerebral dissemination (e.g. melanoma), a cerebral MRI or CT if not available is indicated to exclude the presence of brain metastases[10].

Identification of the number of lung metastases

Preoperative lung radiology is crucial to determine whether the patient can benefit from a complete resection of lung metastases and to plan the type of intervention[15]. Metastases may have various radiologic appearances but generally are round, well deliniated, and peripherally located in the lower lobes due to a better vascularization of these areas (Figure 17.1). The chest CT scan is the standard for the evaluation of pulmonary nodules and invasion of adjacent structures (great vessels, chest wall, spinal column, and esophagus). It should be performed within 4 weeks of the pulmonary metastasectomy[15]. Nevertheless, despite the progress of radiologic imaging with thin-slice multidetectorrow CT scans, the ability to detect all metastatic nodules is uncertain, and many surgeons still recommend bimanual palpation of the lung to detect metastases that are not visible on the preoperative CT[17,18]. Various studies have shown that 16 to 46% of pulmonary lesions discovered during the bimanual palpation of the lung were not identified on preoperative chest CT[19–21]. Most of these studies have involved a helical CT with 5-mm thin-section reconstructions. More recent thin-slice CT scanners allow better spacial resolution and seem to achieve a level of metastasis detection comparable to bimanual palpation. Thus, the thoracoscopic approach to these diseases is more and more defendable. Recently, Kang et al. have reported 27 patients by comparing the pathology reports with preoperative radiologic report[22]. The thin slice (1-mm) chest CT scan was compared with bimanual palpation by thoracotomy. The sensitivity and negative predictive value were 97 and 96%, respectively, in patients with a nonsarcomatous tumor.

Pulmonary reserve

Complete pulmonary function and a cardiac evaluation should be performed prior to the pulmonary metastasectomy according to the European Respiratory Society/European Society of Thoracic Surgeons guidelines[23]. Postoperative pulmonary reserve of the patient must be estimated considering the number and locations of lung metastases. Peripheral lesions are generally removed by nonanatomic resection (wedge resection). But centrally located or larger metastases may require anatomic resections (segmentectomy, lobectomy, or pneumonectomy). In case of bilateral involvement with multiple metastases, the estimation of postoperative pulmonary function may be particularly difficult if lesions are centrally located and multiple anatomic resections are required[10]. In this situation, sternotomy with palpation of the two lungs may be necessary to assess the resectability of bilateral pulmonary lesions. In general, it is recommended to use the most parenchyma-sparing approach because metastases can be multiple and can recur.

Surgical resection
Extent of surgical resection

The goal of pulmonary metastasectomy is the complete resection of the metastases while preserving as much pulmonary parenchyma as possible. Most of the pulmonary metastatic lesions are generally located at the periphery of the lung and easily accessible to wedge resection. In contrast to primary lung cancer

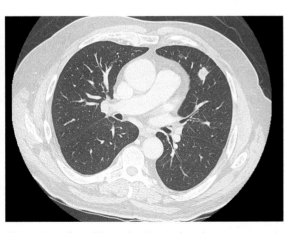

Figure 17.1 Chest CT scan showing single pulmonary metastasis located in the left superior lobe originating from colorectal carcinoma excised by thoracoscopic wedge.

Table 17.3 Preoperative exams

Primary tumor	CT Scan MRI Colonoscopy
Extrathoracic disease	Thoracoabdominal CT PET scan/CT Brain MRI
Pulmonary metastases	Chest CT (number, localization)
Lymph node involvement	PET scan/CT Mediastinoscopy EBUS/EUS
Cardiopulmonary function	Spirometry Echocardiography Stress test

Table 17.4 Technique used in lung metastasectomy

Staplers

Cautery resection (precision resection)

Laser resection (Nd:YAG laser)

Ligasure system

Ultracision scalpel

Image-guided ablatives therapy:

- Radiofrequency
- Microwave
- Cryoablation

that generally requires anatomic resection, wedge resection is as effective as anatomic resection to manage metastasis to the lung parenchyma[10]. Pulmonary metastases are easily managed by wedge resections using a standard stapler. This approach has the advantage of achieving clear surgical margins and efficient aerostasis. Other techniques have been developed as an alternative to staplers to allow maximal sparing of lung parenchyma, especially when lesions are multiple[24] (Table 17.4). Cautery resection (precision resection), initially described by Perelman, may be proposed for deeply located or peripheral lesions in patients who are not candidates for anatomic resection[25]. The technique consists of nodule resection by cautery and individual ligation of small vessels and bronchi. Another approach uses lasers. This is usually performed by thoracotomy and allows a superficial limited excision without deformation of the pulmonary parenchyma. It can also allow complete resection for lesions located close to major bronchi and/or vessels[21]. The 1,318-nm Nd:YAG laser is the only laser device capable of dissecting lung parenchyma due to its high absorption of water[26,27]. The disadvantages of laser systems are the financial investment and staff education. Moreover, this expensive technique has not proven a clear benefit in comparison to cautery resection. The Ligasure Vessel Sealing System, which is an electrothermal bipolar tissue sealing system, and the Ultracision scalpel using ultrasonic waves promoting coagulation have been proposed recently for wedge resection, but data are lacking in thoracic surgery on lung parenchyma with these techniques[28,29].

For large or central lesions, segmentectomy, lobectomy, or occasionally pneumonectomy may be required. Within the International Registry of Lung Metastases, pulmonary metastasectomy was achieved with wedge resection in 67%, segmentectomy in 9%, lobectomy in 21%, and pneumonectomy in 3%[9]. Some authors consider pneumonectomy to be a relative contraindication to pulmonary metastasectomy that should be reserved for solitary centrally located tumors with a long tumor-free-interval without previous pulmonary resection. Resection extended to other structures (chest wall, great vessels) may be justified if complete resection can be achieved[30,31].

Surgical approach

Surgical approach is determined by the number of metastases, their location, the functional reserves of the patient, and whether or not the disease is limited to one hemithorax. The choice of surgical approach should permit complete resection while saving as much pulmonary parenchyma as possible[32]. There are different approaches, each with their advantages and disadvantages: thoracotomy (anterior or posterolateral), median sternotomy, bilateral transsternal thoracotomy (Clamshell incision), and thoracoscopy. The optimal approach still remains controversial (Table 17.5)[10,32,33].

In a recent survey of the European Society of Thoracic Surgeons (ESTS), the approaches and

Table 17.5 Summary of the different surgical approaches

Surgical approach	Advantages	Disadvantages
Thoracotomy	Good unilateral exposure Bimanual palpation	Painful Second intervention if bilateral lesion
Sternotomy	Bilateral exposure Less painful	Poor exposure to lower lobe
Clamshell incision	Bilateral exposure	Painful Sacrifice of both internal mammary arteries
Video-assisted thoracoscopic surgery	Less painful Low morbidity Faster recovery	No bimanual palpation, detection of centrally located lesion

preferences were recorded and included anterolateral thoracotomy (36.3%), video-assisted thoracoscopic surgery (28.8%), posterior muscle-sparing thoracotomy (26%), posterolateral thoracotomy (22.6%), axillary thoracotomy (17.2%), sternotomy (1.4%), bilateral staged thoracotomy (66.2%), single-stage sternotomy (26.9%), single-stage bilateral sequential thoracotomy (19.3%), bilateral staged versus single-stage VATS (12.4 vs 7.6%), and single-stage clamshell incision (7.6%)[34].

The most commonly used approach is the lateral or posterolateral thoracotomy via the fourth or fifth intercostal space, which allows optimal exposure of the lung with the opportunity to perform bimanual palpation of the entire lung to find additional nodules not noticeable on the pre-operative CT scan. Postoperative pain and the inability to reach the contralateral lung are major disadvantages. Systematic one-stage bilateral thoracotomies provide no survival advantage when unilateral disease is evident on radiologic findings[35]. Most centers propose staged posterolateral thoracotomies for patients with bilateral disease. Median sternotomy offers the advantage to reach both lungs, allowing bilateral resection[36]. Postoperative pain is less important than a bilateral thoracotomy. However, access to the lower lobes, lymph node dissection, and anatomic resections are more difficult than with a classical thoracotomy.

Clamshell incision (bilateral anterior thoracotomy with transverse sternotomy) allows excellent visualization and palpation of the lung but involves a sacrifice of two mammary arteries and important postoperative pain and is nowadays considered of historical interest[10].

Video-assisted thoracoscopic surgery has gained progressive interest for pulmonary metastasectomy[37,38]. The potential benefits of the VATS approach are numerous: less pain, faster recovery, smaller incisions, decreased length of hospital stay, good visualization of the pleural space, less adhesions in the event of reintervention, and better compliance for adjuvant treatment[39]. However, these advantages do not allow bimanual palpation of the entire lung to detect nodules that are not visible on preoperative radiologic exams. Some studies have demonstrated that an open approach with manual palpation allows identification of additional nodules in 16 to 46% of patients in comparison with the VATS approach[19–21,40]. These series were conducted with old-generation CT scans with thick slices of more than 5 mm. Even if there are no prospective, randomized studies comparing the thoracoscopic approach to open bimanual thoracotomy, numerous series have demonstrated comparable survival rates between the two approaches for patients with less than three lesions[41–45]. These results appear to be partly explained by the fact that there is no evidence that the absence of immediate detection of nodules of <5 mm influences tumor disease[46]. Microscopic metastases, undetectable by VATS, can often be resected later if they become detectable on a follow-up CT with no deletary effect on patient survival. In fact, as long as patients can regularly be screened by repeat high-resolution CT scans, new nodules can be detected and additional resections performed (more easily than following a previous thoracotomy). Moreover, the resection of recurrent metastases does not interfere with overall survival in case of metachronous metastases. Many curable patients benefit from repeated resection, and repeated thoracoscopies are better tolerated than repeated thoracotomies. Finally, VATS resection is less traumatic and significantly decreases the immune response with a possible effect on the progression of the disease. Several adjunctive procedures have been suggested to help in the localization of nodules during VATS approach. Needle localization, methylene blue injection, and sonographic evaluation have been used to identify nodules not easily palpable on the visceral pleural surface[47–49]. However, these maneuvers may help for the resection of solitary radiologically detectable lesions and will not allow for detection of lesions less than 5 mm.

Even without any randomized, controlled trial or meta-analysis available, an ESTS workgroup proposed some recommendations on an optimal surgical approach: for bilateral lesions, staged thoracotomy with an interval of 3 to 6 weeks and an interval CT are recommended. A VATS approach seems appropriate for diagnostic procedures and is not still accepted as a therapeutic modality. At this time, there is no alternative to bimanual palpation.

In conclusion, the optimal approach for pulmonary metastasectomy continues to evolve, and the patient must be informed of the different surgical and interventional options with their advantages and limitations. Given continued advancement in both imaging and operative technology, the role of VATS is expected to grow.

Lymph node involvement

Although mediastinal lymph node dissection or sampling is currently performed during pulmonary resection for primary lung cancer, many surgeons do not routinely perform this procedure during lung metastasectomy. In a recent ESTS survey, 56% of surgeons performed mediastinal sampling, 13% completed dissection, and 32% did no lymph node biopsy[34]. There are two distinct clinical scenarios: (1) lymph node involvement discovered on preoperative imaging or invasive mediastinal staging and (2) incidental lymph node involvement discovered during surgery after mediastinal sampling or complete dissection. When systematic or sampling lymph node dissection is performed, lymph node metastases are identified in 12 to 32%[50–52]. Systematic mediastinal lymph node dissection has been reported to have a significant difference in survival between patients with positive lymph nodes versus negative lymph nodes. Pfannschmidt reported 245 patients who underwent systematic lymph node dissection during pulmonary metastasectomy and found hilar or mediastinal lymph node involvement in 32%[52]. Median survival was 64 months for patients without nodal metastases and 33 and 21 months for patients with hilar and mediastinal metastases, respectively. Other series have

reported that hilar or mediastinal lymph node involvement has worse survival in various primary tumors, including colorectal, renal or head and neck cancers[53–56]. The morbidity after complete mediastinal lymphadenectomy has been reported to be low and does not require much extra operative time[57]. Even though survival benefit after lymph node dissection is unclear, most authors consider that complete mediastinal lymphadenectomy or sampling should be recommended during pulmonary metastasectomy to achieve accurate staging and guide additional chemotherapy[16].

When mediastinal lymph node involvement is suspected in preoperative findings, more formal mediastinal evaluation should be performed, including mediastinoscopy, EBUS, or EUS. Pulmonary metastasectomy is questionable for preoperative histologically proven mediastinal involvement, and some authors propose to exclude patients with positive mediastinal lymph nodes from pulmonary metastasectomy[16].

Resection of recurrent metastases

Recurrence of pulmonary metastasis is a common situation occurring in approximately 50% of cases. Within the International Registry of Lung Metastases, recurrent disease was found in 53%, and patients who underwent a second metastasectomy had a survival at 5 years of 44%[9]. A longer time interval between the first metastasectomy and recurrent metastases appears to have a more favorable prognosis. Surgical resection of recurrent pulmonary metastases has been studied particularly in patients with colorectal cancer, with 5-year survivals ranging from 29 to 85%[58–60]. These results suggest that the biology of the tumor is more important than the strategy of resection, biology allowing some lesions that are not detected by CT scans to be resected later without significant impact on overall survival. Conversely, in the case of biologically aggressive tumors, complete resection of all pulmonary lesions may not improve prognosis. No controlled studies are available to define the optimal imaging protocol after metastasectomy. Even if palpation at the time of metastasectomy was performed, regular follow-up is recommended. The interval for follow-up is not defined, but an ESTS workgroup's recent recommendation was chest CT in the postoperative period, which will be repeated every 6 months for the first 2 years, then yearly[15]. If the lung has not been palpated or the tumor doubling time is short, a more frequent radiologic monitoring should be discussed.

Other ablative techniques

Alternative, less aggressive therapies are currently under investigation. Radiologic ablation under guidance has been proposed using three different techniques: radiofrequency[61], microwave[62], and cryoablation[63]. These CT-guided techniques have some potential limitations. It is impossible to ensure complete destruction of the lesion and resection margins cannot be obtained with histologic evidence. These techniques are still under investigation and may present serious complications (pneumothorax, hemoptysis, hemorrhage, bronchopleural fistula) and are usually reserved for nonoperable patients or patients who choose them.

Specific situations (different primary tumors)

Colorectal cancer

Lung metastases develop in 5 to 15% of colorectal cancer patients, and pulmonary metastasectomy is a treatment option in 1 to 2% of all patients with colorectal carcinoma[64]. Colorectal cancer is currently the most common primary tumor for patients with potentially resectable pulmonary metastases. Pulmonary metastases may develop along four different types of scenarios: (1) synchronous with the primary colorectal cancer; (2) development of lung metastases in a patient who had previously developed liver metastases, (3) development of isolated lung metastases; and (4) recurrent pulmonary metastases after previous lung metastasectomy. Multiple studies have investigated the outcome of colorectal cancer patients who underwent resection of lung metastasis, with 5-year survival varying from 24 to 68% and with median survival of 18 to 67 months[64–67]. Several survival prognostic factors have been identified: (1) disease-free interval between colonic tumor and lung metastasis identification of >12 months, (2) CEA preoperatively normal, (3) absence of hilar or mediastinal lymph node infiltration, and (4) single pulmonary metastasis. Patients presenting with both hepatic and pulmonary metastases have a 5-year survival rate after lung metastasectomy ranging from 11 to 61%[64]. These results are comparable with patients who underwent only pulmonary metastasectomy. Nevertheless, none of these factors is an absolute contraindication to pulmonary resection. Repeated pulmonary resections also have encouraging results, with survival at 5 years between 29 and 85%[58–60]. With the development of new chemotherapeutic agents, the progression-free survival and overall survival have been dramatically increased in stage IV colorectal cancer, and pulmonary metastasectomy is currently questioned. Cancer Research UK has began recently a randomized, controlled trial PulMiCC (Pulmonary Metastasectomy in Colorectal Cancer) in patients with pulmonary metastases comparing treatment with chemotherapy alone versus surgery combined with chemotherapy[68]. Moreover, in metastatic colorectal cancer, additional systemic chemotherapy should be considered. The exact role of combined liver and lung metastasectomy in the context of modern chemotherapeutic modalities is also currently under discussion.

Soft tissue sarcoma

Between 20 and 50% of patients with soft tissue sarcoma will develop pulmonary metastases. Frequently, the lung is the only metastatic site of sarcoma, and death usually occurs due to uncontrolled intrathoracic disease. Many studies have suggested a survival benefit in patients who undergo pulmonary metastasectomy. These tumors are generally poorly chemosensitive, and pulmonary metastasectomy is recommended as long as complete surgical resection is feasible. Survival at 5 years varies from 29 to 52%[69–73]. The principal prognostic factor of survival is the completeness of resection. Poor prognostic factors found are (1) high-grade tumor, (2) tumor of >5 cm, (3) multiple metastases, (4) a bilateral disease and (5) a short disease-free interval.

Osteosarcoma

Treatment of osteosarcoma is nowadays multidisciplinary. It includes the combination of chemotherapy and surgery. If lung metastases are synchronous, chemotherapy is started, and lung metastasectomy is performed after resection of the primary tumor. Postoperatively, surgery is usually combined with systemic chemotherapy. The 5-year survival rate varies from 7 to 65%[74–76]. Completeness of resection, long disease-free survival interval, and number of metastases have been described as prognostic factors for survival. Repeat pulmonary metastasectomy for osteosarcoma is also considered a viable option, and remissions or possible cure may be obtained even in patients who experience two or more lung relapses.

Renal cell carcinoma

Several studies have shown survival benefit after pulmonary metastasectomy in renal carcinoma[77]. Two studies have shown a 5-year survival of 45 and 42% after complete resection in comparison with 8 and 22% in the case of incomplete resection[55,78]. Hilar or mediastinal lymph node invasion indicated poorer prognosis. A recent study published by the Mayo Clinic showed a 5-year survival of 74% after pulmonary metastasectomy compared to 19% for incomplete resection[77]. Current indications for systemic chemotherapy following metastasectomy are questionable in this nonchemosensitive disease. To date, targeted therapy have some effectiveness for palliation.

Melanoma

More than 30% of patients with a malignant melanoma will develop lung metastases, associated with a poor prognosis[79]. In solitary pulmonary lesions, pulmonary metastasectomy may offer a benefit on survival, with 5-year survival ranging from 21 to 35%. Complete resection is also an important prognostic factor of survival, with 5-year survival of 21% and median survival of 19 months in comparison with 13% and 11 months, respectively, for incomplete resection[80]. Disease-free interval of less than 12 months and invasion of thoracic lymph nodes confer poorer prognosis. Systemic chemotherapy following surgery has not proven efficient.

Nonseminomatous testicular germ cell tumor

Pulmonary metastases are frequently encountered in patients with nonseminomatous testicular germ cell tumors[81,82]. Resection of the residual pulmonary lesion is indicated after chemotherapy when there is normalization of tumor markers (beta-HCG, alpha-fetoprotein). Residual pulmonary lesions after chemotherapy may result in three distinct lesions which cannot be differentiated radiologically: (1) necrotic lesions, (2) viable tumor, and (3) mature teratoma. Nevertheless, complete resection of viable tumor or mature teratoma is associated with a 5-year

survival if from 79 to 94%. Viable tumor and an absence of tumor marker normalization after chemotherapy are associated with poorer prognosis. Pulmonary metastasectomy may also be indicated in cases of poor response to chemotherapy when complete resection is feasible.

Breast cancer

Metastatic disease in breast cancer is often widespread, and pulmonary metastasectomy is rarely indicated. However, some patients will develop solitary isolated lung metastases amenable to lung metastasectomy. Complete resection, solitary metastasis, and long disease-free interval have a better prognosis. Nonetheless, breast cancer is treated as systematic disease, and prolonged survival is probably attributed to systemic chemotherapy or hormone therapy[83].

Other tumors

Pulmonary metastasectomy may also be considered for patients with other histologic types such as head and neck[84], uterine[85], pancreatic[86], or hepatocellular[87] carcinoma. Unfortunately, criteria of pulmonary resection are rarely indicated for these tumors. Glandular metastases from head and neck cancer have a much better prognosis than squamous cell cancer.

Conclusion

Isolated pulmonary metastases are common in patients with cancer and can be found with different types of primary tumors. Various studies suggest that pulmonary metastasectomy has an impact on overall survival and should be proposed if the primary tumor is controlled, if there are no extrathoracic metastasis, and if complete resection can be performed (adequate pulmonary and cardiac functional reserves). Several prognostic factors may influence survival (single metastasis, unilateral, long diseasefree interval, type of primary cancer). The major prognostic and survival factor is the achievement of complete resection. Pulmonary resection should be lung sparing. Thus, wedge resections are the preferred approach. VATS with high-resolution CT scan before and after seems to offer equivalent oncologic results to the classical thoracotomy with bimanual palpation of the lung and allows a more easy reoperation, which can occur along the course of these diseases.

References

1 Downey RJ. Surgical treatment of pulmonary metastases. *Surg Oncol Clin North Am* 1999; 8:341.

2 Putnam JB Jr. New and evolving treatment methods for pulmonary metastases. *Semin Thorac Cardiovasc Surg* 2002; 14:49–56.

3 Harvey JC, Lee K, Beattie EJ. Surgical management of pulmonary metastases. *Chest Surg Clin North Am* 1994; 4:55–66.

4 Rusch VW. Pulmonary metastasectomy: current indications. Chest 1995; 107: 322S-31S.

5 Treasure T. Pulmonary metastasectomy: a common practice based on weak evidence. *Ann R Coll Surg Engl* 2007; 89:744–8.

6 Casiraghi M, De Pas T, Maisonneuve P, et al. A 10-year single-center experience on 708 lung metastasectomies: the evidence of the "international registry of lung metastases". *J Thorac Oncol* 2011; 6:1373–8.

7 Robert JH, Ambrogi V, Mermillod B, et al. Factors influencing long-term survival after lung metastasectomy. *Ann Thorac Surg* 1997; 63:777–84.

8 Younes RN, Fares AL, Gross JL. Pulmonary metastasectomy: a multivariate analysis of 440 patients undergoing complete resection. *Interact Cardiovasc Thorac Surg* 2012; 14:156–61.

9 Long-term results of lung metastasectomy: prognostic analyses based on 5206 cases. The International Registry of Lung Metastases. *J Thorac Cardiovasc Surg* 1997; 113:37–49.

10 Erhunmwunsee L, D'Amico TA. Surgical management of pulmonary metastases. *Ann Thorac Surg* 2009; 88:2052–60.

11 Pastorino U. Lung metastasectomy: why, when, how. *Crit Rev Oncol Hematolo* 1997; 26:137–45.

12 Pastorino U, Veronesi G, Landoni C, et al. Fluorodeoxyglucose positron emission tomography improves preoperative staging of resectable lung metastasis. *J Thorac Cardiovasc Surg* 2003; 126:1906–10.

13 Dalrymple-Hay MJ, Rome PD, Kennedy C, et al. Pulmonary metastatic melanoma – the survival benefit associated with positron emission tomography scanning. *Eur J Cardiothorac Surg* 2002; 21:611–4; discussion 4–5.

14 Fortes DL, Allen MS, Lowe VJ, et al. The sensitivity of 18F-fluorodeoxyglucose positron emission tomography in the evaluation of metastatic pulmonary nodules. *Eur J Cardiothorac Surg* 2008; 34:1223–7.

15 Detterbeck FC, Grodzki T, Gleeson F, Robert JH. Imaging requirements in the practice of pulmonary metastasectomy. *J Thorac Oncol* 2010; 5:S134–9.

16 Garcia-Yuste M, Cassivi S, Paleru C. Thoracic lymphatic involvement in patients having pulmonary metastasectomy: incidence and the effect on prognosis. *J Thorac Oncol* 2010; 5:S166–9.

17 Margaritora S, Porziella V, D'Andrilli A, et al. Pulmonary metastases: can accurate radiological evaluation avoid thoracotomic approach? *Eur J Cardiothorac Surg* 2002; 21:1111–4.

18 Kayton ML, Huvos AG, Casher J, et al. Computed tomographic scan of the chest underestimates the number of metastatic lesions in osteosarcoma. *J Pediatr Surg* 2006; 41:200–6; discussion 200–6.

19 McCormack PM, Bains MS, Begg CB, et al. Role of video-assisted thoracic surgery in the treatment of pulmonary metastases: results of a prospective trial. *Ann Thorac Surg* 1996; 62:213–6; discussion 6–7.

20 Cerfolio RJ, McCarty T, Bryant AS. Non-imaged pulmonary nodules discovered during thoracotomy for metastasectomy by lung palpation. *Eur J Cardiothorac Surg* 2009; 35:786–91; discussion 91.

21 Nakas A, Klimatsidas MN, Entwisle J, et al. Video-assisted versus open pulmonary metastasectomy: the surgeon's finger or the radiologist's eye? *Eur J Cardiothorac Surg* 2009; 36:469–74.

22 Kang MC, Kang CH, Lee HJ, et al. Accuracy of 16-channel multi-detector row chest computed tomography with thin sections in the detection of metastatic pulmonary nodules. *Eur J Cardiothorac Surg* 2008; 33:473–9.

23 Brunelli A, Charloux A, Bolliger CT, et al. ERS/ESTS clinical guidelines on fitness for radical therapy in lung cancer patients (surgery and chemo-radiotherapy). *Eur Respir J* 2009; 34:17–41.

24 Venuta F, Rolle A, Anile M, et al. Techniques used in lung metastasectomy. *J Thorac Oncol* 2010; 5:S145–50.

25 Cooper JD, Perelman M, Todd TR, et al. Precision cautery excision of pulmonary lesions. *Ann Thorac Surg* 1986; 41:51–3.

26 Rolle A, Pereszlenyi A, Koch R, et al. Laser resection technique and results of multiple lung metastasectomies using a new 1,318-nm Nd:YAG laser system. *Lasers Surg Med* 2006; 38:26–32.

27 Rolle A, Pereszlenyi A, Koch R, et al. Is surgery for multiple lung metastases reasonable? A total of 328 consecutive patients with multiple-laser metastasectomies

with a new 1,318-nm Nd:YAG laser. *J Thorac Cardiovasc Surg* 2006; 131:1236–42.

28 Shigemura N, Akashi A, Nakagiri T, et al. A new tissue-sealing technique using the Ligasure system for nonanatomical pulmonary resection: preliminary results of sutureless and stapleless thoracoscopic surgery. *Ann Thorac Surg* 2004; 77:1415–8; discussion 9.

29 Eichfeld U, Tannapfel A, Steinert M, Friedrich T. Evaluation of ultracision in lung metastatic surgery. *Ann Thorac Surg* 2000; 70:1181–4.

30 Migliore M, Jakovic R, Hensens A, Klepetko W. Extending surgery for pulmonary metastasectomy: what are the limits? *J Thorac Oncol* 2010; 5:S155–60.

31 Putnam JB Jr., Suell DM, Natarajan G, Roth JA. Extended resection of pulmonary metastases: is the risk justified? *Ann Thorac Surg* 1993; 55:1440–6.

32 Kaifi JT, Gusani NJ, Deshaies I, et al. Indications and approach to surgical resection of lung metastases. *J Surg Oncol* 2010; 102:187–95.

33 Davidson RS, Nwogu CE, Brentjens MJ, Anderson TM. The surgical management of pulmonary metastasis: current concepts. *Surg Oncol* 2001; 10:35–42.

34 Internullo E, Cassivi SD, Van Raemdonck D, et al. Pulmonary metastasectomy: a survey of current practice amongst members of the European Society of Thoracic Surgeons. *J Thorac Oncol* 2008; 3:1257–66.

35 Younes RN, Gross JL, Deheinzelin D. Surgical resection of unilateral lung metastases: is bilateral thoracotomy necessary? *World J Surg* 2002; 26:1112–6.

36 Roth JA, Pass HI, Wesley MN, et al. Comparison of median sternotomy and thoracotomy for resection of pulmonary metastases in patients with adult soft-tissue sarcomas. *Ann Thorac Surg* 1986; 42:134–8.

37 Liu HP, Lin PJ, Hsieh MJ, et al. Application of thoracoscopy for lung metastases. *Chest* 1995; 107:266–8.

38 Dowling RD, Keenan RJ, Ferson PF, Landreneau RJ. Video-assisted thoracoscopic resection of pulmonary metastases. *Ann Thorac Surg* 1993; 56:772–5.

39 Petersen RP, Pham D, Burfeind WR, et al. Thoracoscopic lobectomy facilitates the delivery of chemotherapy after resection for lung cancer. *Ann Thorac Surg* 2007; 83:1245–9; discussion 50.

40 Ellis MC, Hessman CJ, Weerasinghe R, et al. Comparison of pulmonary nodule detection rates between preoperative CT imaging and intraoperative lung palpation. *Am J Surg* 2011; 201:619–22.

41 Gossot D, Radu C, Girard P, et al. Resection of pulmonary metastases from sarcoma: can some patients benefit from a less invasive approach? *Ann Thorac Surg* 2009; 87:238–43.

42 Mutsaerts EL, Zoetmulder FA, Meijer S, et al. Long term survival of thoracoscopic metastasectomy vs metastasectomy by thoracotomy in patients with a solitary pulmonary lesion. *Eur J Surg Oncol* 2002; 28:864–8.

43 Nakajima J, Murakawa T, Fukami T, Takamoto S. Is thoracoscopic surgery justified to treat pulmonary metastasis from colorectal cancer? *Interact Cardiovasc Thorac Surg* 2008; 7:212–6; discussion 6–7.

44 Chao YK, Chang HC, Wu YC, et al. Management of lung metastases from colorectal cancer: video-assisted thoracoscopic surgery versus thoracotomy – a case-matched study. *Thorac*

Cardiovasc Surg 2012 Sep; 60(6):398–404. doi: 10.1055/s-0031-1295574. Epub 2012 Jan 7.

45 Carballo M, Maish MS, Jaroszewski DE, Holmes CE. Video-assisted thoracic surgery (VATS) as a safe alternative for the resection of pulmonary metastases: a retrospective cohort study. *J Cardiothorac Surg* 2009; 4:13.

46 Sonett JR. Pulmonary metastases: biologic and historical justification for VATS. Video assisted thoracic surgery. *Eur J Cardiothorac Surg* 1999; 16(Suppl 1):S13–5; discussion S5–6.

47 Pittet O, Christodoulou M, Pezzetta E, et al. Video-assisted thoracoscopic resection of a small pulmonary nodule after computed tomography-guided localization with a hook-wire system: Experience in 45 consecutive patients. *World J Surg* 2007; 31:575–8.

48 Sortini D, Carrella G, Carcoforo P, et al. Sonographic evaluation for peripheral pulmonary nodules during video-assisted thoracoscopic surgery. *Surg Endosc* 2004; 18:563.

49 Wang YZ, Boudreaux JP, Dowling A, Woltering EA. Percutaneous localisation of pulmonary nodules prior to video-assisted thoracoscopic surgery using methylene blue and TC-99. *Eur J Cardiothorac Surg* 2010; 37:237–8.

50 Ercan S, Nichols FC 3rd, Trastek VF, et al. Prognostic significance of lymph node metastasis found during pulmonary metastasectomy for extrapulmonary carcinoma. *Ann Thorac Surg* 2004; 77: 1786–91.

51 Veronesi G, Petrella F, Leo F, et al. Prognostic role of lymph node involvement in lung metastasectomy. *J Thorac Cardiovasc Surg* 2007; 133: 967–72.

52 Pfannschmidt J, Klode J, Muley T, et al. Nodal involvement at the time of pulmonary metastasectomy: experiences in 245 patients. *Ann Thorac Surg* 2006; 81:448–54.

53 Saito Y, Omiya H, Kohno K, et al. Pulmonary metastasectomy for 165 patients with colorectal carcinoma: prognostic assessment. *J Thorac Cardiovasc Surg* 2002; 124:1007–13.

54 Pfannschmidt J, Muley T, Hoffmann H, Dienemann H. Prognostic factors and survival after complete resection of pulmonary metastases from colorectal carcinoma: experiences in 167 patients. *J Thorac Cardiovasc Surg* 2003; 126:732–9.

55 Pfannschmidt J, Hoffmann H, Muley T, et al. Prognostic factors for survival after pulmonary resection of metastatic renal cell carcinoma. *Ann Thorac Surg* 2002; 74:1653–7.

56 Seki M, Nakagawa K, Tsuchiya S, et al. Surgical treatment of pulmonary metastases from uterine cervical cancer: operation method by lung tumor size. *J Thorac Cardiovasc Surg* 1992; 104:876–81.

57 Allen MS, Darling GE, Pechet TT, et al. Morbidity and mortality of major pulmonary resections in patients with early-stage lung cancer: initial results of the randomized, prospective ACOSOG Z0030 trial. *Ann Thorac Surg* 2006; 81:1013–9; discussion 9–20.

58 Kim AW, Faber LP, Warren WH, et al. Repeat pulmonary resection for metachronous colorectal carcinoma is beneficial. *Surgery* 2008; 144:712–7; discussion 7–8.

59 Watanabe K, Nagai K, Kobayashi A, et al. Factors influencing survival after complete resection of pulmonary metastases from colorectal cancer. *Br J Surg* 2009; 96:1058–65.

60 Welter S, Jacobs J, Krbek T, et al. Long-term survival after repeated resection of pulmonary metastases from colorectal cancer. *Ann Thorac Surg* 2007; 84:203-10.

61 King J, Glenn D, Clark W, et al. Percutaneous radiofrequency ablation of pulmonary metastases in patients with colorectal cancer. *Br J Surg* 2004; 91:217–23.

62 Simon CJ, Dupuy DE, Mayo-Smith WW. Microwave ablation: principles and applications. *Radiographics* 2005; 25(Suppl 1): S69–83.

63 Beland MD, Dupuy DE, Mayo-Smith WW. Percutaneous cryoablation of symptomatic extraabdominal metastatic disease: preliminary results. *AJR Am J Roentgenol* 2005; 184:926–30.

64 Gonzalez M, Ris HB, Krueger T, Gervaz P. Colorectal cancer and thoracic surgeons: close encounters of the third kind. *Expert Rev Anticancer Ther* 2012; 12:495–503.

65 Pfannschmidt J, Hoffmann H, Dienemann H. Reported outcome factors for pulmonary resection in metastatic colorectal cancer. *J Thorac Oncol* 2010; 5:S172–8.

66 Pfannschmidt J, Dienemann H, Hoffmann H. Surgical resection of pulmonary metastases from colorectal cancer: a systematic review of published series. *Ann Thorac Surg* 2007; 84:324–38.

67 Gonzalez M, Poncet A, Combescure C, et al. Risk factors for survival after lung metastasectomy in colorectal cancer patients: a systematic review and meta-analysis. *Ann Surg Oncol* 2012.

68 Treasure T, Fallowfield L, Lees B. Pulmonary metastasectomy in colorectal cancer: the PulMiCC trial. *J Thorac Oncol* 2010; 5:S203–6.

69 Kim S, Ott HC, Wright CD, et al. Pulmonary resection

of metastatic sarcoma: prognostic factors associated with improved outcomes. *Ann Thorac Surg* 2011; 92:1780–6; discussion 6–7.

70 Porter GA, Cantor SB, Walsh GL, et al. Cost-effectiveness of pulmonary resection and systemic chemotherapy in the management of metastatic soft tissue sarcoma: a combined analysis from the University of Texas MD Anderson and Memorial Sloan-Kettering Cancer Centers. *J Thorac Cardiovasc Surg* 2004; 127:1366–72.

71 Pfannschmidt J, Klode J, Muley T, et al. Pulmonary metastasectomy in patients with soft tissue sarcomas: experiences in 50 patients. *Thorac Cardiovasc Surg* 2006; 54:489–92.

72 Canter RJ, Qin LX, Downey RJ, et al. Perioperative chemotherapy in patients undergoing pulmonary resection for metastatic soft-tissue sarcoma of the extremity: a retrospective analysis. *Cancer* 2007; 110:2050–60.

73 Predina JD, Puc MM, Bergey MR, et al. Improved survival after pulmonary metastasectomy for soft tissue sarcoma. *J Thorac Oncol* 2011; 6:913–9.

74 Briccoli A, Rocca M, Salone M, et al. Resection of recurrent pulmonary metastases in patients with osteosarcoma. *Cancer* 2005; 104:1721–5.

75 Briccoli A, Rocca M, Salone M, et al. High grade osteosarcoma of the extremities metastatic to the lung: long-term results in 323 patients treated combining surgery and chemotherapy, 1985–2005. *Surg Oncol* 2010; 19:193–9.

76 Harting MT, Blakely ML. Management of osteosarcoma pulmonary metastases. *Semin Pediatri Surg* 2006; 15:25–9.

77 Alt AL, Boorjian SA, Lohse CM, et al. Survival after complete

177

surgical resection of multiple metastases from renal cell carcinoma. *Cancer* 2011; 117:2873–82.

78 Assouad J, Petkova B, Berna P, et al. Renal cell carcinoma lung metastases surgery: pathologic findings and prognostic factors. *Ann Thorac Surg* 2007; 84:1114–20.

79 Oliaro A, Filosso PL, Bruna MC, et al. Pulmonary metastasectomy for melanoma. *J Thorac Oncol* 2010; 5:S187–91.

80 Petersen RP, Hanish SI, Haney JC, et al. Improved survival with pulmonary metastasectomy: an analysis of 1,720 patients with pulmonary metastatic melanoma. *J Thorac Cardiovasc Surg* 2007; 133:104–10.

81 Pfannschmidt J, Hoffmann H, Dienemann H. Thoracic metastasectomy for nonseminomatous germ cell tumors. *J Thorac Oncol* 2010; 5:S182–6.

82 Pfannschmidt J, Zabeck H, Muley T, et al. Pulmonary metastasectomy following chemotherapy in patients with testicular tumors: experience in 52 patients. *Thorac Cardiovasc Surg* 2006; 54:484–8.

83 Garcia-Yuste M, Cassivi S, Paleru C. Pulmonary metastasectomy in breast cancer. *J Thorac Oncol* 2010; 5:S170–1.

84 Shiono S, Kawamura M, Sato T, et al. Pulmonary metastasectomy for pulmonary metastases of head and neck squamous cell

carcinomas. *Ann Thorac Surg* 2009; 88:856–60.

85 Yamamoto K, Yoshikawa H, Shiromizu K, et al. Pulmonary metastasectomy for uterine cervical cancer: a multivariate analysis. *Ann Thorac Surg* 2004; 77:1179–82.

86 Kitano K, Murayama T, Sakamoto M, et al. Outcome and survival analysis of pulmonary metastasectomy for hepatocellular carcinoma. *Eur J Cardiothorac Surg* 2012; 41:376–82.

87 Arnaoutakis GJ, Rangachari D, Laheru DA, et al. Pulmonary resection for isolated pancreatic adenocarcinoma metastasis: an analysis of outcomes and survival. *J Gastrointest Surg* 2011; 15:1611–7.

Chapter

18

Tube thoracostomy

Evidence-based management of chest drains following pulmonary surgery

Alessandro Brunelli

Management of chest tubes remains a critical aspect in the post-operative course of patients following lung resection. It is traditionally influenced by two factors: presence of air leak and daily pleural fluid output. The combination of these two factors has characterized protocols of chest tube removal.

Prolonged air leak

Figures from the last edition of the European Society of Thoracic Surgeons Database Annual Report (www.ests .org/documents/PDF/Database_ESTS_Report_2012 .pdf) showed that the incidence of an air leak lasting longer than 5 days is about 8.3% after lobectomy, 6.8% after segmentectomy and 3.5% after wedge resection.

These data confirm that prolonged air leak (PAL) remains a bothersome complication. Several authors have shown that PAL is a major determinant of post-operative hospital stay and costs[1,2]. Varela and colleagues[2] have shown that only 10% of patients with PAL are likely to be discharged by the seventh post-operative day, whereas 90% of those without PAL can be sent home by this time. They found that the excess cost attributable to PAL (driven mainly by the increased length of stay) was about 39,000 euros in 21 patients with this complication, an average of 1,860 euros per patient[2].

Although many patients can be safely sent home with a one-way valve or portable chest drainage system, this practice is not always well accepted by patients, is not feasible in all settings and is not possible for patients with medium- to high-grade air leaks.

PAL is not only a financial issue, but it has also been shown to increase the risk of other medical complications, particularly empyema[3].

For this reason, several authors have attempted to predict the occurrence of this complication in an effort to identify high-risk patients in whom to apply preventative measures.

The most consistently reported risk factors are reduced pulmonary function indicative of a damaged and fragile lung parenchyma, use of steroids, performance of an upper lobectomy, low body-mass index (BMI) and presence of pleural adhesions[4]. Together with the group from Salamanca[5], we recently developed an aggregate risk model stratifying the risk of PAL in four risk classes according to the presence of four weighted factors: age > 65, 1 point; presence of adhesions, 1 point; FEV1 < 80%, 1.5 points; and body-mass index < 25.5, 2 points. The sum of the individual points in each patient yields a cumulative score, which may range from 0 to 5.5. For instance, a 75-year-old patient with an FEV1 of 70%, BMI of 24 and pleural adhesions would have the maximum score of 5.5 points. According to the score, four risk classes were derived with an incremental risk of PAL. In the validation set, the risk of PAL was nil in class A (no risk factors present, score 0), 6.7% in class B (score 1), 10.9% in class C (score 1.5–3) and 25.7% in class D (score > 3.5).

The best way to avoid the occurrence of PAL is to prevent this complication during surgery by applying meticulous technique. However, once this complication is evident in the post-operative period, several measures have been tested to reduce the duration of air leak (chest tube management, autologous blood patching, reoperation etc.).

Certainly one of the most studied methods used in the post-operative phase is the application of different protocols of chest tube management. Several randomized clinical trials have been published comparing suction versus 'water seal / no suction'.

Core Topics in Thoracic Surgery, ed. Marco Scarci, Aman Coonar, Tom Routledge and Francis Wells. Published by Cambridge University Press. © Cambridge University Press 2016

Table 18.1 Summary of the randomized trials comparing suction versus no suction

Author	Algorithm	No. of pts.	Favour no suction	Benefit
Cerfolio RJ 2001[22]	No suction on POD2	33	Yes	Larger air leak seal by POD3
Marshall B 2002[23]	No suction on ward arrival	68	Yes	Shorter air leak duration
Brunelli A 2004[24]	No suction on POD1	145	No	No difference in air leak duration, increased trend of complications
Brunelli A 2005[25]	Alternate suction	94	Yes to alternative suction	Shorter tube duration, LOS, less PAL vs full-time no suction
Alphonso N 2005[26]	Immediate no suction	234	No	No difference

LOS = length of stay; PAL = prolonged air leak; POD = post-operative day

There are relative pros and cons in using suction versus no suction. Theoretically, suction promotes pleura-pleura apposition favouring the sealing of air leak and certainly favouring the drainage of large air leaks. However, suction has also been shown to increase the flow through the chest tube proportional to the level of suction applied, and it is assumed that this increased airflow increases the duration of drainage. Further, the use of suction has also historically been associated with reduced patient mobilization, particularly if wall suction is used. On the other hand, the so-called water seal or no-suction approach has been shown to be effective in some circumstances to reduce the duration of air leak, presumably by decreasing the airflow, whilst also favouring mobilization (since the patient is not attached to the wall suction). Nonetheless, the absence of suction makes this approach ineffective in the case of medium to large air leaks (particularly in the presence of a large pneumothorax) and is associated with an increased risk of other complications (particularly pneumonia and arrhythmia).

Table 18.1 is a summary of the findings of the randomized trials published on suction versus no suction in lung resection patients. As evident from the table, these trials yielded mixed results. Some authors found a benefit by using 'water seal'; others did not find any difference between the two modalities.

There are a number of problems with these studies. By comparing suction and no suction, whilst maintaining identical drain removal criteria, the studies automatically favour the no suction group, in that the measurement is the removal of air and not the healing of the fistula. The application of suction would increase the airflow through the fistula; however, there is no evidence to suggest that suction slows the healing of the fistula itself. To truly demonstrate the difference between suction and no suction, it would be necessary to have a higher airflow criterion when removing the chest drain for the suction group – something not possible with traditional systems due to their inaccuracy in measuring the severity of the air leak. This lack of objective data for more sensitive measurement of air leak severity has prevented the standardization of studies, and even test and control groups within studies, resulting in a lack of accurate quantification and reproducibility. Further, a conceptual problem inherent to all these studies is the definition of 'water seal' and suction.

Standardization of terminology

A recent collaborative proposal from the European Society of Thoracic Surgeons (ESTS), American Association for Thoracic Surgery (AATS), Society of Thoracic Surgeons (STS) and General Thoracic Surgical Club (GTSC) on standardization of nomenclature has helped clarify some controversial definitions based on physical and physiological principles[6].

Among others the following terms were discussed and proposed:

- *Passive drainage* occurs when intrapleural pressure rises above atmospheric pressure.
- *Active drainage* occurs when a sub-atmospheric pressure is applied to the pleural space either by an

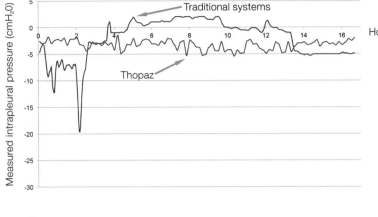

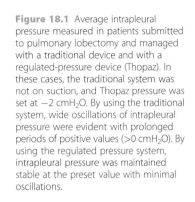

Figure 18.1 Average intrapleural pressure measured in patients submitted to pulmonary lobectomy and managed with a traditional device and with a regulated-pressure device (Thopaz). In these cases, the traditional system was not on suction, and Thopaz pressure was set at -2 cmH$_2$O. By using the traditional system, wide oscillations of intrapleural pressure were evident with prolonged periods of positive values (>0 cmH$_2$O). By using the regulated pressure system, intrapleural pressure was maintained stable at the preset value with minimal oscillations.

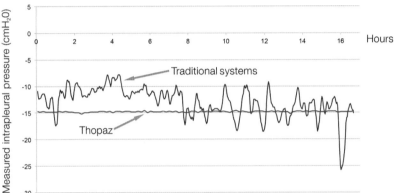

Figure 18.2 Average intrapleural pressure measured in patients undergoing pulmonary lobectomy and managed with a traditional device and with a regulated-pressure device (Thopaz). In these cases, both systems were placed on suction at -15 cmH$_2$O. By using the traditional system, wide oscillations of intrapleural pressure were evident despite the suction, whereas by using the regulated pressure system, the intrapleural pressure was maintained stable at the preset value.

external suction device or by creating a column of liquid within the chest tube that extends below the level of the pleural space (siphoning effect). In this regard, the old term 'water seal' does not always correspond to 'no suction'. It may at times represent a form of uncontrolled, active drainage.

Recent findings from our group[7] have shown large variations of values of pleural pressure measured during the last hour before chest tube removal in a series of uncomplicated pulmonary lobectomies, while the chest tube was maintained on water seal without external suction. Pressure can vary from values above atmospheric pressure, exposing patients to the risk of tension pneumothorax, to values as negative as minus 40 cmH$_2$O in the same patient and during a relatively short period of time (Figure 18.1).

To simplify terminology and understanding of the 'active drainage', the situation where a sub-atmospheric pressure is created by an external suction device has been defined as 'external suction applied'. In all other cases (previously referred as 'water seal'), the definition 'no external suction applied' has been proposed.

Another important definition is the distinction between regulated (variable) suction and unregulated (fixed) suction. *Regulated suction* is a form of active drainage obtained through the application of an external source of suction capable of modifying its level of suction (negative pressure) in response to the feedback coming from the pleural space. In other words, the suction source applied to the chest drainage system is capable of varying its activity to maintain a preset value of pressure. As a consequence, these systems can be best described as suction when needed by the patient and non-suction when not (Figure 18.2). *Non-regulated* or fixed suction is a form of active drainage provided by an external source of suction not capable of varying its level based on the intrapleural pressure level (i.e. wall suction).

Electronic drainage systems

Some companies have recently produced and commercialized chest drainage systems with built in electronics able to measure air flow.

There are several experiences already published in the medical literature reporting on the clinical characteristics and benefits of these novel devices.

In summary, the main features of the commercially available digitalized chest drainage systems are the following:

1. Objective measurement of air leak, which improves reproducibility and interobserver agreement
2. Graphical display of trends of airflow, which assists in chest tube management
3. Recording of data for later export, retrospective analysis and medico-legal purposes
4. Compact, light and portable design
5. Built-in pump, no need to attach to chest wall for suction
6. Provide regulated, variable suction to generate a stable intrapleural negative pressure (Figures 18.1 and 18.2)
7. Intelligent systems, which work only when needed to mantain preset negative levels in the presence of air leak (suction when needed, non-suction when not)
8. Unaffected by gravity and the position of the system relative to the patient

One the most important studies about digital systems is the one published from the Salamanca group[8]. They found a high inter-observer variability among staff surgeons in deciding when to remove a chest tube when using a traditional device. On the other hand, the inter-observer agreement was almost perfect when a digital system was used to assess air leak. The main reason explaining the difference is the availability of objective data about air leak upon which to base the decision on whether to remove the chest tube.

The objective unequivocal quantification of the air leak is likely the most important factor explaining the clinical benefits found in two randomized clinical trials comparing digital versus traditional devices[9,10].

Cerfolio and colleagues[9] found that patients connected to a digital system had a shorter duration of chest tube (0.8 days less) and hospital stay (0.7 days less) than those connected to a traditional device. One interesting aspect of this study was the crossover of patients with an air leak on both devices, which made it possible to correlate the readings obtained from both systems.

The authors were able to find a certain linear correlation between the median airflow measured by the digital device and the intensity of the bubbling.

The other randomized trial showing the efficacy of digital systems over traditional ones was the one published by our group[10]. Only lobectomy patients were included in the study, with 160 patients randomized into two groups. The group connected to a digital system had a significantly shorter duration of chest tube placement, which resulted in a reduced hospital stay of about 1 day. Consequently, we were able to find a cost reduction of about 500 euros per patient. Additionally, 51% of patients with the digital drainage device had their chest tube removed by the second post-operative day compared to only 12% of those with the analog device. One of the most important aspects of this study was the use of a standardized fast-track chest tube removal protocol, taking advantage of the objective information about air leak recorded in the system. We did not rely on instantaneous assessment of air leak anymore but rather on average values of air leak, expressed in ml/min, recorded during the last 3–6 hours.

Both of these randomized trials were conducted using a system, called Digivent, no longer available on the market.

Pleural pressure

Some new electronic chest drainage systems are not only able to measure the airflow but also the pleural pressure. Little is known about the influence of the pleural pressure on the duration of air leak and even less on the importance of it to the recovery of the lung after surgery.

A recent paper combining patients from Ancona and Mayo Clinics has shown that the differential pressure (difference between minimum pressure and maximum pressure) calculated from measurements taken during the 6 post-operative hours following lobectomy was associated with the duration of air leak and the risk of a PAL[11].

Patients with an airflow greater than 50 ml/min and a differential pressure greater than 10 cmH$_2$O have a risk of PAL > 72 hours as high as 52%.

This work may have clinical implications insofar as by modifying the differential pressure (narrowing the 'swing' between maximum and minimum pressure), there may be the possibility to influence the duration of air leak.

These findings were derived from data recorded by using the Digivent system, which is no longer

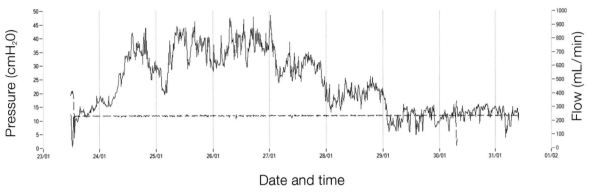

Figure 18.3 Airflow–pleural pressure graph downloaded from a regulated-pressure chest drainage system in a patient undergoing pulmonary lobectomy. The red line represents airflow, and the blue line the pleural pressure recorded at the chest. In this patient there was a prolonged period of air leak. The device worked to maintain the pleural pressure stable at the preset value without oscillations in spite of the airflow.

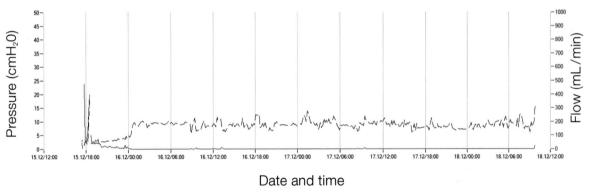

Figure 18.4 Airflow–pleural pressure graph downloaded from a regulated-pressure chest drainage system (Thopaz) in a patient undergoing pulmonary lobectomy. The red line represents airflow, and the blue line the pleural pressure recorded at the chest. There was an initial period of a few hours with some air leak and in which the pleural pressure was maintained stable at −2 cmH$_2$O (which was the preset value in this case). Once the airflow stopped, the patient stabilized his own pleural pressure within physiological values. The device simply observed without exerting any suction.

available on the market. That system featured separate flow and pressure sensors located at the canister level, which allowed for influence by external factors such as siphoning effects and positioning of the patient.

New systems, such as the Thopaz (Medela Healthcare, Switzerland), provide more sophisticated data and clinical results. They feature a pressure sensor that measure the intrapleural pressure of the chest and contain an intelligent algorithm that controls the pump, meaning they are capable of reacting to the feedback coming from the sensor. The airflow is accurately measured (with 1% error rate) by the activity of the pump to maintain a preset level of pressure. In a sealed environment and in the case of no air leak, the pump function ceases to work once the preset negative pressure is reached, turning the

system into a non-suction device. Nevertheless, it never stops measuring and recording pressure data. In the absence of air leak, Thopaz will simply observe and record the pressure of the intrapleural space.

One of the great potential advantages of regulated suction devices (i.e. Thopaz) is the capability to maintain a stable pressure even in the case of air leak with minimal variability in the range of 0.1 cmH$_2$O (Figure 18.3). Furthermore, when the preset pressure is at or below −8 cmH$_2$O and there is no air leak, the device works passively, as a one-way valve, only monitoring and recording the pleural pressure driven by the patient himself or herself (Figure 18.4).

What you set in the device is what you really get inside the pleural space. In contrast to a traditional chest drainage system, the oscillations around the preset value are minimal (Figure 18.1), which may contribute to reducing the duration of air leak, according to the aforementioned paper[11]

The introduction of these types of novel electronic chest drainage systems in clinical practice has been shown to be effective and safe. In a previous investigation, Pompili and colleagues[12] used propensity score case-matched analysis to compare the first consecutive 51 lobectomy patients managed with Thopaz with 51 counterparts managed with a traditional device.

Patients managed with Thopaz had chest tube durations approximately 2 days shorter and hospital stays 1.5 days shorter, with a consequent saving of approximately 750 euros per patient.

Moreover, compared to patients managed with a traditional system, those connected to the novel electronic device had a consistently shorter duration of chest tube since the very first cases. The 'learning curve' sloped down for the first 40 patients before reaching a plateau, when the maximum benefit of the electronic device was evident.

Modern chest drain devices, which are able to apply regulated suction to maintain the preset intrapleural pressure, represent the ideal instruments to reliably assess the effect of different levels of negative pressure on the duration of air leak. They may overcome the main limitation of previous trials using traditional devices and comparing suction versus no suction: the impossibility of controlling whether the preset level of suction was indeed maintained inside the chest.

In this regard, we[13] recently compared the effect of different levels of pleural pressure on the duration of air leak under controlled conditions by using a regulated chest drainage system (Thopaz). One hundred patients undergoing pulmonary lobectomy were randomized to receive two different types of chest drainage management: group 1, regulated individualized suction mode, with different pressure levels depending on the type of lobectomy and ranging from −11 to −20 cmH$_2$O based on a previous investigation[7]; group 2, regulated seal mode (−2 cmH$_2$O). At this low level of suction, the system works only to compensate the occurrence of values more positive than −2 cmH$_2$O in case of air leak. Otherwise, it works passively as a regulated, nonsuction device. We found that the average air leak duration and the number of patients with PAL were similar between the groups, showing that a regulated

seal is as effective and safe as regulated suction in managing chest tubes following lobectomy. Although this experience can be refined with the application of different levels of suction or different endpoints, it will contribute to set the basis for future investigation on active pleural management based on regulated pleural pressure.

Pleural effusion

The other factor influencing the timing of chest tube removal is the amount of pleural fluid output observed daily from the chest tubes. Traditionally, most surgeons accepted the cutoff of about 200 ml/day as a safe threshold below which to pull out a chest tube. However, this value is based more on tradition than on scientific data or physiology.

The pleural fluid turnover is fully regulated by the lymphatic drainage system located at the parietal level. This system is particularly developed at the diaphragmatic and mediastinal surfaces, and the visceral pleura is substantially excluded from this mechanism since its permeability is in physiological conditions at least 10-fold less than that of parietal pleura. The hourly turnover of the pleural fluid is about 0.2 ml/kg, leading in physiological conditions to its complete renewal in about 1 hour[14].

Lymphatics act as an efficient negative-feedback system to regulate pleural fluid dynamics as they can markedly increase draining flow (20–30 fold) in response to increased filtration, such as the one occurring after lung surgery as a result of postoperative inflammation. Studies on experimental hydrothorax have shown that pleural lymphatics are able to generate a pressure to bring the lung close to the chest with minimal residual pleural liquid volume[15]. Another important factor of the equation is that hydrothorax may be actually favoured by the presence of the chest tube because excessive sub-atmospheric pressure (above physiological range, such as −20 cmH$_2$O) may cause an increase in fluid filtration. Also, the presence of a chest tube itself is an irritant to the pleural lining, creating an inflammatory effect, thereby increasing fluid filtration.

These physiologic principles seem to support the concept that it is not really necessary to drain all the fluid in pleural space by chest tube, since the pleura can absorb this excess fluid physiologically. But how much fluid can we safely leave behind? There is really

Table 18.2 Summary of the randomized trials comparing single versus double chest tubes

Author	Protocol	CT Duration	Pl Effusion	Pain	Residual Pl effusion or new drain
Alex J 2003[17]	RCT	Same	Same	Reduced	Same
Gomez-Caro A 2006[18]	RCT	Same	Same	Reduced	Same
Okur E 2009[19]	RCT	Reduced	Reduced	Reduced	Same

scant information in the literature about pleural fluid management after lung surgery.

Probably the most important study in this regard is the one from Cerfolio and colleagues[16]. In more than 2,000 patients submitted to lung resection, they found that a fluid threshold of less than 450 ml/day (provided that the presence of cerebrospinal fluid, chylothorax or hemothorax has been ruled out) was safe and that only 11 patients (<1%) needed to be readmitted for recurrent symptomatic pleural effusion.

Since that paper, several thoracic surgeons have started changing their attitude in pleural fluid management to being more aggressive in pulling a chest tube even with a high pleural fluid output.

In our unit, we currently remove a chest tube in the absence of air leak when the daily amount of pleural fluid is less than 400 ml/day. Using this policy, we did not observe any significant increase in readmissions for symptomatic pleural effusion or need for chest tube re-insertion.

Single versus double chest tube

Traditionally, thoracic surgeons have used two chest tubes to drain the pleural space after lobectomy. The dogma, learned from school and mentors, is that one tube should be placed at the apex to drain air and the other at the base to drain fluid. Once again, this practice has never been challenged and has been accepted for granted as the best practice in thoracic surgery.

In the last 10 years, however, there have been several randomized trials that have demonstrated that the use of a single chest tube after lobectomy is safe and effective. Further, as the presence of the chest tube is an irritant and encourages fluid secretion, the presence of only a single tube will reduce the incidence of drains being left in situ due to measured fluids in the drainage device.

Table 18.2 summarizes the randomized trials comparing single versus double chest tubes after pulmonary lobectomy[17–19].

All authors found an advantage of using a single chest tube in terms of pain. No differences were detected in terms of residual pleural effusion or a need to re-insert a chest tube.

Okur and colleagues found that the use of a single tube reduced the duration of chest drains in place and the amount of drained pleural fluid[19].

We also found that the pressure exerted and measured within the pleural space when applying suction to a single chest tube was not different from the intrapleural pressure measured when two chest tubes were used[20]. In this regard, the concern that a single chest tube may not be sufficient to promote adequate lung re-expansion does not appear to be supported by this finding.

The practice of using a single chest tube is corroborated by recent findings from our group[21] about the influence of chest tubes on respiratory function and static and dynamic chest pain. We measured forced expiratory volume and chest pain (by numeric pain scale) immediately before and 1 hour after chest tube removal in 104 patients submitted to lung resection.

The static and dynamic pain scores decreased by approximately 40% after chest tube removal. Compared to the pre-removal value, the average FEV1 increased by 13% after tube removal (about 200 ml). After chest tube removal, 67% of patients showed an FEV1 improvement. Similar results were observed in patients operated on through video-assisted thoracic surgery (VATS) or thoracotomy.

These findings indicate that the chest tube has an impact not only on pain but also on respiratory function. Therefore, in this regard, the use of a single chest tube appears even more warranted.

The current practice in our unit is to use a single 24-French chest tube placed in a mid-position through the apex. We adopted this practice more than 4 years ago, and we did not notice any increase in recurrent symptomatic pleural effusion requiring tube re-insertion.

185

References

1   Irshad K, Feldman LS, Chu VF, et al. Causes of increased length of hospitalization on a general thoracic surgery service: a prospective observational study. *Can J Surg* 2002 Aug; 45 (4):264–8.

2   Varela G, Jiménez MF, Novoa N, Aranda JL. Estimating hospital costs attributable to prolonged air leak in pulmonary lobectomy. *Eur J Cardiothorac Surg* 2005 Feb; 27(2):329–33.

3   Brunelli A, Xiume F, Al Refai M, et al. Air leaks after lobectomy increase the risk of empyema but not of cardiopulmonary complications: a case-matched analysis. *Chest* 2006 Oct; 130(4):1150–6.

4   Brunelli A, Cassivi SD, Halgren L. Risk factors for prolonged air leak after pulmonary resection. *Thorac Surg Clin* 2010 Aug; 20(3):359–64.

5   Brunelli A, Varela G, Refai M, et al. A scoring system to predict the risk of prolonged air leak after lobectomy. *Ann Thorac Surg* 2010 Jul; 90(1):204–9.

6   Brunelli A, Beretta E, Cassivi SD, et al. Consensus definitions to promote an evidence-based approach to management of the pleural space: a collaborative proposal by ESTS, AATS, STS, and GTSC. *Eur J Cardiothorac Surg* 2011 Aug; 40(2):291–7.

7   Refai M, Brunelli A, Varela G, et al. The values of intrapleural pressure before the removal of chest tube in non-complicated pulmonary lobectomies. *Eur J Cardiothorac Surg* 2012 Apr; 41(4):831–3.

8   Varela G, Jiménez MF, Novoa NM, Aranda JL. Postoperative chest tube management: measuring air leak using an electronic device decreases variability in the clinical practice.

Eur J Cardiothorac Surg 2009 Jan; 35(1):28–31.

9   Cerfolio RJ, Bryant AS. The benefits of continuous and digital air leak assessment after elective pulmonary resection: a prospective study. *Ann Thorac Surg* 2008 Aug; 86(2):396–401.

10 Brunelli A, Salati M, Refai M, et al. Evaluation of a new chest tube removal protocol using digital air leak monitoring after lobectomy: a prospective randomised trial. *Eur J Cardiothorac Surg* 2010 Jan; 37(1):56–60.

11 Brunelli A, Cassivi SD, Salati M, et al. Digital measurements of air leak flow and intrapleural pressures in the immediate postoperative period predict risk of prolonged air leak after pulmonary lobectomy. *Eur J Cardiothorac Surg* 2011 Apr; 39(4):584–8.

12 Pompili C, Brunelli A, Salati M, et al. Impact of the learning curve in the use of a novel electronic chest drainage system after pulmonary lobectomy: a case-matched analysis on the duration of chest tube usage. *Interact Cardiovasc Thorac Surg* 2011 Nov; 13(5):490–3.

13 Brunelli A, Salati M, Pompili C, et al. Regulated tailored suction vs regulated seal: a prospective randomized trial on air leak duration. *Eur J Cardiothorac Surg* 2012 Sep 28. [Epub ahead of print] PubMed PMID:23024236.

14 Miserocchi G, Beretta E, Rivolta I. Respiratory mechanics and fluid dynamics after lung resection surgery. *Thorac Surg Clin* 2010 Aug; 20(3):345–57.

15 Miserocchi G. Mechanisms controlling the volume of pleural fluid and extravascular lung water. *Eur Respir Rev* 2009; 18(114):1–9.

16 Cerfolio RJ, Bryant AS. Results of a prospective algorithm to remove chest tubes after pulmonary resection with high output. *J Thorac Cardiovasc Surg* 2008 Feb; 135(2):269–73.

17 Alex J, Ansari J, Bahalkar P, et al. Comparison of the immediate postoperative outcome of using the conventional two drains versus a single drain after lobectomy. *Ann Thorac Surg* 2003 Oct; 76(4):1046–9.

18 Gómez-Caro A, Roca MJ, Torres J, et al. Successful use of a single chest drain postlobectomy instead of two classical drains: a randomized study. *Eur J Cardiothorac Surg* 2006 Apr; 29(4):562–6.

19 Okur E, Baysungur V, Tezel C, et al. Comparison of the single or double chest tube applications after pulmonary lobectomies. *Eur J Cardiothorac Surg* 2009 Jan; 35(1):32–5.

20 Brunelli A, Cassivi SD, Fibla J, Di Nunzio L. Pleural pressure immediately after pulmonary lobectomy: single versus double chest tubes for suction. *J Thorac Cardiovasc Surg* 2010 Sep; 140(3): e52–3.

21 Refai M, Brunelli A, Salati M, et al. The impact of chest tube removal on pain and pulmonary function after pulmonary resection. *Eur J Cardiothorac Surg* 2012 Apr; 41(4):820–2.

22 Cerfolio RJ, Bass C, Katholi CR. Prospective randomized trial compares suction versus water seal for air leaks. *Ann Thorac Surg* 2001 May; 71(5):1613–7.

23 Marshall MB, Deeb ME, Bleier JI, et al. Suction vs water seal after pulmonary resection: a randomized prospective study. *Chest* 2002 Mar; 121(3):831–5.

24 Brunelli A, Monteverde M, Borri A, et al. Comparison of water

seal and suction after pulmonary lobectomy: a prospective, randomized trial. *Ann Thorac Surg* 2004 Jun; 77(6):1932–7.

25 Brunelli A, Sabbatini A, Xiumé F, et al. Alternate suction reduces

prolonged air leak after pulmonary lobectomy: a randomized comparison versus water seal. *Ann Thorac Surg* 2005 Sep; 80(3):1052–5.

26 Alphonso N, Tan C, Utley M, et al. A prospective randomized

controlled trial of suction versus non-suction to the under-water seal drains following lung resection. *Eur J Cardiothorac Surg* 2005 Mar; 27(3):391–4.

Chapter 19

Primary spontaneous pneumothorax

Giuseppe Cardillo, Gerard Ngome Enang, Francesco Carleo, Bernardo Ciamberlano, Pasquale Ialongo, Aldo Morrone and Massimo Martelli

Pneumothorax is a relatively common clinical problem which usually occurs in young healthy males, but anyone can be affected. Irrespective of aetiology (primary, or secondary to pre-existing lung disorders or injury), immediate management depends mainly on the extent of cardiorespiratory impairment and degree of symptoms.

Definition

Pneumothorax is defined as the presence of air in the pleural space[8]. This is due to one of the following reasons: (1) the existence of communication between alveolar spaces and pleura; (2) direct or indirect communication between the atmosphere and the pleural space; (3) presence of gas-producing organisms in the pleural space; (4) trauma involving bowel and diaphragm; of (5) oesophageal perforation. Clinically, pneumothorax is classified as spontaneous (no obvious precipitating factor present) and secondary (in the presence of pre-existing lung disease) (Table 19.1)[20]. Nevertheless, different national guidelines (BTS, British Thoracic Society; Belgian Society of Pneumology; SEPAR, Sociedad Espanola de Neumologia y cirugia toracica)[3,17,20,21,22,23] and a consensus statement (Delphi Consensus Statement) have been published. There are still a lot of discrepancies about the treatment of spontaneous pneumothorax among the different specialists involved. A new consensus statement by the European Respiratory Society (ERS) was delivered in 2015[27].

Spontaneous pneumothorax (SP) is divided into primary spontaneous pneumothorax (PSP) and secondary spontaneous pneumothorax (SSP). PSP is defined as the spontaneously occurring presence of air in the pleural space in patients without clinically apparent underlying lung disease. It is usually caused

Table 19.1 Clinical classification of pneumothorax

Spontaneous
Primary: no apparent underlying lung disease
Secondary: clinically apparent underlying disease (e.g. chronic obstructive pulmonary disease and cystic fibrosis)

Catamenial
in conjunction with menstruation

Traumatic
Iatrogenic: secondary to transthoracic and transbronchial biopsy, central venous catheterization, pleural biopsy and thoracentesis
Non-iatrogenic: secondary to blunt or penetrating chest injury

by ruptured pleural blebs or bullae. SSP is caused by a variety of respiratory disorders. The most frequent underlying disorders are chronic obstructive pulmonary disease with emphysema, cystic fibrosis, tuberculosis, lung cancer and HIV-associated *Pneumocystis carinii* pneumonia, followed by rarer disorders such as lymphangioleiomyomatosis and histiocytosis X (Table 19.2).

Epidemiology

PSP has an incidence of 7.4 to 18 cases (age-adjusted incidence) per 100,000 population each year in males and 1.2 to 6 cases per 100,000 population each year in females[4,7]. PSP typically occurs in tall, thin subjects. Smoking plays a role in the development of PSP. The lifetime risk in healthy smoking men may be as much as 12% compared with 0.1% in non-smoking men. PSP recurs in up to 25% of the cases after a first episode and up to 50% after a second episode,

Core Topics in Thoracic Surgery, ed. Marco Scarci, Aman Coonar, Tom Routledge and Francis Wells. Published by Cambridge University Press. © Cambridge University Press 2016

Table 19.2 Frequent and/or typical causes of secondary spontaneous pneumothorax

Hyperinflation
Emphysema

Airway disease
Cystic fibrosis
Severe asthma

Infectious lung disease
Pneumocystis carinii pneumonia
Tuberculosis
Necrotizing pneumonia

Interstitial lung disease
Idiopathic pulmonary fibrosis
Sarcoidosis
Histiocytosis X
Lymphangioleiomyomatosis

Connective tissue disease
Rheumatoid arthritis, scleroderma and ankylosing spondylitis
Marfan's syndrome
Ehlers-Danlos syndrome

Malignant disease
Lung cancer
Sarcoma
Metastases to lung

especially in the first 2 years after the initial episode. There are, therefore, two distinct epidemiological forms: (1) primary pneumothorax, with a peak incidence in young people between 20 and 40 years old, especially if the person is very tall and underweight, and (2) secondary pneumothorax, which has a peak incidence in those aged above 55 years. Because lung function in these patients is already compromised, SSP can be more serious. The general incidence is almost similar to that of PSP.

Pathogenesis

The pathogenesis of the spontaneous occurrence of a communication between the alveolar spaces and the pleura remains unknown. Subpleural blebs and bullae are found at the lung apices at thoracoscopy and on computed tomographic (CT) scanning in up to 90% of cases of PSP[5,14,15].

Smoking is implicated. The risk increases with the length of time and the number of cigarettes smoked. It has been associated with a 12% risk of developing pneumothorax in healthy smoking men compared with 0.1% in non-smokers. The risk of recurrence of PSP is as high as 54% within the first 4 years and in 80–86% of young patients who continue to smoke after their first episode of PSP.

Signs and symptoms

Symptoms in PSP may be minimal or absent. In contrast, symptoms are often greater in SSP, even if the pneumothorax is relatively small in size. The typical symptoms are chest pain and dyspnoea. Almost all patients with PSP report a sudden ipsilateral chest pain. Dyspnoea may be present but is usually mild. In SSP, dyspnoea is the most prominent clinical feature; chest pain, cyanosis, hypoxemia and hypercapnia, sometimes resulting in acute respiratory failure, can also be present. Physical examination can be normal in a small pneumothorax. In a large pneumothorax, breath sounds and tactile fremitus are typically decreased or absent, and percussion is hyper-resonant. Severe symptoms and signs of respiratory distress suggest the presence of tension pneumothorax, which is, however, extremely rare in PSP. These signs include

- Dyspnoea, tachypnea, increased work of breathing
- Hypoxia
- Abnormal pulse or blood pressure
- Poor perfusion
- Distended neck veins, muffled heart sounds
- Depressed mental state

Clinical evaluation should probably be the main determinant of the management strategy.

Diagnostic approaches of SP

The diagnosis of pneumothorax is usually confirmed by imaging techniques. The following imaging modalities are employed for the diagnosis and management of pneumothorax:

- Standard postero-anterior (PA) chest X-ray
- Lateral X-rays
- CT scanning

Standard erect PA chest radiographs in inspiration are recommended for the initial diagnosis of pneumothorax rather than expiratory films. The diagnostic characteristic is displacement of the pleural line. If uncertainty exists, then CT scanning is highly desirable.

Lateral X-rays may provide additional information when a suspected pneumothorax is not confirmed by a PA chest film.

CT scanning can be regarded as the 'gold standard' in the detection of small pneumothoraces and in size estimation. It is generally performed before surgery in patients >40 years old (either smokers or non-smokers). The 2010 British Thoracic Surgery guidelines recommend using CT when required to differentiate between pneumothorax and bullous lung disease, when aberrant tube placement is suspected and when the plain chest radiograph is difficult to read owing to the presence of subcutaneous emphysema (grade C recommendation).

Treatment

The chief objective of the management of primary spontaneous pneumothorax is elimination of the intrapleural air, either by observation in the case of partial pneumothorax or by evacuation using any of several different methods when the pneumothorax is complete and/or there is total lung collapse.

The secondary aim is to prevent recurrence when there is a high probability of recurrence or when recurrence could potentially be serious.

Treatment options for PSP include

- Non-surgical: observation, needle aspiration (thoracentesis), chest (intercostal) tube drainage, and
- Surgical (video-assisted thoracoscopy, and thoracotomy) approaches.

Observation. This should be the first-line treatment for patients who have a partial pneumothorax and no dyspnoea (grade B recommendation). If the lung is less than 20% collapsed, monitoring of the patient's condition with a series of chest X-rays can be done, until the air in the pleural space is completely absorbed and the lung has re-expanded. The reabsorption rate is 1.25 to 1.8% per day. A 25% pneumothorax will take 20 days to resolve.

Needle aspiration (thoracentesis). When the lung is more than 20% collapsed, the air in the pleural space can be removed by inserting a needle or hollow tube (chest tube). This can be done even when the pneumothorax is small and non-threatening, because it may take weeks for it to heal on its own[18]. Thoracentesis is associated with less pain, and patients do not have to be admitted to hospital. The rate of immediate resolution ranges between 50 and 88%. Several randomized clinical trials have shown this procedure to be as effective in both the short and long term as chest tube drainage (grade A recommendation).

Chest (intercostal) tube drainage. This is the most common approach, even if there is a trend towards a non-surgical approach in most countries. Small-bore catheters (14F) are easier to insert and cause less discomfort (grade B recommendation). Intercostal tube drainage (16F–24F) are very popular. During this procedure, chest (intercostal) tubes are connected to a one-way valve system that allows air to escape but not to re-enter the chest cavity and may be left in place for several hours to several days[6].

Indications for surgery:

- Second ipsilateral pneumothorax,
- First contralateral pneumothorax,
- Bilateral spontaneous pneumothorax,
- Spontaneous hemothorax,
- Persistent air leak (>4–5 days of chest tube drainage),
- Incomplete lung re-expansion after chest (intercostal) drainage, and
- Professions at increased risk (aircraft personnel, sportsmen, scuba divers).

The aforementioned professions are considered unsafe unless permanent treatment of spontaneous pneumothorax has been achieved; in some instances, professional guidelines suggest that pleurodesis is performed on both lungs and that lung function tests and CT scan must be normal before normal activity is resumed.

There are two objectives in the surgical management of pneumothorax. The first widely accepted objective is resection of blebs or the suture of apical perforations to treat the underlying defect. The second objective is to create a pleural symphysis (pleurodesis) to prevent recurrence. There are three options: pleurectomy, abrasion, and talc poudrage.

Video-assisted thoracoscopy (VATS) is the 'gold standard' for surgical treatment of PSP. It is a less invasive approach and has the benefits of less postoperative pain, better wound cosmetics, shorter duration of drainage and hospital stay, better functional recovery, better short- and long-term patient satisfaction, and at least equivalent cost-effectiveness to the open approach. Video-assisted magnification allows easier identification of the bullae or blebs, which can be managed through VATS in different ways: stapling and resection, which is the commonest approach; by no-knife stapling, useful in emphysematous-like lung; or by endoloop ligation, which has been shown by Cardillo et al. to be less effective than the previous techniques[11]. However, bullectomy without additional pleurodesis does not prevent recurrence as effectively as combining the two techniques. Horio and Naunheim have shown that recurrence rate diminished from 16 to 1.9% and from 20 to 1.5%, respectively, when a pleurodesis was added to bullectomy[13,16]. Cardillo has shown bullectomy to be superior to bulla ligation (endoloop) with a drop of recurrence rate from 4.54 to 0%. Bullectomy with pleural abrasion or with talc poudrage is the technique most often used by most thoracic surgeons (grade D recommendation)[1,2,20].

The different pleurodesis techniques (pleurectomy, pleural abrasion and talc poudrage) have all shown to be effective in preventing recurrences[19]. Parietal pleurectomy is often extended from the apex to the fifth–sixth intercostal space or lower. Pleural abrasion is usually performed with a pad. Talc pleurodesis is performed by instilling 2–4 g of sterile talc in the pleural cavity. It is a very fast technique, with the lowest rate of related complications, compared to the risk of bleeding reported for pleurectomy, and sometimes, even for pleural abrasion. Talc poudrage has been shown to be efficacious and safe with a success rate of 95% in the largest series. No concern exists regarding the oncological safety of talc and about the long-term lung function after talc poudrage. Graded talc, with a very low percentage (4–5%) of particles with a diameter of less than 5 microns, has been extensively and safely used in Europe for more than 70 years for pleurodesis in recurrent spontaneous pneumothorax and has been shown to be well tolerated without long-term sequelae[9–12].

Follow-up

The need for follow-up in patients following an episode of pneumothorax is unclear. No data are available in the world literature.

Prevention

Although it's often not possible to prevent a pneumothorax, stopping smoking is an important way to reduce the risk of a first pneumothorax episode and to avoid a recurrence[2]. Most recurrences occur within 2 years from the first episode.

References

1 Tschopp JM et al. Management of spontaneous pneumothorax: state of the art. *Eur Respir J* 2006; 28:637–50.

2 Cardillo G et al. Videothoracoscopic talc poudrage in primary spontaneous pneumothorax: a single-institution experience in 861 cases. *J Thorac Cardiovasc Surg* 2006; 131:322–8.

3 MacDuff A, Arnold A, Harvey J. Management of spontaneous pneumothorax: British Thoracic Society Pleural Disease Guidelines, 2010.

4 Miller A. Spontaneous pneumothorax. In: Light RW, Lee YCG, eds., *Textbook of Pleural Diseases*. 2nd edn. London: Arnold Press, 2008: 445–63.

5 Light RW, Lee YCG. Pneumothorax, chylothorax, hemothorax and fibrothorax. In: Murray J, Nadel J, Mason R, et al., eds., *Textbook of Respiratory Diseases*. 5th edn. Philadelphia: Saunders Elsevier, 2010: 1764–91.

6 Chan SS. The role of simple aspiration in the management of primary spontaneous pneumothorax. *J Emerg Med* 2008; 34:131–8.

7 Noppen M. Spontaneous pneumothorax: epidemiology, pathophysiology and cause. *Eur Respir Rev* 2010; 19:117, 217–21.

8 Jantz MA, Anthony VB. Pathophysiology of the pleura. *Respiration* 2008; 75:121–33.

9 Janssen J, Cardillo G. Primary spontaneous pneumothorax: towards outpatient treatment and abandoning chest tube drainage. *Respiration* 2011; 82:201–3.

10 Bridevaux PO, Tschopp JM, Cardillo G, et al. Safety of large-particle talc pleurodesis after talc poudrage under thoracoscopy for primary spontaneous pneumothorax: a European multicentre prospective study. *Eur Respir J* 2011; 38:770–3.

11 Cardillo G, Facciolo F, Giunti R, et al. Videothoracoscopic treatment of primary spontaneous pneumothorax: a 6-year experience. *Ann Thorac Surg* 2000; 69:357–61.

12 Cardillo G, Carleo F, Carbone L, et al. Long-term lung function following videothoracoscopic talc poudrage for primary spontaneous recurrent pneumothorax. *Eur J Cardiothorac Surg* 2007; 31:802–5.

13 Horio H, Nomori H, Kobayashi R, et al. Impact of additional pleurodesis in video-assisted thoracoscopic bullectomy for primary spontaneous pneumothorax. *Surg Endosc* 2002; 16:630–4.

14 Hatz RA, Kaps MF, Meimarakis G, et al. Long-term results after video-assisted thoracoscopic surgery for first time and recurrent spontaneous

neumothorax. *Ann Thorac Surg* 2000; 70:253–7.

15 Loubani M, Lynch V. Video-assisted thoracoscopic bullectomy and acromycin pleurodesis: an effective treatment for spontaneous pneumothorax. *Respir Med* 2000; 94:888–90.

16 Naunheim KS, Mack MJ, Hazelrigg SR, et al. Safety and efficacy of video-assisted thoracic surgical techniques for the treatment of spontaneous pneumothorax. *J Thorac Cardiovasc Surg* 1995; 109:1198–1204.

17 Harvey J, Prescott RJ. Simple aspiration versus intercostal tube drainage for spontaneous pneumothorax in patients with normal lungs: British Thoracic Society Research Committee. *BMJ* 1994; 309:1338–9.

18 Ayed AK, Chandrasekaran C, Sukumar M. Aspiration versus tube drainage in primary spontaneous pneumothorax: a randomized study. *Eur Respir J* 2006; 27:477–82.

19 Noppen M, Alexander P, Driesen P, et al. Manual aspiration versus chest tube drainage in first episodes of primary spontaneous pneumothorax: a multicenter, prospective, randomized pilot study. *Am J Respir Crit Care Med* 2002; 165:1240–4.

20 Baumann MH, Strange C, Heffner JE, et al. Management of spontaneous pneumothorax: an American College of Chest Physicians Delphi Consensus Statement. *Chest* 2001; 119:590–602.

21 Henry A, Arnold T, Harvey J. BTS guidelines for the management of spontaneous pneumothorax. *Thorax* 2003; 58 (Suppl 2):39–52.

22 De Leyn P, Lismonde M, Niname V, et al. Belgian Society of Pneumology: guidelines on the management of spontaneous pneumothorax. *Acta Chir Belg* 2005; 105:265–7.

23 Rivas de Andrés JJ, Jiménez López FM, Laureano Molins LR, et al. SEPAR guidelines for the diagnosis and treatment of spontaneous pneumothorax. *Arch Bronconeumol* 2008; 44(8):437–48.

24 Allanah Barker, Eleni C Maratos, Lyn Edmonds, Eric Lim. Recurrence rates of video-assisted thoracoscopic versus open surgery in the prevention of recurrent pneumothoraces: a systematic review of randomised and non-randomised trials. *Lancet* 2007 July; 370 (9584): 329–35.

25 Humaid. *Interact Cardiovasc Thor Surg* 2008; 7:673–7.

26 Treasure T. Minimal access surgery for pneumothorax. *Lancet* 2007 July; 370 (9584):294–5.

27 Tschopp JM. ERS task force statement: diagnosis and treatment of primary spontaneous pneumothorax. *Eur Respir J* 2015 Aug; 46(2):321–35. doi: 10.1183/09031936.00219214. Epub 2015 Jun 25.

Bronchopleural fistula management

Steven M. Woolley and Susannah M. Love

A bronchopleural fistula (BPF) is an abnormal connection between the bronchial tree and the pleural space. The development of a fistula following pulmonary resection due to a bronchial stump dehiscence is a rare and potentially fatal complication. The incidence is reported as between 1 to 20% following pneumonectomy and 0.5% after lobectomy, and reported mortality varies between 20 and 70%[1,2,3,4,5]. The risk of death is highest when a fistula presents within the first 2 weeks after surgery, and the main cause of death is aspiration pneumonia[4].

The most common aetiology of a bronchopleural fistula is a complication of pulmonary resection, either segmentectomy, lobectomy or pneumonectomy. This chapter will focus upon post-operative fistulae, but they can occur in the non-operative setting. Non-operative fistulae can be caused by a necrotizing pneumonia or empyema and neoplasms of lung, thyroid, oesophagus or the lymphatic system. Also, they can be secondary to blunt or penetrating chest trauma or as a complication of medical procedures such as radiotherapy, lung biopsy or chest drain insertion. The 'air leak' responsible for causing a pneumothorax is often erroneously referred to as a bronchopleural fistula, but these leaks are alveolar-pleural fistulae, rather than the more proximally located bronchopleural fistulae.

The risk factors for post-resection fistula formation can be classified into pre-operative, intra-operative and post-operative factors. Table 20.1 shows a list of risk factors which have been suggested to predispose to BPF after lung resection. Pre-operative factors focus upon co-morbidities, drug history and any pre-operative oncological treatment. Algar et al. found a significant association between development of BPF and COPD, hyperglycaemia, hypoalbuminaemia,

steroid therapy and low predicted post-operative FEV1[6]. A multivariate analysis by Asamura et al. of risk factors for BPF in 1,360 pulmonary resections for lung cancer reported similar findings but in addition found an increased risk associated with liver cirrhosis and pre-operative radiotherapy in excess of 5,000 Gy[3].

Intra-operatively, Asamura et al. identified right-sided resection, pneumonectomy (especially right-sided), mediastinal lymph node dissection and residual carcinoma at the bronchial stump as technical factors predisposing to fistula formation[3]. Also, long and devascularized bronchial stumps are reported as risk factors[2]. The mechanisms for the increased risk related to right-sided resections are two-fold. Firstly, the right main bronchus is usually supplied by one bronchial artery, whereas the left is supplied by two bronchial arteries. Secondly, the left main bronchus, after resection, retracts up behind the aortic arch, where it is surrounded by the richly vascularized mediastinal tissue. The right main bronchus is left exposed without any natural protective covering within the pleural cavity.

Post-operative risk factors include prolonged positive-pressure ventilation and the development of infection within the bronchial stump or an empyema in the pleural space which can break down the bronchial stump. Post-operative management should aim at early extubation followed by early mobilization and physiotherapy to reduce the risk of re-intubation. In clinical scenarios where post-operative mechanical ventilation is unavoidable, ventilator settings should be weaned to decrease peak airway pressures and positive end-expiration pressure, and the endotracheal tube cuff and tip should be as proximal as possible from the bronchial stump[7]. Airway suctioning of

---

Core Topics in Thoracic Surgery, ed. Marco Scarci, Aman Coonar, Tom Routledge and Francis Wells. Published by Cambridge University Press. © Cambridge University Press 2016

Table 20.1 Risk factors for development of a bronchopleural fistula

Pre-operative	Age
	Diabetes mellitus
	Steroid therapy
	Hypoalbuminaemia
	Pre-operative radiotherapy
	Liver cirrrhosis
	COPD
	Low predicted post-operative FEV1
	Surgery for ongoing infection
Operative	Right pneumonectomy
	Long bronchial stump
	Devascularization of the bronchus
	Positive resection margin
Post-operative	Mechanical ventilation
	Empyema

(a)

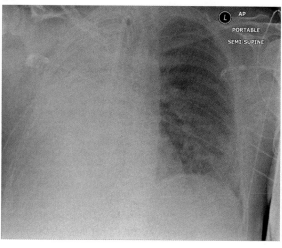

Figure 20.1A CXR of a patient 2 weeks after pneumonectomy ventilated via a tracheostomy.

ventilated patients after pneumonectomy should be carried out cautiously as vigorous instrumentation can cause fistula formation.

Post-operative fistulae can present with a broad spectrum of signs, symptoms and times of onset. Several classification systems have been suggested to describe post-operative fistulae based upon time between surgery and onset of symptoms. Varoli et al. suggested that fistulae should be classified depending on time of onset after the operation: early (1–7 days), intermediate (8–30 days) and late fistulae (>30 days)[8]. Hollaus et al. recommended that fistulae after pneumonectomy should be classified on a I–III scale (I: <14 days where risk of aspiration and mortality is high; II: 14–90 days, where fibrothorax is in a state of formation which prevents massive aspiration, but mortality is high as patients will have already been discharged and may fail to seek adequate and prompt treatment; and III: >90 days, where a fibrothorax has formed, making massive aspiration impossible, and mortality is much decreased)[4].

Early presentation is most likely due to a technical failure due to misfired staples, poor suture technique or a closure performed with excessive tension with poor apposition of tissues. Intermediate or late presentation suggests a secondary cause such as weak bronchial tissues, residual or recurrent tumour or infection within the bronchial stump or from within the pleural cavity such as an empyema within the pleural space.

Clinical presentation of a BPF is variable depending upon the time of onset since the initial operation. Early fistula can present with sudden cardiovascular collapse either due to a tension pneumothorax or a large aspiration of pleural contents into the contralateral lung and, if the patient survives the initial insult, subsequent acute respiratory distress syndrome (ARDS). Early fistulae can present in a less dramatic fashion, such as a cough productive of clear or purulent sputum, a prolonged or new-onset air leak or development of surgical emphysema. A late fistula classically presents with a cough productive of frothy, serosanguinious sputum; often patients describe coughing this fluid up on waking in the morning or when they lie flat. If the fistula is due to an empyema, the patient may have symptoms associated with sepsis such as pyrexia and rigors.

Radiologically, a fistula should be suspected if there is a fall in the air-fluid level by more than 2 cm on the chest radiograph or the appearance of a new air-fluid level within a previously opacified hemithorax. Figure 20.1 shows a marked drop in the fluid level in a right pneumonectomy space in a ventilated patient. When a fluid level does drop in a patient after pneumonectomy, unfortunately, BPF is a common cause; other causes include breakdown of the wound and fluid draining percutaneously or iatrogenic drainage of fluid from the space. A rare cause can be dehydration. Bronchoscopy allows direct visualization of the bronchial tree, often enabling identification and localization of a fistula. However, small

(b)

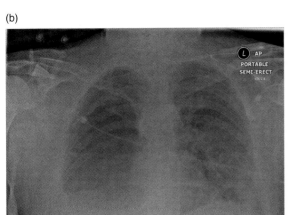

Figure 20.1B The same patient 12 hours later after developing a BPF; the fluid level in the pneumonectomy space has dropped dramatically.

fistulae are not always seen with bronchoscopy. If a suspected fistula is not identified via plain bronchoscopy, a suspicious site can be irrigated with saline, and the presence of continuous bubbling can help confirm the location of a fistula. In addition, injection of methylene blue into the lumen of a suspected bronchi can confirm the presence of a fistula if the dye subsequently appears within the chest drainage tube. More recently, CT bronchography has also been described as a useful technique in the evaluation of patients with a suspected BPF[9]. Of course, some of these more complex imaging procedures may not be appropriate in an unstable patient requiring critical care, and bronchoscopy remains the 'gold standard' for diagnosis of BPF.

Surgical techniques to avoid BPF

As mentioned earlier, risk factors for BPF include leaving a long bronchial stump and devascularization of the bronchial stump by excessive diathermy or skeletonization. These factors are avoided relatively easily. When comparing handsewn or stapled bronchial stumps, there is no clear advantage to either technique with experienced operators[6]. Though, as a stapled technique is very reproducible and simple to teach, it is now the most commonly used method in UK centres. Further measures to avoid fistula formation include covering the bronchial stump at the time of resection. Most authors agree that a vascularized

tissue should be used to promote early healing of the bronchial stump, and a wide variety of tissues have been used for this purpose, including pleura, intercostal muscle, diaphragm, pericardium, azygous vein and omentum[5,10,11]. Asamura and Naruke as well as Klepetko have all suggested that a pedicled pericardial flap covering the bronchial stump is a good method to decrease incidence of BPF in their reported series[3,14]. There is reasonable agreement that following a right pneumonectomy the bronchial stump should be covered due to the increased risk of BPF on this side. With a left pneumonectomy, however, some surgeons do not routinely cover the stump as the stump tends to retract behind the aorta and is surrounded by well-vascularized mediastinal tissues which can be closed over the stump.

Treatment strategies for BPF

As mentioned earlier, in early BPFs, aspiration of pleural fluid into the contralateral lung is a common problem which leads to a high mortality rate. This means that in such patients thorough early drainage of the pleural space on the side of the BPF must be achieved to avoid contamination of the contralateral lung. Drainage is commonly closed via intercostal drains. Antibiotics to treat any pleural space infection are also normally given as the pleural space associated with a BPF must be presumed to be infected unless proven otherwise. Bronchoscopy is performed both to attempt to identify the fistula and to clear any secretions or suction-contaminated pleural fluid from the contralateral lung and airways. In patients requiring ventilation, this may be necessary via a double-lumen tube or a long ET tube selectively intubating the contralateral bronchus to protect the unaffected side from aspiration of pleural fluid. The immediate management of an early BPF can be summarized as protection of the airway (by drainage, clearance of fluid secretions and possible selective ventilation) and treatment of infection by appropriate antibiotic cover.

Large fistulae that present early after lung resection are often best managed by exploration and operative repair as long as the patient is stable enough to tolerate the procedure and there is not heavy contamination of the pleural cavity[12,13]. When repaired early like this, techniques such as stump resection or revision can be used, and in the case of post-lobectomy BPF, completion pneumonectomy may

195

be an option. Khan et al. suggested that direct closure is possible in around 80% of patients, and it is suggested that the stump be covered in a vascularized pedicle flap, as mentioned earlier[16]. Thorough washout of the space together with antibiotics delivered by continous irrigation and systemically have rarely prevented the development of post-pneumonectomy empyema.

Where there is an established empyema associated with a bronchopleural fistula, this is more difficult to treat, and treatment has two main goals: to close the fistula and to sterilize or obliterate the pleural space. It is commonly suggested that definitive surgical repair is not carried out until the pleural space infection is cleared and the patient is in the best possible condition for surgery[15]. Various methods have been used to attempt to clear infection from the pleural space, including irrigation with saline, dilute iodine solution or antibiotic installations along with continued administration of IV antibiotics[15,16]. Even with these strategies, it is often not possible to clear the pleural space infection with closed drainage, and open thoracostomy drainage can be necessary. A commonly used technique to deal with BPFs associated with empyema is the Clagett procedure; this is a two-stage procedure consisting of open pleural drainage, closure of the BPF, removal of the necrotic tissue and then secondary closure or obliteration of the pleural cavity with antibiotic solution[14,15]. This procedure was developed at the Mayo Clinic and modified there by Pairolero et al. to include intrathoracic muscle flap transposition to reinforce the closed BPF[16]. With this technique, they reported 84% of patients in whom the procedure was completed having a healed chest wall with no evidence of recurrent infection and the BPF remaining closed in 86%[19]. Though these techniques report good outcomes, they can involve multiple surgical procedures, prolonged hospital stays and extended periods of open chest drainage and packing[17]. Gharagozloo et al. have suggested that pleural space irrigation can speed up this process; however, they also suggest that this is only appropriate for early-stage BPFs, not those with established indurated pleural tissue[18].

Where there is still a large pleural space present, other techniques can be used to obliterate this space. Historically, thoracoplasty was commonly used for this purpose, but increasingly now, the space is filled with muscle flaps or omentum. Muscles flaps which

can be used to fill the pleural space include latissimus dorsi, pectoralis major, serratus anterior, pectoralis minor, rectus abdominis and intercostal muscle[19–21]. Omentum is especially good for filling irregularly shaped cavities and is normally very vascular promoting rapid healing[15]. In malnourished patients, however, it can have little bulk and become less useful. Sometimes for very large spaces a combination of limited thoracoplasty and muscle transposition may be useful.

There have also been a variety of bronchoscopic techniques which have been employed to attempt to deal with BPFs. These have generally been carried out in patients either deemed to unwell to undergo surgical correction under general anaesthetic or in patients with small BPFs who are quite well and wish to avoid invasive surgery. Many materials and devices have been used to try to close fistulae including ethanol silver nitrate, cyanoacrylate compounds, coils, lead plugs, balloons, fibrin or tissue glue, antibiotics, gel foam, spigots, autologous blood patches and more recently Amplatzer-type devices[22–24]. All of these techniques have had variable success rates and in general seem to work best on smaller and more peripheral fistula. It has been suggested they work best with fistulae around 1 mm and have no real use in fistulae above 8 mm[25]. As mentioned earlier, they are often used in patients where major surgery is not an option. In summary, the principles of treatment of a BPF are protection of the airway and treatment of infection initially, then closure of the fistula and management of the pleural space. Though endobronchial techniques have been used successfully, the most commonly employed methods of treatment with the highest success rates all involve major surgical intervention.

More recently, treatment strategies using some of the elements described earlier plus negative pressure wound therapy have been reported. Schneiter et al. have reported an accelerated treatment for post pneumonectomy empyema comprising multiple debridements and packing the chest with iodine soaked swabs with negative-pressure therapy and antibiotics[25]. In this report, they describe successfully treating 97% of 75 patients with a post-pneumonectomy BPF. Similar treatment has also been described by Perentes et al. with repeated intrathoracic VAC dressings until granulation tissue covered the entire chest cavity[26]. The current evidence regarding negative-therapy dressing for treatment of post–lung resection BPF and empyema was reviewed by Haghshenasskashani et al.[27]. The conclusions of this review were that negative-pressure therapies can potentially alleviate the morbidity and decrease hospital stay in patients with empyema after lung resection. As evidence grows regarding their use, they may play an important role in the treatment of BPF.

References

1   McManigle JE, Fletcher GL, Tenholder MF. Bronchoscopy in the management of bronchopleural fistula. *Chest* 1990 May; 97(5): 1235–8.

2   Cerfolio RJ. The incidence, etiology, and prevention of postresectional bronchopleural fistula. *Semin Thorac Cardiovasc Surg* 2001 Jan; 13(1):3–7.

3   Asamura H, Naruke T, Tsuchiya R, et al. Bronchopleural fistulas associated with lung cancer operations. Univariate and multivariate analysis of risk factors, management, and outcome. *J Thorac Cardiovasc Surg* 1992 Nov; 104(5):1456–64.

4   Hollaus PH, Lax F, el-Nashef BB, et al. Natural history of bronchopleural fistula after pneumonectomy: a review of 96 cases. *Ann Thorac Surg* 1997 May; 63(5):1391–6.

5   Taghavi S, Marta GM, Lang G, et al. Bronchial stump coverage with a pedicled pericardial flap: an effective method for prevention of postpneumonectomy bronchopleural fistula. *Ann Thorac Surg* 2005 Jan; 79(1): 284–8. Review.

6   Algar FJ, Alvarez A, Aranda JL, et al. Prediction of early bronchopleural fistula after pneumonectomy: a multivariate analysis. *Ann Thorac Surg* 2001 Nov; 72(5):1662–7.

7   Liberman M, Cassivi SD. Bronchial stump dehiscence: update on prevention and management. *Semin Thorac Cardiovasc Surg* 2007 Winter; 19(4):366–73.

8   Varoli F, Roviaro G, Grignani F, et al. Endoscopic treatment of bronchopleural fistulas. *Thorac Surg* 1998 Mar; 65(3):807–9.

9   Sarkar P, Patel N, Chusid J, et al. The role of computed tomography bronchography in the management of bronchopleural fistulas. *J Thorac Imaging* 2010; 25:W10–3.

10 Deschamps C, Bernard A, Nichols FC, et al. Empyema and bronchopleural fistula after pneumonectomy: factors affecting incidence. *Ann Thorac Surg* 2001; 72:243–7.

11 Klepetko W, Taghavi S, Pereslenyi A, et al. Impect of different coverage techniques on incidence of postpneumonectomy stump fistula. *Eur J Cardiothorac Surg* 1999; 15:758–63.

12 Puskas JD, Mathisen DJ, Grillo HC, et al. Treatment strategies for bronchopleural fistula. *J Thorac Cardiovasc Surg* 1995 May; 109(5):989–95; discussion 995–6.

13 Khan JH, Rahman SB, McElhinney DB, et al. Management strategies for complex bronchopleural fistula. *Asian Cardiovasc Thorac Ann* 2000; 8:78–84.

14 Clagett OT, Geraci JE. A procedure for the management of postpneumonectomy empyema *J Thorac Cardiovasc Surg* 1963; 45:141–5.

15 Stafford EG, Clagett OT. Postpneumonectomy empyemaneomycin instillation and definitive closure. *J Thorac Cardiovasc Surg* 1972; 63:771–5.

16 Pairolero PC, Arnold PG, Trastek VF, et al. Postpneumonectomy empyema: the role of intrathoracic muscle transposition *J Thorac Cardiovasc Surg* 1990; 99:958–68.

17 Zaheer S, Allen MS, Cassivi SD, et al. Postpneumonectomy empyema: results after the Clagett procedure. *Ann Thorac Surg* 2006 Jul; 82(1): 279–86; discussion 286–7.

18 Gharagozloo F, Trachiotis G, Wolfe A, et al. Pleural space irrigation and modified Clagett procedure for the treatment of early postpneumonectomy empyema. *J Thorac Cardiovasc Surg* 1998 Dec; 116(6):943–8.

19 Meland NB, Arnold PG, Pairolero PC, Trastek VF. Refinements in intrathoracic use of muscle flaps. *Clin Plast Surg* 1990; 17:697–703.

20 Zimmermann T, Muhrer KH, Padberg W, Schwemmle K. Closure of acute bronchial stump insufficiency with a musculus latissimus dorsi flap. *Thorac Cardiovasc Surg* 1993; 41:196–8.

21 Arnold PG, Pairolero PC. Intrathoracic muscle flaps: an account of their use in the management of 100 consecutive patients. *Ann Surg* 1990; 211:656–62.

22 Lois M, Noppen M. Bronchopleural fistulas: an overview of the problem with special focus on endoscopic management. *Chest* 2005; 128:3955–65.

23 West D, Togo A, Kirk AJ. Are bronchoscopic approaches to post-pneumonectomy bronchopleural fistula an effective alternative to repeat thoracotomy? *Interact Cardiovasc Thorac Surg* 2007 Aug; 6(4):547–50. Epub 2007 May 30.

24 Spiliopoulos S, Krokidis M, Gkoutzios P, et al. Successful

exclusion of a large bronchopleural fistula using an Amplatzer II vascular plug and glue embolization. *Acta Radiol* 2012 May 1; 53(4): 406–9.

25 Schneiter D, Grodzki T, Lardinois D, et al. Accelerated treatment of postpneumonectomy empyema: a binational long-term study. *J Thorac Cardiovasc Surg* 2008 Jul;

136(1):179–85. doi: 10.1016/j.jtcvs.2008.01.036

26 Perentes JY, Abdelnour-Berchtold E, Blatter J, Lovis A, et al. Vacuum-assisted closure device for the management of infected postpneumonectomy chest cavities. *J Thorac Cardiovasc Surg* 2015 Mar; 149(3):745–50. doi: 10.1016/j.jtcvs.2014.10.052. Epub 2014 Oct 14.

27 Haghshenasskashani A, Rahnavardi M, Yan TD, McCaughan BC. Intrathoracic application of a vacuum-assisted closure device in managing pleural space infection after lung resection: is it an option? *Interact Cardiovasc Thorac Surg* 2011 Aug; 13(2):168–74. doi: 10.1510/icvts.2011.267286. Epub 2011 May 20.

21   Surgery for pectus and other congenital chest wall disorders

Jakub Kadlec, Jean-Marie Wihlm and Aman S. Coonar

Congenital chest wall disorders represent a broad spectrum of abnormalities. Their physiological implications vary from concerns about the cosmetic appearance to life-threatening conditions. Pectus excavatum and carinatum are the commonest, representing 97% of all chest wall deformities. Rare conditions include Poland syndrome, sternal defects, and Jeune's and Jarcho-Levin syndromes. The incidence, sex ratio and familial occurrence of all these abnormalities are depicted in Table 21.1[1,2].

Pectus excavatum (funnel chest)

An early portrayal of a patient with pectus excavatum was found among the works of Leonardo da Vinci from 1510[3]. The deformity presents as a depression of the lower anterior chest wall as a result of posterior deviation of the sternum and usually the third to seventh ribs and costal cartilage. It represents nearly 90% of all congenital chest wall abnormalities and has high familial occurrence. Despite this, no clear genetic basis has been established. It is more frequently seen in patients with Marfan and Ehler-Danlos syndromes, and these patients comprise about 2% of all patients with pectus excavatum (Figure 21.1).

Table 21.1 The incidence, sex ratio and familial occurrence of congenital chest wall deformities

Abnormality	Incidence	M:F ratio	Familial occurrence
Pectus excavatum	1:200	4–5:1	40%
Pectus carinatum	1:1 500	3–4:1	25%
Poland syndrome	1:30 000	2–3:1	1%
Sternal defects	<1:100 000	1:1.5	Unknown
Jeune's syndrome	<1:100 000	1:1	Unknown
Jarcho-Levin syndrome	<1:200 000	1:1	Unknown

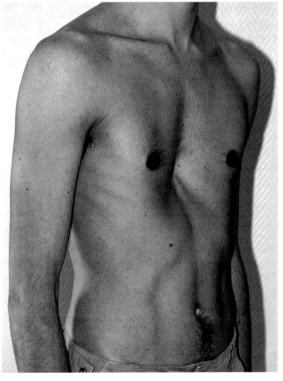

Figure 21.1 Pectus excavatum.

Core Topics in Thoracic Surgery, ed. Marco Scarci, Aman Coonar, Tom Routledge and Francis Wells. Published by Cambridge University Press. © Cambridge University Press 2016

The deformity is usually noted soon after birth or in early childhood and often becomes more marked during the period of rapid growth in puberty. It may be symmetrical or asymmetrical and sometimes associated with scoliosis or kyphoscoliosis. If asymmetrical, the depression is usually more marked on the right, and the sternum is rotated rightward and angled posteriorly[1,2].

There are several hypotheses behind the development of pectus excavatum. These include intrauterine external pressure, muscular imbalance, thickened substernal ligament and, most commonly accepted, (in some cases asymmetrical) sternocostal cartilage overgrowth. In some cases the ultrastructural and biochemical studies of cartilage from affected patients revealed decreased level of zinc and increased level of magnesium and calcium[4]. Given the association with Marfan syndrome and similar phenotypes and the familial nature of some cases of pectus, it is likely that there is an important genetic component.

The affected individuals seek medical attention due to embarrassment over the appearance, exertional dyspnea, poor stamina, pain and occasionally palpitation. Apart from the depression of the lower sternum, a typical posture of a tall, thin patient with a 'pot-belly', forward, drifted shoulders and flaring of the costal margin is often seen. Severe scoliosis with a Cobb angle[1] of more than 15° and usually rightward curvature between the fourth and ninth thoracic vertebrae is found in approximately 15% of patients.

Patients often develop nipple and, in females, breast asymmetry. A systolic murmur might be present in severe cases due to compression of the heart and mitral regurgitation secondary to valve prolapse. Echocardiographical studies revealed mitral valve prolapse in 18–65% of patients with severe deformity and compression of the ventricle in up to 95% of patients during exercise, with significant reduction of prolapse and ventricular compression after

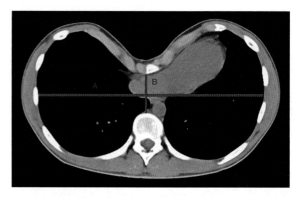

Figure 21.2 Haller index evaluated by CT scan.

correction of the deformity[5,6]. Pulmonary function tests may show a moderate restrictive pattern with a reduced forced vital capacity. Interestingly, despite subjective improvement of patients post-operatively, some patients do not show significant improvement in pulmonary function tests[7]. However, there is some evidence showing that correction of pectus excavatum can have a positive impact on cardiac function during exercise[8,9].

The psychological impact of the deformity on patients cannot be underestimated. Patients are often teased by their peers and siblings or overprotected by parents. This leads to avoidance of swimming, sports and situations when the shirt would be removed in front of others. Lower self-esteem and social anxiety are frequent consequences.

Several radiological indexes were developed to objectively measure the severity of pectus deformity. The most commonly used Haller (pectus) index is a ratio between transverse chest diameter (A) and distance from the posterior aspect of the sternum to the anterior surface of the spine (B) at the level of the deepest part of the deformity (Figure 21.2). The diameters are taken from axial computed tomography or lateral and postero-anterior chest radiographs. This ratio for normal individuals is around 2.5, and it is more than 3.2 in patients with severe pectus excavatum[10].

Treatment

Open repair

The first surgical repair with resection of rib cartilages was attempted by Meyer in 1911, but his operation did not improve the deformity. German surgeon Sauerbruch is credited with the first successful repair in 1913, and the 'Sauerbruch procedure' comprises

---

1 The Cobb angle is used to quantify the magnitude of spinal deformities. To measure the Cobb angle, one must first decide which vertebrae are the end vertebrae of the curve deformity (vertebrae at the upper and lower limits of the curve), and the Cobb angle is formed by the intersection of two lines: one parallel to the endplate of the superior end vertebra and the other parallel to the endplate of the inferior end vertebrae. Scoliosis is defined as a lateral spinal curvature with a Cobb angle of 10° or more.

bilateral resection of the third to fifth costal cartilages, sternal osteotomy and external traction of the sternum for 6 weeks after the operation. Mark Ravitch in 1949 further developed the open repair. The main feature of the original 'Ravitch procedure' (Figure 21.3) was an intra-perichondrial resection of the abnormal costal cartilages, perichondrial repair, resection of the xiphisternal junction, release of substernal ligament, transverse cuneiform osteotomy of sternum and its fixation in a corrected position with Kischner wires or sutures[11]. Modifications were made by different surgeons to prevent possible complications, the most important modifications being more limited cartilage resection with preservation of lateral and medial cartilage to retain the growing centres and mobility of sternocostal joints, use of metal struts for stabilization of the sternum to prevent recurrence of deformity and use of Marlex mesh to avoid second operation for removal of strut, which is usually performed about 1 year after correction (Figure 21.4)[12].

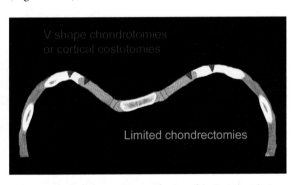

Figure 21.3 Cartilage-sparing modification of the Ravitch technique.

In the sternal turnover technique, the cartilages are resected, and the sternum is mobilized and rotated by 180°. This procedure was popular in Japan, but a high incidence of osteonecrosis and fistula formation in 46% of patients precluded widespread use of this technique[13].

Minimally invasive repair (MIRPE)

Donald Nuss introduced a less invasive procedure for correction in 1998[14]. Cartilage resections, sternal osteotomy and liberation are not required. The correction of deformity is achieved by the placement of a semi-customized stainless steel curved bar which moves the sternum to the correct position, leading to cartilage remodelling over time (Figure 21.5). The bar is inserted via relatively small lateral incisions through a tunnel created between the pericardium and maximal sternal depression. Once in place, the bar is turned over by 180° with the convexity pointing anteriorly and secured with lateral stabilizers. There is a potential risk of injury to the heart, so thoracoscopic guidance was added to the original operation to decrease such a risk. The bar is usually removed after 3 years[15]. In some cases, two or more bars may be needed.

Prosthetic reconstruction and nonsurgical treatment

In milder deformities, purely cosmetic techniques with the use of a custom-made silicone prosthesis have been reported as well as use of a vacuum bell or bracing as an alternative to surgical treatment.

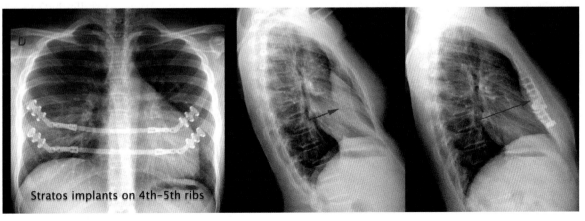

Figure 21.4 Titanium implants maintaining the correction and cardiopulmonary decompression.

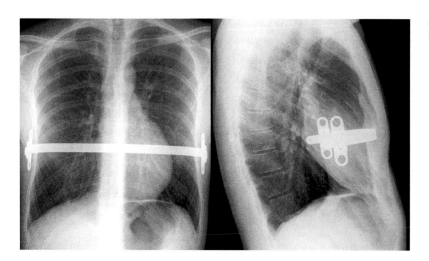

Figure 21.5 Front and lateral chest X-rays of a Nuss bar in place.

Complications and results of surgery

There is a spectrum of possible complications either early or late after repair. The obvious complications include pain, infection, seroma, bleeding, haemothorax and pneumothorax, atelectasis, pneumonia, injury to the heart and great vessels, liver injury, residual deformity, recurrence of deformity, allergy to metals, dislodgement or fracture of the substernal bars, pericarditis, keloid formation and psychological problems. The more specific complications include floating sternum due to extensive resection of costal cartilages and liberation of the sternum, acquired restrictive thoracic dystrophy (acquired Jeune's syndrome) due to injury to the growing centres of costal cartilages in children, sternal necrosis, acquired scoliosis secondary to biomechanical forces after minimally invasive repair of asymmetrical forms and acquired pectus carinatum due to overcorrection, especially in patients with connective tissue disorders. There are also unfortunate cases of asymmetry and retarded growth of the breasts due to injury of developing breast tissue as a result of poorly placed skin incisions in pre-pubescent girls[16]. This complication must, of course, be considered and avoided.

Despite the aforementioned complications, the results of open and minimally invasive procedures are very good, with minimal recurrence and patient satisfaction around led 95%. Although there are no randomized, controlled trials comparing the Ravitch and Nuss procedures, a recent meta-analysis of prospective and retrospective studies showed no significant differences in the overall complication rate in both procedures[17].

However, rates of re-operation for bar migration, persistent deformity, pneumothorax and haemothorax were significantly higher with the Nuss procedure. Duration of surgery was significantly longer by 70 minutes for the Ravitch procedure. There was no difference in length of hospital stay, time to ambulation or patient satisfaction[18].

Specific considerations

Age of repair

Pectus excavatum is often noticed early after birth, but it may not be evident till later in childhood. It tends to progress to at least mid-teens. The timing of corrective surgery remains a matter of debate. Earlier repair has the potential advantage of flexibility of the chest and a lower risk of costal flaring developing. Psychological and physiological impacts may also be minimized if repair is performed before commencing school. The development of an acquired restrictive thoracic defect in the original Ravitch cohort discouraged early repair with a recommendation not to operate before the age of 8. An increasing age of repair is seen in large paediatric registries, in which the mean age for operation has increased to 14 years[19]. This is challenged by some, who state that the Ravitch procedure can be performed safely in patients from 3 years of age if the medial and lateral fourths of costal cartilages are spared.

The situation is different in patients with Marfan and other connective tissue disorders due to a higher risk of recurrence or acquired pectus carinatum. In these patients, it is recommended to perform the operation after the patient is fully grown. Operation should also consider the needs of other problems that these patients may have, for example, surgery for aortic disease.

In general, the Ravitch procedure is the preferred option for fully grown adults due to the less compliant chest wall and risk of costal flaring (which may be treated at the same time if already present), although recently published data show good mid-term results with the Nuss procedure if more than one bar is used for correction[20]. Consequently, in the future there may be more use of the Nuss in older patients[21].

Symmetry of deformity

Asymmetry of chest deformity usually develops or progresses during growth of a child and is thus more common in adolescents and adults. The Ravitch procedure is usually preferred for asymmetrical forms, although specific techniques of morphology-tailored bar shaping for correction by Nuss procedure also provide good results[22,23].

Incision

Two small lateral chest incisions are generally used in the Nuss procedure, which gives excellent cosmetic results. Horizontal or vertical incisions can be used in the Ravitch procedure. The advantage of a vertical incision is of an easier approach to deformed cartilages with shorter length of scar. In contrast, subpectoral transverse incisions allow better access to inferior costal flaring and an easier positioning of bars, which can also be removed through the lateral parts of the same incision. Submammary incisions are cosmetic and also allow combined or staged breast augmentation or reconstruction. It is essential that the incision is placed appropriately to avoid injury to breast tissue.

Resuscitation

With new procedures, new issues develop. The bar in the Nuss procedure requires a modified approach if cardiopulmonary resuscitation is required. It is argued that the bar prevents effective chest compression. Chest depressions should be performed with higher force, and early chest opening or bar removal should be considered if soon after surgery. Anterior and posterior placement of defibrillation pads is also necessary to provide effective defibrillation[24].

Internal mammary artery injury and patency

There is risk of direct injury to mammary arteries during dissection in both the open and Nuss procedure, which can have implications if future coronary artery bypass grafting is required. Interestingly, recent data show that even without direct injury, the bar in the Nuss procedure compromises flow in the mammary artery by pressure against the sternum in 44% of patients, usually with bilateral mammary occlusion[25].

Cardiac surgery and pectus excavatum

Congenital and acquired cardiac diseases in patients with pectus excavatum present challenges during cardiac surgery. These include exposure, positioning the sternal retractor, harvesting the mammary artery, aortic cannulation and difficulty in closing the chest. Simultaneous repair is advantageous in that it avoids two operations but also due to an early improvement in right ventricular function[26]. A modified Ravitch procedure is an option but is time-consuming and requires additional dissection and cartilage resections. So, recently, several authors have advocated an 'open Nuss' technique, easy to perform under visual control, before closing the sternotomy[27,28].

Multidisciplinary approach

Due to the complexity of problems in some patients, advice and cooperation with other specialities are of great importance to allow optimal timing and results of corrective surgery. These include paediatricians, physiotherapists, orthopaedic surgeons, plastic surgeons, cardiologists, cardiac surgeons, geneticists and psychotherapists.

Pectus carinatum (Pigeon chest)

Pectus carinatum is characterized by an anterior projection of the sternum with adjacent anterior ribs and represents nearly 10% of all congenital chest wall abnormalities. A geographical difference is described. One of the author's personal experiences is that this is 15–20% in Europe and up to 50% in parts of South America. The shape of the deformity has a similar shape to the keel of a ship, hence the Latin word 'carinatum'. It usually develops between 11 and 15 years of age, and its aetiology is thought to be similar to pectus excavatum. It is associated with scoliosis in approximately 15% of patients and with an increased incidence of congenital heart disease especially in Marfan patients.

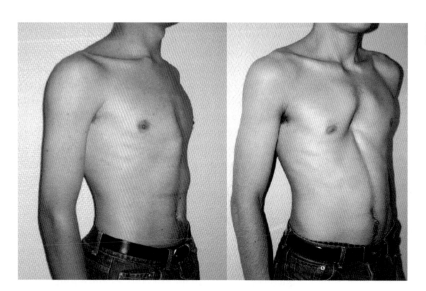

Figure 21.6 Pectus carinatum (**A**) and pectus arcuatum (**B**).

Two types are included in this category according to the affected part and shape of the sternum and to a different aetiology: pectus carinatum of vertical type (chondrogladiolar or 'chicken breast'; Figure 21.6A) and pectus arcuatum (chondromanubrial or 'pouter pigeon breast' or Currarino-Silverman syndrome) sometimes associated with an excavatum shape of the lower sternum (Figure 21.6B).

The pectus carinatum type is the most frequent, occurring in about 90% of all cases. The sternum projects anteriorly to a point corresponding to the bottom of the sternal body with the xiphoid process and the adjacent lower cartilages angling posteriorly and a slightly concave shape of the anterior ribs laterally. One-third of patients have an asymmetrical form with anterior displacement of usually the lateral part of the sternum and anterior ribs on only one side leading to rotation of the sternum. The Haller index is measured in the same way as described for pectus excavatum and is usually less than 1.9. The aetiology is similar to pectus excavatum due to an excessive length of sternocostal cartilages, mainly in the middle and lower parts of the deformity[1,2].

Pectus arcuatum is the least common type, occurring in about 10% of all carinatum deformities, with a relative anterior protrusion of the angle of Louis and second and third costal cartilages (sometimes described as 'horn of Steer') associated with an inferior depression of the lower part of the sternum in some cases. In this case, there is a premature fusion of the manubrium and segmental pieces of the sternum, leading to a characteristic short and broad

flat bone without cartilage at the manubriosternal junction.

Presentation is usually with embarrassment over appearance, breathing difficulties and pain when lying prone or inadvertently bumping into objects. Many patients avoid swimming and sports activity with similar psychological consequences as pectus excavatum. Severe forms have an impact on pulmonary function with a restrictive pattern and also impaired diaphragmatic function at exercise due to diaphragmatic flattening. Some patients report improvement of breathing difficulties after operation, although objective evidence for this improvement is equivocal.

Treatment for pectus carinatum

Open repair

Surgical repair is performed by a modified Ravitch procedure, usually comprising a third to seventh sub-perichondrial cartilage resection or division and partial sternal osteotomy usually comprising a small wedge to correct the inferior sternal protrusion and rotational abnormality. The correction may be secured by pre-sternal titanium bridging implants or plates (Figure 21.7).

Correction of the pectus arcuatum type requires resection or division of the second to fourth costal cartilages with resection of the prominent manubriosternal junction. The inferior pectus excavatum component requires further osteotomy and support by mesh or bar[12,29]. The operative results are good, with 90% patient satisfaction and low morbidity.

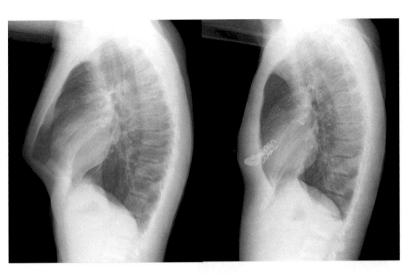

Figure 21.7 Pre- and post-operative lateral chest X-ray view of an open correction of pectus carinatum.

Minimally invasive repair (MIRPC)

This procedure preserves cartilages, and sternal osteotomy is not performed. The principle is similar to the Nuss procedure with a bar implanted subcutaneously in front of the sternum, pushing back the deformity. Results of long-term follow-up are awaited[30].

Self-adjustable bracing

Conservative correction with self-adjustable bracing is becoming a popular choice before skeletal maturity is achieved. Treatment consists of 6 months of correction and 18 months of maintenance phase. Mid-term results are promising[31–34].

Poland's syndrome

This syndrome is named after Poland, who as a medical student in 1841 described this condition, characterized by a congenital absence of pectoral muscle. Subsequent reports described other possible components of this syndrome. These include a lack of subcutaneous tissue and absence of the breast, ribs and axillary hairs. Reported extra-thoracic features are syndactyly, hypoplasia and rarely absence of digits, palm or arm (Figure 21.8)[1,2]. Unilateral palsy of abducens oculi muscles or facial muscles is occasionally observed (Möbius syndrome).

The cause of this pathology is unknown. There are various theories that there may be a genetic component, as the more severe Holt-Oram syndrome is due to mutation in a gene responsible for segmental body development[35,36].

Surgical repair is warranted for paradoxical chest wall movement with lung herniation and also for cosmetic reasons, especially in women with breast aplasia. The correction is usually performed in conjunction with a plastic surgeon. This is a rare condition. The authors have used semi-rigid contoured chest wall prosthesis made of polypropylene mesh and methyl methacrylate and in other cases titanium implants. Missing rib reconstruction with titanium implants and parietal defect covering with polytetrafluoroethylene (PTFE) is another recent option[37]. Soft tissue coverage can be provided with a rotational latissimus dorsi muscle flap and the breast augmented with use of a silicone prosthesis. A period of tissue expansion may be needed prior to placement of the breast prosthesis.

Sternal defects

Sternal defects are rare conditions which are caused by a failure of anterior fusion of the two sternum halves. These abnormalities range from a relatively simple sternal cleft to absence of the sternum and chest wall, creating thoracic or thoracoabdominal ectopia cordis[1,2].

Sternal cleft

The cleft primarily involves the upper half of the sternum and may be associated with cervicofacial haemangiomas. The soft tissue of the chest wall, pericardium and diaphragm are well developed, and there is no obvious association with congenital heart

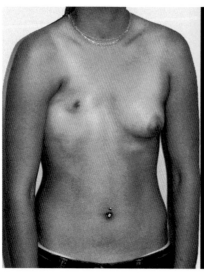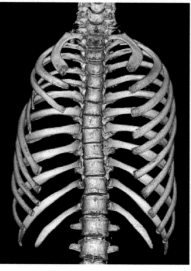

Figure 21.8 Poland syndrome with absence of breast and missing ribs.

abnormalities or omphalocele. Lung herniation via the cleft during crying or Valsalva's manoeuvre is the most common presentation, usually without any compromise of respiratory function. Surgical repair is recommended to protect underlying structures and is usually performed in newborns with direct closure of the cleft by posterior periosteal flaps and chondral grafts[38].

Thoracic ectopia cordis

In this condition, the abnormality consists of a lower sternal cleft or absent sternum, and the heart protrudes anteriorly from the chest without coverage by soft tissue or pericardium. The chest cavity is underdeveloped, and congenital heart disease is often present, especially tetralogy of Fallot and, atrial and ventricular septal defect. Surgical repair with survival to adulthood is possible. This is usually staged.

Thoracoabdominal ectopia cordis (Cantrell's pentalogy)

The thoracoabdominal ectopia cordis differs from thoracic ectopia cordis by coverage of the heart by a thin omphalocele-like membrane or skin and, lack of anterior rotation of the heart and associated defects in the diaphragm and abdominal wall. The most frequent congenital heart defect is left ventricular diverticulum associated with tetralogy of Fallot or atrial and ventricular septal defects. The sternum has a cleft that is present in its lower half, with part of the heart protruding via a diaphragmatic defect.

This condition is less frequent than thoracic ectopia cordis, and surgical repair is also possible.

Jeune's disease (asphyxiating thoracic dystrophy, short rib thoracic dysplasia)

Jeune described this condition in 1954. It is an autosomal recessive disease presenting with a narrow, bell-shaped thorax and protuberant abdomen. The underlying genetic problem leads to abnormal cilia function. This causes a variety of abnormalities including abnormal rib development. It is one of a group of rare related conditions known as 'short rib thoracic dysplasias' (STRD). The pathology is based on poor endochondrial ossification leading to wide and short ribs with abundant and irregular costal cartilage. The thorax is narrow in transverse and sagittal axes, with a horizontal direction of the ribs leading to decreased respiratory movements and hypoplastic lungs. Short limbs, hypoplastic pelvis, phalange abnormalities, renal microcystic disease and liver dysfunction might also be present. The patients usually die in infancy due to respiratory insufficiency or pneumonia, but patients with less severe forms may live into adulthood.

There are reports of surgical attempts to expand the chest and allow growth of hypoplastic lungs. These include expandable prosthetic titanium ribs, sternal split and expansion, Nuss procedure and, most effective, lateral thoracic expansion. The latter consists of division of lateral parts of ribs and underlying tissue in a staggered fashion and plating them together in an expanded manner with titanium struts[39,40].

This procedure may need to be repeated to accommodate growth of the child and thorax.

Pathophysiology of acquired Jeune's disease is different. This condition develops as a consequence of excessive resection of growing costal cartilages during open pectus excavatum repair in very young children, and use of the term 'acquired restrictive thoracic dystrophy' is also seen.

Jarcho-Levin syndrome (spondylothoracic dysplasia and spondylocostal dysostosis)

Spondylocostal dysostoses are a varied group of axial skeletal disorders characterized by multiple segmentation defects of the vertebrae (SDV), rib malalignment with variable points of intercostal fusion and often a reduction in rib number. Jarcho-Levin syndrome was described in 1938. Many of the published patients are from Puerto Rican families. It is a rare disease existing in two distinct subtypes: (1) spondylothoracic dysplasia and (2) spondylocostal dysostosis.

Spondylothoracic dysplasia is an autosomal recessive disease with very abnormal and very short vertebral bodies of the thoracolumbar spine, leading to a close proximity of origin of ribs and their bilateral posterior fusion. The primary pathology in spinal and rib bone formation is preserved. The posterior thorax is severely shortened with hypoplastic lungs as a consequence. This condition has typical crab-like appearance on chest radiograph. Prognosis is poor due to underdeveloped lungs, and the majority of patients die in infancy as a result of respiratory insufficiency or pneumonia.

Spondylocostal dysostosis has both autosomal recessive and dominant inheritance with a variable degree of asymmetrical spinal and rib abnormalities but no symmetrical costal fusion. Spinal scoliosis is typical, and lung pathology is usually less prominent. These patients are usually treated by orthopaedic surgeons by means of implantation of expandable prosthetic titanium inserts for correction of spinal abnormality and growth, with life expectancy into adulthood and in some cases normal.

References

1　Huddleston CB. Chest wall deformities. In: Patterson GA, Cooper JD, Deslauries J, Lerut AEMR, Luketich JD, Rice TW, eds., *Pearson's Thoracic & Esophageal Surgery*, Vol. 1: *Thoracic*, 3rd edn. Philadelphia: Elsevier, 2008:1236–42.

2　Kucharczuk JC, Kaiser LR. Surgery of pectus deformities. In: Patterson GA, Cooper JD, Deslauries J, Lerut AEMR, Luketich JD, Rice TW, eds., *Pearson's Thoracic & Esophageal Surgery* Vol. 1 *Thoracic*, 3rd edn. Philadelphia: Elsevier, 2008:1329–39.

3　Ashrafian H. Leonardo da Vinci and the first portrayal of pectus excavatum. *Thorax* 2013; 68:1081.

4　Rupprecht H, Hümmer HP, Stöss H, Waldherr T. Pathogenesis of chest wall abnormalities – electron microscopy studies and trace element analysis of rib cartilage. *Z kinderchir* 1987; 42:228–9.

5　Saint-Mezard G, Duret J, Chanudet X, et al. Mitral valve prolapse and pectus excavatum: fortuitous association or syndrome? *Presse Med* 1986; 15:439.

6　Coln E, Carrasco J, Coln D. Demonstrating relief of cardiac compression with the Nuss minimally invasive repair for pectus excavatum. *J Pediatr Surg* 2006; 41:683–6.

7　Malek MH, Berger DE, Marelich WD, et al. Pulmonary function following surgical repair of pectus excavatum; a meta-analysis. *Eur J Cardiothorac Surg* 2006; 30:637–43.

8　Beiser GD, Epstein SE, Stampfer M, et al. Impairment of cardiac function in patients with pectus excavatum, with improvement after operative correction. *N Engl J Med* 1972; 10:267–72.

9　Sigalet DL, Montgomery M, Harder J. Cardiopulmonary effects of closed repair of pectus excavatum. *J Pediatr Surg* 2003; 38:380–5.

10　Haller JA Jr, Kramer SS, Lietman SA. Use of CT scans in selection of patients for pectus excavatum surgery: a preliminary report. *J Pediatr Surg* 1987; 22:904–6.

11　Ravitch MM. The operative treatment of pectus excavatum. *Ann Surg* 1949; 129:429–44.

12　Robicsek F, Folkin A. Surgical correction of pectus excavatum and carinatum. *J Cardiovasc Surg* 1999; 40:725–31.

13　Wada J, Ikeda K, Ishida T, Hasegawa T. Results of 271 funnel chest operations. *Ann Thorac Surg* 1970; 10:526–32.

14 Nuss, D, Kelly RE Jr, Croitoru DP, Katz ME. A 10 year review of a minimally invasive technique for the correction of pectus excavatum. *J Pediatr Surg* 1998; 33:545–52.

15 Park HJ, Lee SY, Lee CS. Complications associated with the Nuss procedure: analysis of risk factors and suggested measures of prevention of complications. *J Pediatr Surg* 2004; 39:391–5.

16 Robicsek F, Fokin AA, Watts LT. Complications of pectus deformity repair. In: Patterson GA, Cooper JD, Deslauries J, Lerut AEMR, Luketich JD, Rice TW, eds., *Pearson's Thoracic & Esophageal Surgery*. Vol. 1: *Thoracic*, 3rd edn. Philadelphia: Elsevier, 2008:1340–50.

17 Coelho MS, Kuenzer RF, Neto NB, et al. Pectus excavatum surgery: sternochondroplasty versus Nuss procedure. *Ann Thorac Surg* 2009; 88:1773–9.

18 Nasr A, Fecteau A, Wales PW. Comparison of the Nuss and Ravitch procedure for pectus excavatgum repair: a meta-analysis. *J Pediatr Surg* 2010; 45:880–6.

19 Papandria D, Arlikar J, Sacco Casamassina MG, et al. Increasing age at time of pectus excavatum repair in children: emerging consensus? *J Pediatr Surg* 2013; 48:191–6.

20 Hanna WC, Ko MA, Blitz M, et al. Thoracoscopic Nuss procedure for young adults with pectus excavatum: excellent midterm results and patient satisfactioin. *Ann Thorac Surg* 2013; 96:1033–6.

21 Pilegaard HK. Extending the use of Nuss procedure in patients older than 30 years. *Eur J Cardiothoracic Surg* 2011; 40:334–8.

22 Park HJ, Lee IS, Kim KT. Extreme eccentric canal type pectus excavatum: morphological study and repair. *Eur J Cardiothorac Surg* 2008; 34:150–4.

23 Park HJ, Jeong JY, Jo WM, et al. Minimally invasive repair of pectus excavatum: novel morphology-tailored, patient-specific approach. *J Thorac Cardiovasc Surg* 2010; 139:379–86.

24 Zoeller GK, Zallen GS, Glick PL. Cardiopulmonary resuscitation in patients with a Nuss bar: a case report and review of the literature. *J Pediatr Surg* 2005; 40:1788–91.

25 Yüksel M1, Özalper MH, Bostanci K, et al. Do Nuss bars compromise the blood flow of the internal mammary arteries? *Interact Cardiovasc Thorac Surg* 2013; 17:571–5.

26 Hasegawa T, Yamaguchi M, Ohshima Y, et al. Simultaneous repair of pectus excavatum and congenital heart disease over the past 30 years. *Eur J Cardiothorac Surg* 2002; 22:874–8.

27 Jarosewsky DE, Fraser JD, DeValeria PA. Simultaneous repair of cardiac pathology and severe pectus excavatum in Marfan patients using a modified minimally invasive repair. *Chest Dis Rep* 2011; 1:e3 5–6.

28 Dimitrakakis D, Von Oppell UO, Miller C, Kornaszewska M. Simultaneous mitral valve and pectus excavatum repairwith a Nuss bar. *Eur J Cardiothorac Surg* 2012; 42:e86–e88.

29 Brichon PY, Wihlm JM. Correction of a severe pouter pigeon breast by triple sternal osteotomy with a novel titanium rib bridge fixation. *Ann Thorac Surg* 2010; 90:97–9.

30 Abramson H, D'Agostino J, Wuscovi S. A 5-year experience with a minimally invasive technique for pectus carinatum repair. *J Pediatr Surg* 2009; 44:116–23.

31 Haje SA, Bowen JR. Preliminary results of orthotic treatment of pectus deformities in children and adolescents. *J Pediatr Orthop* 1992; 12:795–800.

32 Martinez-Ferro M, Fraire C, Bernard S. Dynamic compression system for the correction of pectus carinatum. *Semin Pediatri Surg* 2008; 17:194–200.

33 Lee RT, Moorman S, Schneider M, Sigalet DL. Bracing is an effective therapy for pectus carinatum: interim results. *J Pediatr Surg* 2013; 48:184–90.

34 Emil S, Laberge JM, Sigalet D, Baird R. Pectus carinatum treatment in Canada: current practices. *J Pediatr Surg* 2012; 47:862–6.

35 Li QY, Newbury-Ecob RA, Terrett JA, et al. Holt-Oram syndrome is caused by mutations in TBX5, a member of the Brachyury (T) gene family. *Nat Genet* 1997; 15:21–9.

36 Basson CT, Bachinsky DR, Lin RC, et al. Mutations in human TBX5 [corrected] cause limb and cardiac malformation in Holt-Oram syndrome. *Nat Genet* 1997; 15:30–5.

37 Coonar AS, Qureshi N, Welle FC, et al. A novel titanium rib bridge system for chest wall reconstruction. *Ann Thorac Surg* 2009; 87:e46–8.

38 Milanez de Campos JR, Das Neves Pereira JC, Velhote MCP, Jatene FB. Twenty-seven-year experience with sternal cleft repair. *Eur J Cardiothorac Surg* 2009; 35:539–41.

39 Davis JT, Heistein JB, Castile RG, et al. Lateral thoracic expansion for Jeune's syndrome: midterm results. *Ann Thorac Surg.* 2001; 72:872–7.

40 Muthialu N, Mussa S, Owens CM, et al. One-stage sequential bilateral thoracic expansion for asphyxiating thoracic dystrophy (Jeune syndrome). *Eur J Cardiothorac Surg* 2014; 46: 643–7.

Chapter 22

Eventration, central bilateral diaphragmatic paralysis and congenital hernia in adults

Françoise Le Pimpec-Barthes, Pierre Mordant, Alex Arame, Alain Badia, Ciprian Pricopi, Anne Hernigou and Marc Riquet

Introduction

Diaphragm surgery concerns various rare disorders with radically different functional consequences ranging from the absence of respiratory symptoms to the absence of spontaneous ventilation. Diaphragmatic disorders may also be associated with digestive troubles, cardiac arrhythmia or chest pain. The aetiologies may be traumatic, congenital or degenerative, concerning the diaphragm itself or its innervation from the cortex to the muscle[1,2]. Morphological analysis and specific neuromuscular explorations are often required to refine the diagnosis and to evaluate the need for a specific treatment. This chapter will discuss the diagnostic features and treatment options of the three main diaphragmatic pathologies, including (i) congenital and acquired eventration in adults, (ii) central bilateral paralysis in adults or adolescents, and (iii) hernia in adults or adolescents.

Eventration of hemidiaphragm

'Unilateral eventration' is defined as an elevation of the hemidiaphragm due to the lack or the lengthening of peripheral muscular fibres with normal peripheral attachments. It can affect either all or only a portion of the hemidiaphragm[3]. Unilateral eventrations can be congenital or acquired. True diaphragmatic eventrations are congenital and result from an incomplete development of the muscular portion during the embryonic period. They are usually diagnosed in the neonatal period but sometimes also in young adults. Acquired forms are the result of phrenic nerve paralysis due to traumatic, tumoural, infectious or neuromuscular diseases[4]. Every level of the neuromuscular axis may be involved. However, in nearly 60% of diaphragmatic paralysis (DP) cases,

no specific cause is identified. These DP cases are called 'a frigore' and may follow a previously unnoticed viral infection.

Regarding traumatic causes, it is difficult to evaluate the real frequency of unilateral DP (UDP) apart from iatrogenic causes in surgical series. In adult cardiac surgery, the incidence of irreversible UDP ranges from 2 to 31%[5,6]. The main suspected causes are cold myocardial protection and use of mammary arteries for bypass grafts[5,6]. Among non-surgical traumatic causes, cervical traumas are often reported to induce UDP. However, the neuromuscular junction is also a particularly fragile area which can be torn in sudden and dramatic deceleration. Such lesions happen more on the left side because of anatomic considerations (Figure 22.1).

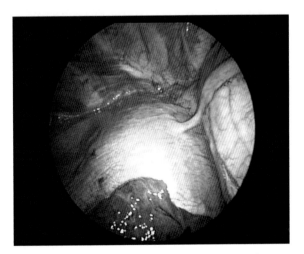

Figure 22.1 Intra-operative views of a left pleural cavity: the phrenic pedicle passes from the pericardium's left side to the left hemidiaphragm's upper part. In case of sudden deceleration, a rupture may occur at the neuromuscular junction.

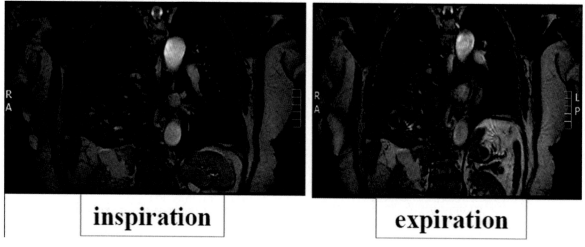

Figure 22.2 Magnetic resonance imaging of the diaphragm showing the movement of the two hemidiaphragms during inspiration and expiration. The fixed right eventration of the hemidiaphragm contrasts with the good mobility on the left side.

Clinical presentation

A UDP may be unnoticed in 50% of patients with moderate to low activity and revealed on chest X-ray. Postural or effort dyspnoea is the most commonly observed symptom. Antepnoea, also called the 'shoe-lace sign', almost formally proves the diaphragmatic damage. In a lying position during sleep, the elevation of the hemidiaphragm is increased, giving hypoventilation and hypoxemia. A ventilatory support using non-invasive ventilation may be proposed to improve the apnoeic syndrome. Recurrent bronchopulmonary infections or cardiac dysrhythmias may occur, being directly linked to the local compression and mediastinal shift. The stomach horizontalization leads to digestive disorders including epigastric pain, strong and painful eructations and gastro-oesophageal reflux disease. Co-morbidity factors such as obesity, cardiomyopathy or pre-existing underlying bronchopulmonary disease potentiate the functional consequences of eventration[3].

Morphological and functional assessments

- **Chest radiography (profile and front)** associated with dynamic X-ray (inspiration and expiration) views are enough to diagnose the eventration and to appreciate its severity. The mediastinal shift shows a major amyotrophied form which is always very symptomatic. In major forms, a paradoxical cranial movement of the distended hemidiaphragm is observed during inspiration due to an increase of abdominal pressure.
- **Diaphragm ultrasonography** is a simple test which allows analysis of diaphragm mobility, but its results may depend on the operator, decreasing its relevance for surgeons.
- **Cervicothoracic CT scan** and **magnetic resonance imaging (MRI)** are useful and unavoidable tools in the diagnosis of aetiology and for evaluation of local consequences (Figure 22.2). Performed in the supine position, they increase the elevation of the hemidiaphragm and show what happens during sleep. They allow the detection of a tumour that can be located on the course of the phrenic nerve somewhere between its root and its end. Local compressions may also be evaluated.
- **Pulmonary function tests** usually show a restrictive syndrome of which severity depends on the importance of the elevation and co-morbidity criteria. The vital capacity reduction, which often exceeds 50%, is further aggravated during transition from a sitting to a supine position. The effect is more evident in right-sided DP.
- **Full-night polysomnography** is interesting to detect a possible sleep apnoea syndrome.
- **Electrophysiological study** is essential to evaluate the conduction of the nerve and to measure the capacity of the muscle to get an efficient

contraction[7,8]. It includes **surface electromyography (EMG) of costal diaphragm, needle EMG of the diaphragm** (usually contraindicated in chronic obstructive lung disease and ventilated patients because of the risk of pneumothorax), **gastric and oesophageal catheters** (to measure transdiaphragmatic pressure, commonly considered to be proportional to the force generated by the diaphragm) and **cervical stimulation tests** (magnetic and electric to measure the conduction time of each nerve). The tests can be repeated to follow the evolution over time and detect possible recovery.

- **Indication for surgery:** When an eventration is diagnosed, it is important to avoid unnecessary surgery and to evaluate precisely its reversibility, which can occur months to years later[9]. This reversibility is evaluated according to a set of arguments, including

  ○ The initial mechanism of the trauma: a phrenic nerve section is obviously definitive but a cervical trauma may recover,
  ○ The time since the onset of the paralysis,
  ○ The importance of the hemidiaphragm distension, and
  ○ The results of the stimulation tests. One should keep in mind that a significant distension of the hemidiaphragm with a thinning of the muscular part is usually the sign of an irreversible amyotrophy even if the nervous conduction has already recovered.

Surgery can be proposed in case of a significant elevation of the hemidiaphragm (more than two or three intercostal spaces on chest X-ray) if the tests show a major dysfunction of the diaphragm, with important functional consequences for the patient and no hope of spontaneous recovery. Before surgery, co-morbidity factors must be controlled – tobacco weaning, active bronchial physiotherapy, weight reduction and sleep apnoeic syndrome.

Asymptomatic or minimally symptomatic eventrations do not require any prophylactic surgical treatment, even in complete hemidiaphragm paralysis confirmed by stimulation tests. A simple follow-up must be proposed to these patients.

Formal contraindications

Morbid obesity is a contraindication because of the high risk of post-operative morbidity and mortality, technical challenge and poor functional results. For these patients, a strict slimming diet is the first measure to propose, sometimes associated with non-invasive ventilation and/or even bariatric surgery. Diffuse neuromuscular disorders (i.e. amyotrophic lateral sclerosis) and pleural tumour represent a contraindication because of short-term pejorative vital prognosis and poor functional benefits. General co-morbidity factors (cardiac or renal failure) must also contraindicate this surgery, temporarily or definitively.

Objective and principles of the surgical treatment of unilateral eventration

Tightening the distended hemidiaphragm using plication[3,10] is the only accepted surgical treatment for a symptomatic eventration. Suggested by Wood in 1916, this technique was used successfully for the first time by Morrison in 1923[11]. Since then, hemidiaphragm plication has only been infrequently performed and reported in the medical literature[10,12–18]. The objective of this treatment is to improve symptoms by pulling down the hemidiaphragm and restoring its anatomical position. This procedure does not restore the active contraction of the muscle; however, it restores the position of both abdominal and thoracic organs, decreases compression and stops the paradoxical movements of the diaphragm, improving the function of the healthy contralateral hemidiaphragm.

When should plication be used?

There is no consensus regarding the time between diagnosis and plication. To plan surgery, the key elements are a good understanding of the mechanism of the lesion and the importance of symptoms. Surgery should be proposed without delay in case of irreversible respiratory decompensation requiring assisted ventilation.

Three different approaches have been described to perform plication. To date, the reference technique is a plication of the hemidiaphragm performed via a limited lateral thoracotomy approach[10,13,16–18]. More recently, plication via video-assisted thoracoscopic approach (VATS) has been proposed by Mouroux and colleagues[15] and later done by other expert centres[14]. In 2004, Huttl[19] first described the laparoscopic approach, and other rare successful cases were reported[20].

Open thoracic approach associated with thoracoscopy

Technical aspects

Under general anaesthesia with double-lumen intubation, the patient is placed in a lateral position. A nasogastric tube is positioned to completely empty the stomach. The thoracoscope is inserted to determine the exact level of thoracotomy. A small lateral thoracotomy is performed (usually through the seventh or eighth intercostal space), and a rib retractor is positioned. After removal of the pleural symphysis, if necessary, a complete local exploration is done. It concerns the thickness of the peripheral muscle, the general aspect of the hemidiaphragm and the whole phrenic nerve all along its course from the apex to its end on the muscle. The hemidiaphragm is then manually tensioned and folded to determine the exact level of the plication plane. This suture area must be chosen on the peripheral muscular parts, thus preserving the phrenic nerve and its branches. It is most often a transverse fold, lined up from the pericardial region (in front of or behind the phrenic pedicle) to the lateral chest wall. We suggest to perform a short opening of the central tendon in order to control the position of the abdominal organs and thus to avoid injuring them when passing the suture through (Figure 22.3). The re-tensioning of the hemidiaphragm allows one to determine the exact position of the U stitches placed on both sides of the fold. The eventrated diaphragm is grasped with Babcock clamps, and the excess portion is sutured at the base

with non-absorbable mattress sutures (with or without pledgets). These stitches are not tied but put on hold on a clamp. Then, when all stitches are positioned, they are tied up while checking the quality of the whole re-tensioning and shape of the hemidiaphragm. If necessary, some stitches may be added to avoid any organ strangulation inside the suture. The opening performed inside the central tendon at the beginning of the procedure is then closed by a non-absorbable continuous suture (Mersuture; Johnson & Johnson, New Brunswick, NJ) with threads. The fold is then sutured laterally to reinforce the first plication (Figure 22.4). In case of major amyotrophia, we systematically reinforce the diaphragm using a prosthetic mesh in non-absorbable mattress, using additional stiches positioned on the peripheral muscle at the beginning of the surgical procedure (Figure 22.5). To reinforce the plication, several rows of double-armed non-absorbable sutures parallel to the sagittal plane may be used without any opening of the central tendon.

Results

Observational retrospective studies and few studies of unpaired control cases[12,13] have been reported. Respiratory functional improvement is almost always observed earlier and sustained in the long term[10,12–14,16,17]. The subjective benefit is measured using different criteria according to the series. It may be a simple questioning, a measure of dyspnoea score using an analog scale or a more complex scale such as the Medical Research Council (MRC) dyspnoea

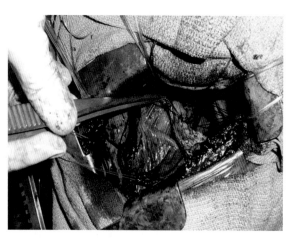

Figure 22.3 The short opening of the central tendon allows control of the position of the abdominal organs, avoiding injury, when passing the sutures.

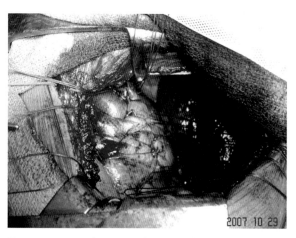

Figure 22.4 Lateral suture reinforcing the first row of hemidiaphragm's plication.

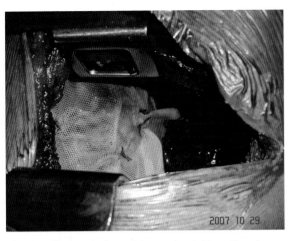

Fig. 22.5 The prosthetic mesh in non-absorbable mattress is sutured laterally to reinforce the muscular plication.

score. The objective results are measured on post-operative flow and volume improvements. The mean improvements of the vital capacity (VC) and the forced expiratory volume in 1 second (FEV1) are in the range of 10 to 20%[13,16,17,21], also assessed in the supine position[21]. In Versteegh's series, all the patients could sleep again in the supine position, and non-invasive ventilation was stopped in the three patients who had it before operation[21]. This benefit persists on long-term follow-up despite a downward trend, as reported in Higgs's series, where 15 of the 19 operated patients had a mean follow-up of 10 years[16]. The blood exchanges also improve, with a significant arterial pressure in oxygen ranging from 7 to 13 mmHg[10,17]. The advantages of thoracotomy are to allow an excellent approach of the whole diaphragm and to apply re-tensioning of the hemidiaphragm with maximal security for all intra-peritoneal organs.

Thoracoscopic plication

History

The first successful VATS approach to treat diaphragm eventration in adults was described in 1996 by Mouroux and colleagues[22]. Then it was developed in paediatry, even in newborns, to avoid the constant disadvantages of thoracotomy. In adults, few centres performed the diaphragm plication using this approach[14,15].

Technical aspects

Under general anaesthesia with double-lumen intubation, a nasogastric tube is inserted to completely empty the stomach. The patient is positioned in the full lateral position. Two 5-mm ports are inserted in the fifth intercostal space on the posterior axillary line (for 5-mm 30-degree angled scope) and on the mammary line (for the grasper), respectively. A short thoracotomy 5-cm working incision is performed in the nineth intercostal space on the posterior axillary line. No rib retraction is generally required, and conventional surgical instruments are introduced through the thoracotomy. An endoscopic clamp introduced through the anterior port is used to grasp and invaginate the apex of the eventration downward into the abdomen. A transverse fold is thus created from the periphery to the cardiophrenic angle behind the phrenic nerve. This fold is first closed using a non-absorbable running suture beginning at the periphery of the diaphragm. The first row is superficial to avoid injury to the abdominal organs. Once at the cardiophrenic angle, the suture is drawn tight, while the clamp used to push the diaphragm downward is removed. A row of return stitches is created along the same axis, and the suture is tied with the free end of the first knot. During the placement of these return stitches, the assistant keeps the suture material taut using forceps introduced through the posterior port. The tension applied in this manner facilitates grasping of the edges of the fold to be sutured. This first back-and-forth series of running suture allows maintenance of the excess of diaphragm within the abdomen, and care is taken to avoid applying tension to this first series of suture. A second back-and-forth series of running suture is carried out similarly, thus burying the first series of suture lines: stitches are inserted through a more peripheral portion of the diaphragm to obtain the desired tension of the hemidiaphragm. Chest drainage is achieved using a single chest tube introduced through the anterior port.

Results

Significant improvements in the functional status were reported in short series[14,15]. At 6-month follow-up in the VATS group, mean forced VC, FEV1, functional residual capacity (FRC) and total lung capacity (TLC) improved by 17, 21, 20 and 16%, respectively ($p < 0.005$). Mean MRC dyspnoea scores also improved significantly in the operated cohort ($p < 0.001$). In the short Kim's series including four patients treated by exclusive tidal volume (VT) plication (without minithoracotomy), no eventration recurrence was observed at 6-month follow-up[23]. However, at 12-month follow-up, a slight elevation of the hemidiaphragm was observed in one patient, but no new surgical procedure was necessary. A validation of these results obtained by minimally invasive technique is needed based on larger prospective studies. Such studies are probably difficult to conduct because of scarcity of the disease and the lack of thoracic surgeons experienced in this disease.

Laparoscopic approach

History

Described in 2004 by Hüttl[19], this approach is still a more exceptional and recent procedure[24].

Technical aspects

Under general anaesthesia with a single-lumen tracheal tube, four ports are inserted: the first one for the camera above the umbilicus and 2 cm lateral to the midline (toward the contralateral side of the affected hemidiaphragm), two working ports placed in line with the first port, ipsilateral to the affected hemidiaphragm, and one near the xiphoid process. The creation of pneumoperitoneum displaces the distended hemidiaphragm upward. A pneumothorax is created by a 5-mm defect in the affected hemidiaphragm. It lets the diaphragm drop down, making it easy to grasp and retract caudally. The pneumoperitoneum is still maintained because the opening in the diaphragm is small, and a chest tube is inserted in case of respiratory or hemodynamic compromise. The diaphragm incision is then closed. A T-shaped plication is constructed from the medial to lateral direction with braided, non-absorbable number 2 (curved needle) hand-sewn pledget-reinforced U stitches.

Results

For the authors, the laparoscopic diaphragmatic plication offers several distinct advantages, such as avoidance of single-lung ventilation, ample working space and visualization, potentially less post-operative pain and a reduction of the risk of visceral injury. In the Groth's series including 25 patients, there was one conversion to thoracotomy because of pleural symphysis, a 25% complication rate and no deaths[25]. A significant short- and mid-term improvement in respiratory quality-of-life scores (St George's Respiratory Questionnaire) and pulmonary function

was reported[25]. While the scores of quality of life and dyspnoea were still improving 1 year after operation, the functional tests (VC and FEV1) were noticeably deteriorating compared with the early post-operative ones.

Due to the small amount of data concerning the importance of eventration and the lack of functional evaluation, this technique could not really be well assessed.

In conclusion, the diaphragmatic plication using thoracic approaches is a treatment recommended in case of symptomatic eventration after treating co-morbidities. It is a safe and efficient technique which allows long-term improvement of the respiratory symptoms in selected patients. Thoracoscopic repair is gaining favour, but short lateral thoracotomy remains the reference technique. To date, the laparoscopic approach has not been validated for the treatment of diaphragm eventration.

Central diaphragm paralysis

Some ventilator-dependent patients following central respiratory paralysis can be weaned from their respirator after the implantation of phrenic pacing. This treatment concerns strictly selected patients with damaged central command but with functional phrenic nerves and preserved diaphragm. The main indications for phrenic pacing are upper cervical spinal cord injury (above or at the C3 level) and central alveolar hypoventilation (either congenital or acquired)[26–28].

General considerations

Compared with mechanical ventilation, phrenic pacing provides more natural breathing, reduces the occurrence of respiratory infection and improves the quality of life, in part through restored olfaction[29]. It is also considered to decrease healthcare cost, thanks to earlier home discharge and reduced infection complications[30,31].

For tetraplegic patients, the criteria to indicate phrenic pacing are a persistent electromyographic response of the diaphragm to bilateral cervical magnetic stimulation and an abolished response of the diaphragm to transcranial magnetic stimulation[32,33]. For patients with central hypoventilation, cervical stimulation confirms the functionality of the phrenic nerves.

Technical aspects

Device

We use a quadripolar phrenic pacing system from Atrotech (Jukka, Atrotech, Tampere, Finland) which has two components: an internal part – the permanently implanted device – and two external antennas taped to the skin and connected to the transmitter (Figure 22.6). The internal component consists of quadripolar electrodes positioned around each phrenic nerve connected by wires to subcutaneous radiofrequency (RF) receivers. Each electrode, stuck on Teflon strips, is placed opposite a quarter of the nerve to subsequently stimulate the nerve fibres of that portion (Figure 22.7).

Surgical technique

Under general anaesthesia with double-lumen intubation, VATS is performed successively for each pleural cavity. The endoscopic camera (5 mm in diameter) is inserted laterally into the third intercostal space. A 4-cm incision is made in the first or second intercostal space, 3 cm laterally to the sternum. A careful dissection of the phrenic nerve is done at the end of the vena cava on the right side and in front of the aorta on the left side. For each nerve, two electrodes are located above the nerve and two below. The Teflon strips supporting the electrodes are sutured on the pleura and the pericardium. Each wire is brought out of the pleural cavity through an intercostal space below the main access and is tunnelled under the pectoralis major muscle to a subcutaneous pocket in the lateral chest wall. In this pocket the wires are connected to a subcutaneous RF receiver on each side (Figure 22.8). Intraoperative tests determine the minimum stimulation thresholds of each electrode. A chest drain is inserted into each pleural space exiting through the lateral port.

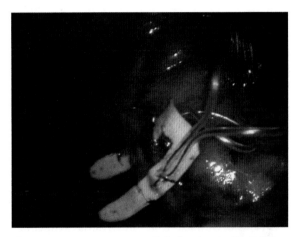

Fig. 22.7 Intra-operative views of left pleural cavity: The Teflon strips supporting the four electrodes are sutured around the phrenic pedicle.

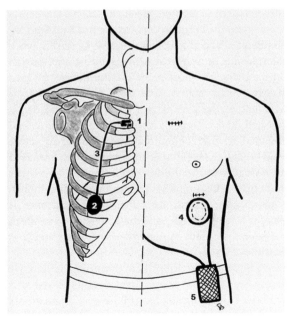

Figure 22.6 Schematic view of the device for phrenic pacing. Internal components on the right side (1 = phrenic electrodes, 2 = subcutaneous radiofrequency receiver, 3 = wires between electrodes and receiver) and external components on the left side (4 = skin antenna, 5 = generator).

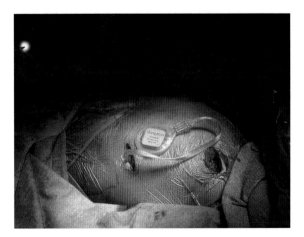

Figure 22.8 The wires between the electrodes and the subcutaneous radiofrequency receiver are tunnelled under the pectoralis major muscle.

215

Reconditioning

Two weeks after surgical implantation, the reconditioning procedure of the diaphragm can start. Short daily stimulation sessions are done initially (only 2 or 5 minutes). The time is progressively increased according to a breath-by-breath monitoring of VT. Intervals of 24 hours between sessions are allowed at the beginning. The intersession intervals are reduced as soon as diaphragmatic contractions are in phase[34]. The reconditioning procedure is considered complete when the patient can spend 8 hours under stimulation alone without a noticeable drop in VT.

Results

When pre-operative electrophysiological tests confirm that the central command is affected but the phrenic nerve conduction is normal, phrenic pacing is successful in all cases without intra-operative complications or peri-operative mortality[26]. In our experience, the only failure was due to a misindication with a compassionate indication because pre-operative tests did not detect any conduction by phrenic nerve. In our series, the level of intra-operative thresholds ranged from 0.05 to 2.9 mA, and ventilatory weaning was obtained after a mean reconditioning time of 6 weeks (2–11 months). Patients with major denutrition had a longer reconditioning and incomplete weaning. All the patients weaned from mechanical ventilation reported an improved quality of life for several reasons. Phrenic stimulation allows one to get a more physiological breathing, recovery of smell and taste and more mobility.

Congenital diaphragmatic hernia

Diaphragmatic hernias are defined as a passage of the abdominal contents through a peripheral orifice of the diaphragm. These congenital hernias are rare but increase in size over time. We will not discuss hiatal hernias, but we will focus on Bochdalek hernias and Morgagni hernias (Larrey and Morgagni hernia). Bochdalek hernias represent 90% of all diaphragmatic hernias. They are due to a closure failure of the posterior pleuroperitoneal track. Morgagni hernias are anterior retrosternal diaphragmatic defects that occur between the xiphoid process of the sternum and costochondral attachments of the diaphragm. In both cases, hernias result from a lack of partitioning between the pleura and peritoneal cavities during the embryonic stage. Anterior hernias are due to an abnormal development of the septum transversum or a failure of fusion of the pleuroperitoneal folds. In neonatal periods, these hernias usually require a treatment in emergency because of respiratory distress. In adults, because of the lack of symptoms, the diagnosis is done later and fortuitously[35].

Bochdalek hernias

Digestive structures may be located and sometimes strangulated (omentum, small or large intestine, stomach or spleen) inside these hernias[36]. In adults, symptoms are usually limited to vague dorsal chest pain or respiratory symptoms. The diagnosis is done on CT scan showing a posterior or lateral defect between the chest wall and the peripheral part of the diaphragm. Except in cases of major co-morbidities, surgery is decided at the time of diagnosis to prevent any organ strangulation. Unlike emergency surgery done in the perinatal period for respiratory failure, the adult form is rarely treated in the emergency setting, except in the case of intestinal obstruction.

The approach mainly depends on the surgeon's habits. Currently, the abdominal access is performed through a short upper midline laparotomy or a sub-costal transverse incision. Detecting the hernial orifice is easy, and the herniated organs are put back into the abdomen. Particular caution must be taken when the spleen is incarcerated while avoiding any traction on its meso. The borders of the hernia sac are then clearly visible, and if necessary, the left triangular ligament of the liver is cut. Then the hernia sac is resected and closed. If the hernial orifice is surrounded by part of the diaphragm, a direct suture may be done using non-absorbable suture. If there is no muscle near the thoracic wall, the sutures may be done by stitching up directly around the ribs. In fact, a too superficial suture runs the risk of recurrence. If there is a too large diaphragmatic defect, a prosthetic mesh may be used. Most of the time direct suture is possible[35,36].

In our thoracic department, a minimally invasive access by VATS is done. The videothoracoscopy is associated with limited lateral lower thoracotomy through the nineth intercostal space to offer a direct intrapleural view. In case of excessive pleuropulmonary adhesion, the small thoracotomy is widened. The content of the hernia sac is reduced towards the abdominal cavity, and the hernia sac is resected. Then the two edges of the diaphragm are sutured with the same recommendation as through abdominal access. This VATS approach represents the first choice over an open or laparoscopic approach in the management of adult patients with Bochdalek or Morgagni hernias because intra-thoracic severe adhesions of digestive structure are easily removed with a direct and secure vision.

Morgagni-Larrey hernias

These hernias are rarely symptomatic and are usually well tolerated even in large size. Exceptionally, they are revealed by an acute episode of intestinal obstruction. On chest X-ray, a filling of the cardiophrenic angle, mostly right-sided, is observed. The diagnosis is determined by CT scan or MRI, especially thanks to sagittal and frontal reconstructions showing the diaphragmatic defect. The risk of incarceration of digestive structures indicates surgery as soon as the diagnosis is determined.

Repair of foramen of Morgagni hernias has been described through the abdomen and through the chest. A short upper midline incision is done to access the hernia. The size of the incision depends on the patient's size, the size of the hernia and the content of the hernia. The most important is to have an excellent visualization of the content. Once the peritoneal cavity is entered, the abdominal viscera are displaced in their normal intra-abdominal position. The limits of the hernia sac can be observed, and the sac is resected. Regarding the size of the diaphragm defect, the repair is done either directly or by placing some prosthetic mesh in case of a large defect[35]. In a small defect, a horizontal mattress using non-absorbable sutures allows a direct closure of the two edges of the muscle. In its anterior part, the suture is fixed to

the posterior part of the chest wall (xiphoid or ribs) to secure the closure. In case of a large defect, a suture of the diaphragm without tension is impossible and requires the use of a synthetic patch. The patch is fixed to the edges of the diaphragm and on the chest wall using non-absorbable interrupted sutures. The prosthetic material used depends on the surgeon's habits and may be polytetrafluoroethylene (PTFE) or various non-absorbable synthetic meshes[37]. The most important aspect of these repairs of diaphragmatic defects is to obtain a suture without tension to avoid recurrence. In fact, the important force applied on the diaphragm during breathing, cough or in effort requires strong sutures that can resist those forces in any circumstances. The transthoracic approach, via thoracoscopy, provides a wide exposure and an easy repair of the hernia defect[38]. The repair is performed as in the transabdominal approach.

Conclusion

Surgery of the diaphragm remains a rare procedure and concerns either central dysfunctions or muscle damage. Surgical indications for central or peripheral paralysis and for eventrations must be reserved to symptomatic patients after complete electrophysiological analysis. In these selected patients, the surgical treatment using a minimally invasive approach gives excellent long-term results. For hernias, surgery is indicated as soon as the diagnosis is determined to avoid the risk of incarceration of digestive structures.

Acknowledgement

We are grateful to Valerie Mege-Lin for her help with English style and grammar.

References

1 Aldrich TK, Tso R. The lungs and neuromuscular disease. In: Masson RJ, Broaddus VC, Murray JF, Nadel JA, eds., *Murray and Nadel's Textbook of Respiratory Medicine*, 4th ed. Philadelphia: Elsevier Saunders, 2005: 2287–90.

2 Wilcox PG, Pardy RL. Diaphragmatic weakness and paralysis: review. *Lung* 1989; 167:323–41.

3 Deslauriers J. Eventration of the diaphragm. *Chest Surg Clin North Am* 1998; 8:315–30.

4 Elefteriades J, Singh M, Tang P, et al. Unilateral diaphragm paralysis: etiology, impact and natural history. *J Cardiovasc Surg (Torino)* 2008; 49:289–95.

5 DeVita JA, Robinson LR, Rehder J, et al. Incidence and natural history of phrenic neuropathy occurring during

open heart surgery. *Chest* 1993; 103:850–6.

6 Efthimiou J, Butler J, Woodham C, et al. Diaphragm paralysis following cardiac surgery: role of phrenic nerve cold injury. *Ann Thorac Surg* 1991; 52:1005–8.

7 Similowski T, Fleury B, Launois S, et al. Cervical magnetic stimulation: a new painless method for bilateral phrenic nerve stimulation in conscious

humans. *J Appl Physiol* 1989; 67:1311–18.

8 Verin E, Straus C, Demoule A, et al. Validation of improved recording site to measure phrenic conduction from surface electrodes in humans. *J Appl Physiol* 2002; 92:967–74.

9 Verin E, Marie JP, Tardif C, Denis P. Spontaneous recovery of diaphragmatic strength in unilateral diaphragmatic paralysis. *Respir Med* 2006; 100:1944–51.

10 Graham DR, Kaplan D, Evans CC, et al. Diaphragmatic plication for unilateral diaphragmatic paralysis: a 10-year experience. *Ann Thorac Surg* 1990; 49:248–52.

11 Morrison JMW. Eventration of the diaphragm due to unilateral phrenic nerve paralysis. *Arch Radiol Electrother* 1923; 28:72–6.

12 McNamara JJ, Paulson DL, Urschel HC, Razzuk MA. Eventration of diaphragm. *Surgery* 1968; 64:1013–21.

13 Ribet M, Linder JL. Plication of the diaphragm for unilateral eventration or paralysis. *Eur J Cardiothorac Surg* 1992; 6:357–60.

14 Freeman RK, Wozniak TC, Fitzgerald EB. Functional and physiologic results of video-assisted thoracoscopic diaphragm plication in adult patients with unilateral diaphragm paralysis. *Ann Thorac Surg* 2006; 81:1853–7.

15 Mouroux J, Venissac N, Leo F, et al. Surgical treatment of diaphragmatic eventration using video-assisted thoracic surgery: a prospective study. *Ann Thorac Surg* 2005; 79:308–12.

16 Higgs SM, Hussain A, Jackson M, et al. Long-term results of diaphragmatic plication for unilateral diaphragm paralysis.

Eur J Cardiothorac Surg 2002; 21:294–7.

17 Wright CD, Williams JG, Ogilvie CM, Donnelly RJ. Results of diaphragmatic plication for unilateral diaphragmatic paralysis. *J Thorac Cardiovasc Surg* 1985; 90: 195–8.

18 Simansky D, Paley M, Refaely Y, Yellin A. Diaphragm plication following chronic nerve injury: a comparison of pediatric and adult patients. *Thorax* 2002; 57:613–6.

19 Huttl TP, Wichmann MW, Reichart B, et al. Laparoscopic diaphragmatic plication, long-term results of a novel surgical technique for postoperative phrenic nerve palsy. *Surg Endosc* 2004; 18:547–51.

20 Groth SS, Andrade RS. Diaphragmatic eventration. *Thorac Surg Clin* 2009; 19(4): 511–9 [review].

21 Versteegh MIM, Braun J, Voigt PG, et al. Diaphragm plication in adult patients with diaphragm paralysis leads to long-term improvement of pulmonary function and level of dyspnea. *Eur J Cardiothorac Surg* 2007; 32:449–56.

22 Mouroux J, Padovani B, Poirier NC, et al. Technique for the repair of diaphragmatic eventration. *Ann Thorac Surg* 1996; 62 (3):905–7.

23 Kim DH, Hwan JJ, Kim KD. Thoracoscopic diaphragmatic plication using three 5-mm ports. *Interact Cardiovasc Thorac Surg* 2007; 6:280–1.

24 Palanivelu C, Rangarajan M, Rajapandian S, et al. Laparoscopic repair of adult diaphragmatic hernias and eventration with primary sutured closure and prosthetic reinforcement: a retrospective study. *Surg Endosc* 2009; 23(5):978–85.

25 Groth SS, Rueth NM, Kast T, et al. Laparoscopic diaphragm plication for diaphragmatic paralysis and eventration:

an objective evaluation of short-term and midterm results. *J Thorac Cardiovasc Surg* 2010; 139:1452–6.

26 Le Pimpec-Barthes F, Gonzalez-Bermejo J, Hubsch JP, et al. Intrathoracic phrenic pacing: a 10-year experience in France. *J Thorac Cardiovasc Surg* 2011; June:1–6.

27 DiMarco AF. Phrenic nerve stimulation in patients with spinal cord injury. *Respir Physiol Neurobiol* 2009; 169 (2):200–9.

28 Weese-Mayer DE, Berry-Kravis EM, Ceccherini I, et al. An official ATS clinical policy statement: congenital central hypoventilation syndrome: genetic basis, diagnosis, and management. *Am J Respir Crit Care Med* 2010; 181:626–44.

29 Adler D, Gonzalez-Bermejo J, Duguet A, et al. Diaphragm pacing restores olfaction in tetraplegia. *Eur Respir J* 2009; 34:365–70.

30 Escların A, Bravo P, Arroyo O, et al. Tracheostomy ventilation versus diaphragmatic pacemaker ventilation in high spinal cord injury. *Paraplegia* 1994; 32:687–93.

31 Hirschfeld S, Exner G, Luukkaala T, Baer GA. Mechanical ventilation or phrenic nerve stimulation for treatment of spinal cord injury–induced respiratory insufficiency. *Spinal Cord* 2008; 46:738–42.

32 Similowski T, Straus C, Attali V, et al. Assessment of the motor pathway to the diaphragm using cortical and cervical magnetic stimulation in the decision-making process of phrenic pacing. *Chest* 1996; 110:1551–7.

33 Luo YM, Polkey MI, Johnson LC, et al. Diaphragm EMG measured by cervical magnetic and electric phrenic nerve stimulation. *J Appl Physiol* 1998; 85:2089–99.

34 Nochomovitz ML, Hopkins M, Brodkey J, et al. Conditioning of the diaphragm with phrenic nerve stimulation after prolonged disuse. *Am Rev Respir Dis* 1984; 130:685–8.

35 Naunheim KS. Adult presentation of unusual diaphragmatic hernias.

Chest Surg Clin North Am 1998 May; 8(2):359–69.

36 Mullins ME, Stein J, Saini SS, Mueller PR. Prevalence of incidental Bochdalek's hernia in a large adult population. *AJR* 2001; 177:363–6.

37 Nasr A, Fecteau A. Foramen of Morgagni hernia: presentation

and treatment [review]. *Thorac Surg Clin* 2009; 19(4): 463–8.

38 Ambrogi V, Forcella D, Gatti A, et al. Transthoracic repair of Morgagni hernia: a 20-year experience from open to video-assisted approach. *Surg Endosc* 2007 Apr; 21(4):587–91.

Benign esophageal disease

Donn H. Spight and Mithran S. Sukumar

Introduction

Benign esophageal disease is widely prevalent and often requires treatment, although the surgical management of the same is less commonly indicated. Surgical treatment of these diseases requires considerable expertise and is best left to those who manage these patients on a daily basis. However, a basic understanding of the diseases and their management is required by all cardiothoracic trainees and practicing thoracic surgeons, and this chapter is an attempt to enable them to do so.

Antireflux surgery

Gastroesophageal reflux disease (GERD) is a very common problem estimated to affect up to 35% of Americans; however, the true prevalence is unknown due to the widespread availability of over-the-counter medications that are able to lessen symptoms without any physician contact. Additionally, lack of consensus on the true constellation of symptoms that constitute the disease makes clinical diagnosis and therapeutic management a challenge. Typical GERD presents with classic symptoms of heartburn or acid regurgitation or both. A broad array of atypical symptoms can also be attributed to GERD, such as vomiting, dysphagia, chest pain, cough, asthma, sore throat, hoarseness, chronic aspiration, or idiopathic pneumonias.

Basic physiology

Heartburn is generally defined as substernal burning or discomfort that radiates upward from the epigastrium. Failure of the zone of high pressure located at the gastroesophageal (GE) junction is the most common etiology of GERD. This area, known as the lower esophageal sphincter (LES), is responsible for preventing retrograde flow of gastric material into the esophageal body. The LES is a region of thickening made up of the collar-sling musculature and clasp fibers of the upper stomach that remain in tonic opposition. Receptive relaxation triggered by the act of swallowing allows passage of a bolus into the stomach. The characteristics that maintain competency of the LES are its resting pressure, the overall length, and the intra-abdominal length subject to positive abdominal pressure. Physiologic or pathologic processes that affect these characteristics often result in GERD.

Median normal manometric values of the LES:

Pressure (mmHg): 13
Overall length (cm): 3.6
Abdominal length (cm): 2

Indications for surgery

A careful assessment of the patient's symptoms is essential before any therapeutic intervention should be undertaken. Many GERD-like symptoms may be associated with other disease processes and will not be relieved by operative intervention. Presentations of typical or atypical symptoms may be related to other disease entities such as achalasia, diffuse esophageal spasm, esophageal carcinoma, pyloric stenosis, peptic ulcer disease, cholelithiasis, or coronary artery disease. Life-threatening entities such as unstable angina must be excluded before proceeding with workup for GERD.

When symptoms point toward GERD, an initial trial of behavior and lifestyle modification is warranted as first-line therapy. These include weight loss, avoiding recumbent position within 2–3 hours after meals, elevating the head of the bed, and smoking

Core Topics in Thoracic Surgery, ed. Marco Scarci, Aman Coonar, Tom Routledge and Francis Wells. Published by Cambridge University Press. © Cambridge University Press 2016

cessation. Patients should avoid acidic or reflux-causing foods such as chocolate, coffee, fatty foods, citrus, and alcohol. Anticholinergic drugs, estrogens, calcium-channel blockers, nitroglycerine, and benzodiazepines should also be avoided if possible.

In the era of proton pump inhibitors (PPIs), patients often move quickly through behavior and lifestyle modifications as well as traditional drug therapy including antacid and histamine-2 receptor antagonists. PPIs suppress acid secretion very effectively. When taken 30 minutes before eating in the morning, a single dose of PPI normalizes esophageal acid exposure in 67% of patients. Adding a second dose before the evening meal increases efficacy to 90%.

In patients who fail medical therapy, have adverse events related to PPIs, have large-volume regurgitation, or do not wish to take PPIs for the rest of their life, surgical alternatives should be considered.

Prior to operative intervention, further diagnostic studies must be obtained to confirm the diagnosis and facilitate operative planning. Esophageal manometry is necessary to evaluate the propulsive force of the esophageal body and identify LES characteristics that may suggest other pathologies. An upper endoscopy is necessary to identify abnormalities such as erosive or eosinophilic esophagitis, esophageal stricture, Barrett's esophagus, or esophageal cancer. An upper GI (gastrointestinal) study is useful to identify esophageal shortening or the presence of a large hiatal hernia.

Operations

The most common antireflux procedure is the 360-degree fundoplication around the lower 4–5 cm of esophagus as described by Nissen. Fundoplications can be performed open or minimally invasively through the abdomen or chest. Typically the minimally invasive approach provides optimal visualization for all but the most complex of reoperative abdomens. Patients who have undergone open foregut operations will often present a significant challenge reentering the region due to dense adhesions to the undersurface of the liver. Right-sided diaphragmatic hernias or large paraesophageal hernias with abdominal contents contained within the right chest are often better approached thoracoscopically due to physical limitations to reduction caused by the liver.

When performed with the patient in a steep reverse Trendelenburg and split leg position, an ergonomic advantage can be gained by the surgeon standing between the legs. Typically a five-trocar setup is employed in a diamond configuration. Utilization of an automatic camera holder and Nathanson liver retractor secured with a bedside retractor system facilitates the creation of a consistent and stable operative field. The ability to work underneath the liver and visualize the vagal nerves in high definition are optimized in the laparoscopic approach.

For patients with severe motility dysfunction, a partial fundoplication can be performed transabdominally as a 270 degree posterior fundoplication (Toupet) or as an anterior fundoplication (Dor). Partial fundoplications can also be performed via a left chest incision (Belsey Mark IV). Typically a Nissen fundoplication is performed for all but the most severe disorders of esophageal peristalsis demonstrated by manometry. In the case of true absence of peristalsis, caution must be taken to rule out achalasia, for which a Heller myotomy would be the indicated operation.

The principles of the transabdominal laparoscopic Nissen fundoplication operation are

1. Crural dissection and identification of left and right vagal nerves. The conduct of the operation begins with division of the pars flaccida to the level of the right diaphragmatic crus. Working bluntly within the avascular plane between the crura and the esophagus, this dissection is carried up and over the esophagus to the crus of the left diaphragm by carefully dividing the phrenoesophageal ligament. The dissection is then carried down the avascular plane between the esophagus and left crus. Blunt dissection can be utilized to mobilize the esophagus anteriorly high into the mediastinum. Care must be taken to identify and avoid violation of the endothoracic fascia (parietal pleura of the lung cavity). Anatomically, the vagal nerves can be identified in the mediastinum in their named positions relative to the esophagus. At the GE junction the left vagus nerve rotates to become an anterior structure and the right a posterior structure. The hepatic branch of the vagus nerve can often be seen coursing toward the liver within the gastrohepatic ligament. Failure to preserve this vagal branch has been reported to cause minor gallbladder emptying dysfunction, although clinically this is rarely significant.

2. Division of the short gastric vessels. This is best accomplished utilizing an ultrasonic dissector or other vessel sealing device. Careful coordination of retraction between the surgeon and first assistant is critical to avoid injury to the stomach or spleen as the dissection approaches the angle of His.

3. Circumferential mobilization of the esophagus and establishment of at least 2.5 cm of intra-abdominal length. This can be accomplished by careful blunt dissection at the base of the right crus outside the mediastinum working toward the left crus, where the angle of His has been previously dissected. Consideration should be made to avoid working too deep away from the esophagus as the celiac axis is nearby. After creation of a posterior window, a 0.25-inch Penrose drain cut 4 inches can be placed around the esophagus and secured with an endoloop. Manipulation of the endoloop by the first assistant allows exposure for mobilization of the entire esophagus high into the mediastinum. If adequate esophageal length cannot be attained after high dissection of the esophagus into the mediastinum, a Collis-type wedge gastroplasty can be performed to tubularize the proximal stomach. This gastric tube is sized with a 48 French (Fr) bougie.

4. Posterior crural closure. Braided permanent suture such as 0-Ethibond or 0-Tycron cut 6–7 inches long provides the optimum strength and handling characteristics to close the crura. The first stitch re-approximates the base of the crura, avoiding the aorta. Pledgets are utilized to prevent shearing of the longitudinally oriented muscle fibers. The highest crural stitch (closest to the esophagus) should not include pledgets to avoid esophageal erosion. Upon closure of the crura, laparoscopic instruments should still be able to enter the mediastinum with minimal effort.

5. Creation of a floppy posterior fundoplication. Various surgeons have reported formal systems by which to construct the fundoplication. To prevent dysphagia, the wrap should be constructed over a 58 or 60Fr bougie. Despite the particular methodology, in general, the wrap should utilize only the fundus of the stomach, with care taken to ensure that no redundancy is created. This is done by a "shoe-shine" maneuver in which the open wrap posterior to the stomach is moved back and forth to show that there is a 1:1 relationship between a pull on one side and a response on the other. The wrap is then secured using a permanent braided 2-0 suture. Rotation or slippage of the wrap is prevented by incorporating a small purchase of esophagus in each bite. The overall length of the wrap should be approximately 3 cm.

Complications

Major complications after laparoscopic Nissen fundoplication are rare and are often related to surgeon experience and technique. In high-volume centers, conversion from laparoscopic to open procedures occurs in less than 2.4% of patients. Death is rare (0.07%). Perioperative complications include wound infection (3%), perforation (4%), pneumothorax (2%), and port-site hernia (0.2–9%). Most common postoperative symptoms include inability to burp, flatulence, bloating (5–34%), and dysphagia (0–25%), which can impact quality of life.

Results

Long-term outcomes evaluating efficacy of Nissen fundoplication demonstrate relief of typical symptoms in more that 90% of patients at 2 years and 80–90% at 5 years or more. Need for antisecretory drugs of some type has been reported widely at 6–62%.

Recurrence of persistent symptoms, inability to swallow, or postprandial discomfort suggests failure of the procedure. Herniation of the wrap into the chest is the most frequent cause of failure after the laparoscopic repair. Creation of a "too tight" or "too loose" fundoplication results in short-term symptomatology. Partial or complete breakdown of the fundoplication may appear later. Careful evaluation of symptoms and a thorough diagnostic evaluation are critical to determining who will benefit from reoperation. Patients with recurrent typical symptoms without dysphagia or evidence of a motility disorder benefit most from a reoperative procedure.

Ingestion of caustics

The extent of esophageal and gastric damage resulting from a caustic ingestion depend upon the properties of the ingested substance (acid or alkali), amount, concentration, physical form (solid or liquid), and the duration of contact with the mucosa.

Typically ingestion occurs in children by accident and the remainder in adults who are psychotic, suicidal, or alcoholic.

Common agents

1. Strong alkali (sodium or potassium hydroxide) in drain cleaners, household cleaning products, or disc batteries. The term "lye" implies substances that contain sodium or potassium hydroxide.
2. Highly concentrated acids (hydrochloric, sulfuric, and phosphoric acid) in toilet bowl cleanenss swimming pool cleaners, and antirust compounds.
3. Liquid household bleach (5% sodium hypochlorite) and dishwasher detergent (alkali).

Pathophysiology

Alkali causes a penetrating injury called "liquefactive necrosis," a process that involves saponification of fats and solubilization of proteins. Cell death occurs from emulsification and disruption of cellular membranes. The injury extends rapidly (in seconds) through the mucosa and wall of the esophagus toward the mediastinum until tissue fluids buffer the alkali. In the stomach, partial neutralization of the ingested alkali occurs by gastric acid and may result in a less severe injury.

Acid ingestion causes a superficial coagulation necrosis that thromboses the underlying mucosal blood vessels, which causes desiccation or denaturation of superficial tissue proteins and forms a protective eschar. Because acid solutions cause pain on ingestion, the amount of acid ingested tends to be limited. The gastric injury is worse in case of acid ingestion because the esophagus is naturally more resistant to acid.

Clinical presentation

Patients may complain of oropharyngeal, retrosternal, or epigastric pain, dysphagia/odynophagia, or drooling. Persistent severe retrosternal or back pain, tachycardia, or crepitus over the neck and chest may indicate esophageal perforation with mediastinitis. These patients may be hemodynamically unstable and in respiratory distress.

Vomiting, hematemesis, abdominal tenderness, rebound, and rigidity suggest peritonitis.

Hoarseness and stridor suggest injury to the larynx and trachea, and dyspnea suggests pulmonary aspiration.

A grading system for esophageal injury to predict clinical outcome has been developed:

Grade 0: Normal
Grade 1: Mucosal edema and hyperemia
Grade 2A: Superficial ulcers, bleeding, exudates
Grade 2B: Deep focal or circumferential ulcers
Grade 3A: Focal necrosis
Grade 3B: Extensive necrosis

Another system is similar to the classification of burns:

First-degree injury: There is superficial mucosal damage with focal or diffuse erythema, edema, and hemorrhage. The mucosal lining subsequently sloughs without scar formation.
Second-degree injury: There is mucosal and submucosal damage, ulceration, vesicle formation, and eventually granulation tissue and scar or stricture.
Third-degree injury: Transmural damage with deep ulcers, black coloration, and perforation.

Initial management

The care of each patient has to be individualized, but most patients will require admission and observation. It is important to establish the type of agent ingested and the amount.

The patient should be managed in a monitored setting with intravenous fluids, supplemental oxygen, PPIs, and adequate analgesics. The use of diluents and induction of emesis are not useful. Blood counts, electrolytes, BUN, and creatinine should be measured. Arterial blood gas provides information on systemic toxicity and gas exchange. Chest and abdominal X-rays assess perforation. CT scan is able to detect other signs of injury such as esophageal thickening, micoperforation, mediastinitis, and intra-abdominal air.

If the patient is unstable (hemodynamic, respiratory, or mental status), then intubation, fluid resuscitation, and invasive monitoring with arterial and central venous lines should be performed. Vasopressors can also be used to maintain hemodynamic stability. The use of steroids is not useful. In patients with perforation or mediastinitis, antibiotics covering both gram-positive and gram-negative organisms should be given.

Upper endoscopy should be performed as quickly as possible to assess the extent and severity of injury.

Observation for 2–4 days may be needed because airway obstruction, delayed perforation, and hematemesis can develop.

In those with evidence of perforation, exploration should be performed. For esophageal perforation, drainage and debridement of the mediastinum via thoracotomy (right or left) with diversion of the esophagus by cervical esophagostomy and gastrostomy should be performed. A jejunostomy is placed to allow for enteral feeding. The perforation should be well drained, and whether repair can be perfomed should be assessed at the time of operation. The use of a covered stent is another option to contain the amount of contamination of the mediastinum.

Rarely, esophagectomy will be needed when there is extensive transmural necrosis of the esophagus. This can be achieved transhiatally or via a thoracotomy; an end-cervical esophagostomy, gastrostomy, and jejunostomy are also constructed. Reconstruction is performed at a later time when the patient has recovered completely from the injury. Depending on the extent of gastric injury, the stomach may be usable. Alternatively, a colon interposition will need to be used. The conduit can be placed substernally with a left neck anastomosis.

For gastric perforation, wide local debridement with primary repair or resection of the damaged tissue can be performed. Depending on the extent of injury the resection can be performed via a simple wedge resection or resection with duodenogastrostomy, gastrojejunostomy, or RY-gastrojejunostomy. Placement of a nasogastric tube for decompression and a feeding jejunostomy tube for enteral access are useful adjuncts.

Long-term management

In patients who have grade 2–3 or second- or third-degree injury, a stricture develops 6 to 8 weeks after the injury. The patient will require endoscopy and dilatation at periodic intervals to allow adequate swallowing.

Rarely, esophagectomy will become necessary.

Gastric outlet obstruction may develop and may be managed with dilatation and ultimately surgical drainage of the stomach by gastrojejunostomy.

Tracheoesophageal fistula may develop, which can be temporized with stenting, but will likely need esophageal resection and reconstruction and repair of the airway with an interposition muscle flap.

Surveillance endoscopy will need to be performed yearly in patients who have a stricture following injury because there is an increased incidence of adenocarcinoma 20 to 40 years after the injury.

Hiatal hernias

The herniation of abdominal contents into the chest through the esophageal hiatus is an increasingly common radiographic finding. Herniation may occur as a result of a congenital defect, trauma, or after antireflux or other hiatal operations. Typically an asymptomatic person will be found to have an air-filled structure behind the heart on plain films. In most cases these abnormalities are asymptomatic and discovered during workup of other problems. The natural history of hiatal hernias is that the pressure gradient between the chest and abdomen results in the enlargement of the hernia over time. Persistent negative intrathoracic pressure and the natural shortening of the esophagus during swallowing result in the thinning out of the phrenoesophageal membrane over time. This stretching is most prominent in anterior and posterior positions resulting in hernia sacs filled with intra-abdominal fat in these common locations.

Types

Hiatal hernias are classified by the relationship of the GE junction and stomach to the diaphragm and surrounding structures.

Type I: Sliding hernia. The GE junction is located above the level of the diaphragm by upward herniation of the cardia into the posterior mediastinum. This is the most common type and frequently associated with GERD.

Type II: The GE junction and cardia of the stomach are located below the level of the diaphragm; however, the fundus of the stomach has entered the mediastinum adjacent to the GE junction. This is a true paraesophageal hernia (PEH) and represents the rarest type.

Type III: The GE junction, cardia, and fundus of the stomach have all entered the mediastinum. This is the most common type found when surgical intervention is required.

Type IV: Similar to type III with the addition of another structure herniated into the mediastinum, such as colon, spleen, small bowel, liver, or pancreas.

Clinical presentation

Patients with hiatal hernias are often asymptomatic; however, symptoms of heartburn or epigastric or chest discomfort are most common. Depending on the size of the hernia, associated symptoms of early satiety, dysphagia, regurgitation, and respiratory complications can be present. These occur due to mass effect of the cardia or fundus within the mediastinum or torsion of the esophagus. Approximately one-third of patients with PEHs are anemic. This is due to friction or pressure-type gastric ulcers (Cameron's lesions) within the herniated portion of the stomach. These patients are often diagnosed as having a PEH on esophagogastroduodenoscopy (EGD). Rarely, cardiac dysfunction can be seen due to compression of the right atrium or ventricle.

Indication for surgery

Traditionally, the presence of a PEH warranted operative repair to mitigate the risk of acute gastric bleeding, obstruction, or strangulation from mesoaxial or organoaxial volvulus. An emergency operation to fix an acute bleed, perforation, or infarction is associated with a significant mortality rate versus less than 1% in elective repairs. However, the incidence of these catastrophic events is relatively low, and gastric strangulation is an exceedingly rare event. With or without the use of mesh, the recurrence rate of hiatal hernias is between 20 and 50% even in large-volume centers. Therefore, the determination to repair a hiatal hernia should be based on the degree of symptomatology within the context of the patient's overall fitness for surgery. Acid reflux symptoms can often be controlled with behavioral or lifestyle modification in conjunction with medications; however, large-volume reflux and mediastinal mass effects will require operative intervention.

Patients should undergo formal evaluation of the hiatal hernia by endoscopy and esophagram prior to surgery to look for ulceration and the presence of strictures, webs, or other abnormalities. Type I hiatal hernias may not be visible on esophagram due to their variable position but will likely be apparent on EGD. Manometry may be challenging in patients with large PEHs due to difficulty in navigating a tortuous distal esophagus or locating the lower esophageal sphincter. pH probe studies are typically not helpful in patients with large, readily apparent pathology.

Operations

PEH repairs can be performed via thoracic or abdominal approaches. The latter is typically favored because it affords quicker recovery due to less postoperative pain and allows easier reduction of torsed GI contents. Gastropexy by placement of a gastrostomy tube can be a useful adjunct in poor operative candidates or in emergency situations. Without dissection of the hernia sac, the patient remains at high risk long term for recurrence or seroma formation. There is no consensus on the need to perform an antireflux operation after a successful PEH repair; however, most experts feel that the requisite complete mobilization of the esophagus to remove the posterior hernia sac requires restoration of the antireflux mechanism through fundoplication. Performance of a fundoplication after the PEH repair also obviates the need to perform a gastropexy or place a gastrostomy tube to prevent reherniation of the stomach.

Principles of hernia repair include hernia reduction, removal of the hernia sac, crural repair, and fundoplication. The ability to successfully reduce the hernia sac depends upon proper camera and trocar positioning. Placing the camera or instruments greater than 15 cm from the xiphoid may make it difficult to visualize or work high into the mediastinum in larger hernias. Abdominal contents herniated into the mediastinum can be returned to the abdomen by gentle grasping by the surgeon and assistant. Typically it is not possible to completely reduce all the contents.

Removal of the hernia sac requires a great degree of skill and experience. This is due to the anatomic complexity of the sac, which has an anterior and posterior peritoneal component as well as lateral elements that are often fused with the blood supply to the stomach. The sac is dissected off the crura initially from the base of the right crus and carried anteriorly. As the sac is dissected, it can be inverted into the abdomen by the assistant. Judicious use of an energy source such as the hook cautery or ultrasonic dissector in conjunction with meticulous dissection is necessary to avoid entry into the pleural cavity through the endothoracic fascia. Inadvertent holes in the endothoracic fascia (parietal pleura) can be closed with an endoloop or sutured. When a pneumothorax becomes clinically significant, placement of a chest tube or conversion to open may be necessary although rare.

With the hernia sac removed, a high dissection of the esophagus in the mediastinum is required to mobilize the GE junction into the abdomen. In up to 5% of cases the minimum of 2.5 cm of intra-abdominal esophageal length cannot be ·obtained even after an extensive circumferential dissection, and a Collis procedure must be performed. Once an adequate esophageal length is established, a posterior crural closure can be initiated. Interrupted placement of pledgeted, permanent sutures allows proper re-approximation. The size of the defect will dictate the number of sutures placed. The placement of sutures closer together allows tension to be reduced as the closure proceeds anteriorly. Rarely, relaxing incisions in the diaphragm are necessary to bring the crura together. When performed on the right side, this newly created defect can be closed primarily or with permanent mesh and covered by the liver. The use of both permanent and absorbable mesh products to reinforce the primary crural closure has been studied extensively with equivocal results regardless of the fixation methods. Placement of reinforcement mesh therefore is largely surgeon dependent.

After closure of the diaphragm a 58Fr soft bougie dilator is passed down the esophagus to assess the tightness of the closure and prevent overtightening of the subsequent fundoplication. Close communication with the anesthesiologist during this maneuver is necessary to prevent perforation of the esophagus or stomach because the posterior closure of the crura will project the esophagus steeply anteriorly. Careful elevation of the stomach as the tip of the bougie passes through the GE junction reduces the traversal angle and thereby reduces the perforation risk.

Performance of a floppy Nissen fundoplication completes the PEH repair.

Complications

Due to the fact that the majority of patients with large PEHs are older, perioperative morbidity relates in large part to underlying medical condition. Major intraoperative complications include pneumothorax, bleeding, esophageal or gastric perforation, and vagal injury. Postoperatively, the extensive mediastinal dissection may lead to significant subcutaneous crepitance in chest, neck, and even head. This usually has little physiologic significance and resolves spontaneously. Early postoperative complications include wound infection, atrial fibrillation, and DVT. Long-term complications include dysphagia, belching, gas bloat, pulmonary symptoms, weight loss, slipped Nissen, and recurrence of PEH.

Results

Despite symptomatic relief in greater than 80% of patients, the recurrence rate of PEHs ranges from 20–40% in large studies. This is independent of the use of mesh or concomitant gastropexy. Failure to recognize a shortened esophagus or poor crural closure with excessive tension has been implicated in the high incidence of recurrence. Most recurrences are asymptomatic. When symptomatic, most patients present with a sliding herniation of their wrap, leading to chest pain or dysphagia.

Diverticuli

These are localized dilatations of the esophagus formed by the mucosa or the entire wall of the esophagus.

Types

- Pharyngoesophageal or Zenker's. An outpouching of esophageal mucosa above the cricopharyngeal spincter in the neck.
- Parabronchial or traction. Localized outpouching of the entire esophageal wall occurring at the level of the carina due to mediastinal scarring from a granulomatous infection.
- Epiphrenic or pulsion. An outpouching of the esophageal mucosa just above the gastroesophageal sphincter in the chest.
- Diffuse intramural diverticulosis. Multiple small (1–3 mm) outpouchings of the esophageal wall, which may be segmental or diffuse.

Clinical presentation

The source of symptoms is usually the underlying pathology that causes the diverticulum. Pharyngeoesophageal diverticula usually cause regurgitation and aspiration, and a left neck mass associated with swallowing may be seen. Parabronchial diverticula are often asymptomatic but may cause dysphagia. Rarely, they may erode into an airway, blood vessel, or pericardium. Epiphrenic diverticula are associated with dysphagia, reflux, regurgitation, and occasionally hematemesis.

Barium swallow establishes the diagnosis, and endoscopy helps rule out other pathology and empty the diverticulum of retained contents. CT scan of the chest adds additional anatomic information regarding location and relation to other structures within the

227

mediastinum. Manometry identifies the underlying esophageal motility disorder.

Nonsurgical management

Management of the underlying motility disorder or mediastinal pathology must be undertaken, and patients who are not symptomatic or are well controlled with medical management of their reflux disease will require no surgical treatment. The isolated presence of an esophageal diverticulum is not an indication for surgery.

Indications for surgery

Patients who have symptoms or complications associated with the diverticulum are to be considered for surgery. Dysphagia, regurgitation, aspiration with pulmonary infection, and reactive airway disease and reflux not controlled with medical management are all reasons to perform surgery. Bleeding, stricture formation, infection, erosion into surrounding structures, perforation, and rarely malignancy are complications that will require surgery.

Operations

Surgery should remove or negate the reservoir effects of the diverticulum, address the underlying motility defect, and treat the resultant reflux.

Pharyngoesophageal: Cricopharyngeal myotomy and diverticulectomy can be performed by open or endoscopic technique. Endoscopic technique usually uses a rigid esophagus and an endoscopic stapler that is used to divide the bridge of tissue between the diverticulum and the esophagus. The use of a flexible endoscopic to coagulate and divide the bridge of tissue between the diverticulum and esophagus is a relatively new technique and is still being evaluated.

Thoracic: Diverticuli within the chest can be managed with a minimally invasive or open approach depending on the surgeon's expertise.

Epiphrenic diverticulum: The open approach is best performed via left thoracotomy through the sixth space with single-lung ventilation and a No. 48 Maloney in the esophagus. The esophagus is circumferentially dissected distal to the carina and then inferiorly to the fundus of the stomach. The diverticulum is dissected from the mediastinum and its neck clearly defined. It is resected at its neck using a stapling device with a staple height of 3.5 mm. The muscular defect is reapproximated with interrupted

4-0 Vicryl. The phrenoesophageal membrane is opened at the hiatus, the cardia is mobilized, and two traction sutures of 2-0 silk are placed through the muscular layer of the distal esophagus on its anterolateral aspect, elevating it from the underlying mucosa. The myotomy is started in between the sutures using cautery set at 10 or sharply. Once most of the muscle has been divided, the remaining fibers can be bluntly separated from the mucosa using a peanut dissector. The myotomy is extended onto the stomach for a few centimeters to ensure destruction of the lower esophageal sphincter. This is then extended superiorly to the level of the aortic arch using a combination of blunt, sharp, or cautery dissection. A vertical strip of muscle is removed from the muscle layer and sent for pathology; this also prevents the muscle from healing to form a circumferential layer around the esophagus. An NG tube is placed and its position confirmed just below the GE junction.

An antireflux repair is performed by placing two rows of vertical mattress sutures through the fundus and muscle of the distal esophagus on each side of the myotomy using 2-0 silk. The second layer of sutures is passed through the diaphragm first to keep the GE junction within the abdomen. The hiatus is recreated by tying previously placed sutures of 0 silk in the crus but allowing for two fingers to pass through along the esophagus. The chest is drained with a No. 28 chest tube.

A Barium swallow is performed on postoperative day 2 (POD2) to assess for leak or obstruction due to the fundoplication.

The minimally invasive approach is performed by a right thoracoscopy and laparoscopy to complete the antireflux procedure.

The camera is placed in the seventh or eighth intercostal space in the line of the antero superior iliac spine, an access incision is placed in the anterior axillary line in the same space, and a working incision is placed in the fifth space between the middle and anterior axillary line. The inferior pulmonary ligament is divided with harmonic scalpel as is the mediastinal pleura over the posterior hilum of the lung until the level of the azygous vein. The pleura posterior to the esophagus is then opened from the level of the azygous vein to the hiatus. The esophagus is circumferentially dissected using the harmonic scalpel at the level of the carina and a 0.5-inch Penrose drain placed around it to aid in traction. The esophagus is then dissected to the hiatus and the diverticulum dissected from the mediastinum. The neck of the diverticulum is clearly identified by sharp and blunt dissection. Using an endoGIA stapler either 45 or 60 mm in length with a 3.5-mm staple height, the diverticulum is divided at its neck. The muscular defect is closed with interrupted sutures of 4-0 Vicryl.

Using stay sutures as described in the open technique, a myotomy is commenced at the distal esophagus and extended superiorly to the level of the carina. The site of the myotomy should be remote from the neck of the diverticulum. Distally, the myotomy is extended to the GE junction. The NG tube is then placed and insufflated with air and the mucosa checked for evidence of perforation. The chest is drained with a No. 28 chest tube.

Next, the patient is placed supine, and laparoscopic partial fundoplication is performed. After placement in the supine split leg position, the esophageal hiatus is mobilized by dividing the gastrohepatic and phrenoesophageal ligament with an ultrasonic dissector. The greater curvature of the stomach is mobilized by dividing the short gastric vessels. It is not necessary to divide the posterior attachments of the esophageal hiatus. The left vagus nerve is mobilized from its anterior position as it comes through the hiatus. The fat pad anterior to the GE junction is removed. The myotomy started in the chest is then carried onto the anterior surface of the stomach for at least 2 cm.

A 58Fr bougie is placed down the esophagus and into the stomach. Creation of the Dor (180-degree anterior) fundoplication begins by placing a permanent 0 suture on the greater curvature fundus 3 cm distal to the angle of His to the left crus of the diaphragm. Sequential sutures are placed between the fundus and left crus folding the stomach anteriorly over the esophagus. A second row of sutures secures the fundus onto the right crus completely covering the myotomy site.

Parabronchial: These diverticuli rarely require surgery, but when performed for complications, they will likely require thoracotomy, excision, and repair of the esophagus with intercostal muscle buttress.

Complications

For pharyngeal diverticulum, mediastinitis, recurrent laryngeal nerve injury, fistula formation, esophageal stenosis, and recurrence or persistence of the diverticulum can occur with an overall incidence of 10%.

Recurrent nerve injury can be managed by observation, aspiration precautions, or temporarily by injection laryngoplasty and permanently by surgical medialization by laryngoplasty or thyroplasty.

Perforation or leak can occur due to the myotomy or at the neck of the diverticulum. If the patient is asymptomatic, it can be managed with NG suction and chest tube drainage with spontaneous healing. For symptomatic patients, reoperation and repair of the leak with intercostal muscle flap buttress should be performed.

Results

Pharyngeal diverticula treated by surgery have good long-term results, and those treated with a rigid endoscopic approach have a shorter hospital stay and recovery. However, exposure fails in approximately 30% of the patients where a rigid endoscope is used.

The incidence of mortality, leak, perforation, and major pulmonary morbidity is very low for operations on thoracic diverticula. Most patients are relieved of their symptoms permanently. Occasional dysphagia and reflux can occur, and the treatment of patients must be individualized.

Motility disorders
Types

Esophageal motility abnormalities (Table 23.1) are usually defined through testing with stationary manometry performed during a series of 10 or more 5-ml liquid swallows under standardized conditions that permit comparison with the data obtained from normal volunteers. Usually sensors are spaced at 5-cm intervals.

Achalasia

There is a loss of peristalsis in the distal esophagus (whose musculature is comprised predominantly of smooth muscle) and a failure of LES relaxation. Although both of these abnormalities impair esophageal emptying, the symptoms of achalasia (e.g. dysphagia and regurgitation) are due primarily to the defect in LES relaxation.

Pathophysiology: degeneration of neurons in the esophageal wall. Histologic examination reveals decreased numbers of neurons (ganglion cells) in the myenteric plexuses. This inflammatory degeneration involves the nitric oxide–producing, inhibitory

229

Table 23.1 Criteria for normal esophageal function and primary motility disorders

Motility pattern	LES resting pressure (10–45 mmHg)	LES relaxation residual (≤8 mmHg)	Effective peristaltic waves (≥30 mmHg)	Ineffective peristaltic waves[a] (<30 mmHg)	Simultaneous contractions (>30 mmHg) propagation rate ≥ 8 cm/s
Normal	10–45 mmHg	≤8 mmHg	≥7 waves	≤2 waves	≤1 contraction
Achalasia	Normal (≤45 mmHg) Abnormal (>45 mmHg)	>8 mmHg	0	0	10 contractions
Distal esophageal spasm	Normal (≤45 mmHg) Abnormal (>45 mmHg)	Normal (≤8 mmHg) Abnormal (>8 mmHg)	1–8	≤2 waves	≥2 contractions ≤9 contractions
Hypercontractile motility Hypertensive LES Nutcracker esophagus	>45 mmHg	≤8 mmHg	7–10 waves[b]	≤2 waves	≤1 contraction
Hypocontractile motility Hypotensive LES Ineffective esophageal motility	<10 mmHg	≤8 mmHg	0–7 waves	3–10 waves	≤1 contraction

[a] 3 and/or 8 cm above the lower esophageal sphincter.
[b] Average amplitude of 10 swallows (20 contractions 3 and 8 cm above the lower esophageal sphincter) greater than 180 mmHg.
LES, lower esophageal sphincter.

neurons that effect the relaxation of esophageal smooth muscle; the cholinergic neurons that contribute to LES tone by causing smooth muscle contraction may be relatively spared. In the smooth muscle portion of the esophageal body, the loss of inhibitory neurons results in aperistalsis.

Etiology

- Primary: Unknown but possible autoimmune.
- Secondary: Chagas disease or infection with *Trypanosome cruzi*, malignancy (gastric, esophageal, lung, pancreatic cancer, and lymphoma), amyloid, sarcoid, eosinophilic esophagitis, MENIIB, Sjögren's syndrome.

Clinical Presentation

- Dysphagia to solids and liquids and difficulty belching occur in 80–90% of patients.

- Weight loss, regurgitation, chest pain, and heartburn occur in approximately 40–60% of patients.

Diagnosis

- Barium swallow. Diagnostic in 95%, shows a dilated esophagus that ends in a beak-like narrowing caused by the LES.
- Manometry. LES pressure higher than 45 mmHg and absent LES relaxation after a swallow, no peristalsis in the smooth muscle portion of the esophagus.
- Endoscopy. To rule out malignancy. The esophagus is usually dilated and contains debri.

Treatment

Calcium channel blockers and nitrates relax the LES and are effective in 70% of patients. Botulinum toxin injection into the LES works in 80%, but the effect lasts for only 6 months. Pneumatic dilation of the LES relieves the obstruction by tearing its fibers. It is effective in 85%, and the effect lasts for up to 3 years.

Surgical: Heller's myotomy of the LES with partial fundoplication by Laparoscopic technique is currently preferred, where the LES is divided and a partial fundoplication performed. Position of the patient and port placement is similar to that for fundoplication. A gastroscope is passed to clear the esophagus and the GE junction and is left crossing the junction. The left lobe of the liver is retracted, exposing the hiatus, and the stomach is retracted inferiorly. This exposes the GE junction, and the gastroheaptic ligament and the peritoneum over the GE junction are then divided. The left crus is completely dissected. The retroesophageal space is then dissected and the esophagus encircled with a vascular tape or penrose drain. The phrenoesophageal ligament is divided, and 6 cm of the esophagus is mobilized. With the cautery on low setting, a myotomy is then performed starting 6–8 cm proximal to the phrenoesophageal ligament and carried through the GE junction and for at least 2 cm onto the stomach. The muscle is swept off the mucosa bluntly with a peanut dissector or graspers for approximately 180 degrees. Care is taken to avoid the vagus nerves. The gastroscope is then used to check for perforation and the GE junction for patency. The left edge of the muscle is then sutured to the left crus and the medial side of the fundus with three 2-0 silk sutures. The tape or drain encircling the esophagus is now removed and the fundus anchored to the apex of the right crus. The rest of the fundus is rolled over the lower esophagus and sutured to the right crus including the right edge of the esophageal myotomy with three sutures of 2-0 silk. The short gastric vessels can be divided if the fundoplication is under tension.

Perforation should be recognized intraoperatively and repaired primarily and covered with the stomach.

Barium swallow is done on POD1 to rule out perforation and assess patency of the GE junction. Clear liquids are started, and the patient is discharged on a liquid diet.

Success rates are higher than dilation, and the recurrence rate is less. The 5-year probability of being asymptomatic is 90%. Recurrence, when it occurs, is usually within 12 months and can be treated by dilatation. Reflux can occur in 30% of patients and is managed medically.

Both balloon dilatation and myotomy have equivalent results over the long term, but younger patients have a higher chance of failure with dilatation. Dilatation has to be performed up to three times over a period of 2 years to yield equivalent results to surgery and has a 4% perforation rate.

Per oral endoscopic myotomy is a new treatment where a myotomy of the LES is performed endoscopically with good initial results.

Patients are managed medically first and then may need dilatation or surgery, with surgery being preferable in patients younger than 40. Botulinum injection is preferred for those who are at higher risk, that is, the elderly or those with many co-morbidities.

Diffuse esophageal spasm

Dysphagia is common in these patients. Chest pain is also common and has to be differentiated from coronary artery disease.

Testing

- Esophageal manometry.
- Endoscopy and barium swallow to rule out other causes of dysphagia. In diffuse esophageal spasm, segmentation of the esophagus may be seen.

Nonsurgical management: Patients whose primary symptom is chest pain – calcium channel blocker, diltiazem 180–240 mg/day or a tricyclic antidepressant, imipramine 25–50 mg at bedtime as the initial treatment. For patients who do not respond to this treatment, isosorbide 10 mg or sildenafil 50 mg taken as needed for pain should be tried. Following which, botulinum toxin injection at the Z-line (100 units given circumferentially in 20-units doses) can be given with relief in 70% of patients and a duration of effect of 7 months. Pneumatic dilatation may also be effective. In patients whose primary symptom is dysphagia, treatment with a calcium channel blocker (diltiazem 180–240 mg/day) is tried initially, followed by botulinum injection or pneumatic dilation.

Indications for surgery: Patients with diffuse esophageal spasm who continue to be symptomatic after medical management, injection, or dilatation with severe dysphagia or chest pain are candidates for surgical treatment. Patient's in whom manometry reveals less than 30% of contractions are effective benefit from surgery. Manometry identifies the proximal extent of the myotomy, which should be high enough to include the entire length of the disordered motility. Surgery for Nutcracker esophagus and hypertensive LES is not clearly beneficial and is probably best avoided.

Operations: A left posterolateral thoracotomy is performed through the sixth space. The inferior pulmonary ligament is divided. The mediastinal pleura is opened over the esophagus from the hiatus to the arch of the aorta and, if needed (based on manometry), to the thoracic inlet. A long myotomy is performed starting where it is easiest, dividing the muscular wall of the esophagus sharply or with cautery on a low setting until the mucosa is seen. The mucosa can then be bluntly or sharply dissected from the muscular layer, and division of the muscle can proceed superiorly and inferiorly to the LES. A strip of muscle can be removed to prevent reapproximation of the muscle layer. The mucosal integrity is tested by air insufflation or methylene blue instillation via the nasogastric tube. A partial fundoplication is then performed. The chest is drained by a single chest tube. A barium swallow can be performed on POD2 prior to allowing the patient to resume oral intake.

A right-sided thoracoscopic approach is preferred because the entire esophagus is readily accessable. A camera incision is placed in the line of the anterosuperior iliac spine in the seventh space, an access incision is placed in the same or sixth space in the anterior axillary line, and the working incision is placed in the fifth space between the middle and anterior axillary line. The inferior pulmonary ligament is divided, and the mediastinal pleura over the esophagus is opened. A myotomy is commenced below the carina dividing the muscle sharply or with cautery on a low setting. The muscle can be held with Hunter graspers or with retraction sutures. The division of the muscle can then be done sharply, bluntly, or with a harmonic scalpel taking care to protect the mucosa. This is carried superiorly to the inlet and distally to the hiatus and the lower esophageal sphincter. A partial fundoplication is then performed laparoscopically.

Complications: Mucosal perforation should be recognized intraoperatively and repaired primarily and buttressed with an intercostal muscle flap.

Results: Relief of symptoms occurs in 80–90% of patients with the myotomy extending to the arch or the thoracic inlet.

References
Literature for antireflux surgery

1 Finks JF, Wei Y, Birkmeyer JD. The rise and fall of antireflux surgery in the United States. *Surg Endosc* 2006; 20: 1698–701.

2 Kahrilas PJ, Shaheen NJ, Vaezi MF, et al. American Gastroenterological Association. American Gastroenterological Association Medical Position Statement on the management of gastroesophageal reflux disease. *Gastroenterology* 2008; 135:1383–91.

3 Morgenthal CB, Shane MD, Stival A, et al. The durability of laparoscopic Nissen fundoplication: 11-year outcomes. *J Gastrointest Surg* 2007 Jun; 11(6):693–700.

4 Terry ML, Vernon A, Hunter JG. Stapled wedge Collis gastroplasty for the shortened esophagus. *Am J Surg* 2004 Aug; 188(2):195–9.

5 Oelschlager BK, Ma KC, Soares RV, et al. A broad assessment of clinical outcomes after laparoscopic antireflux surgery. *Ann Surg* 2012 Jul; 256(1):87–94.

6 Bajbouj M, Becker V, Phillip V, et al. High-dose esomeprazole for treatment of symptomatic refractory gastroesophageal reflux disease: a prospective pH-metry/impedance-controlled study. *Digestion* 2009; 80:112–18. doi:10.1159/000221146

7 Stefanidis D, Hope WW, Kohn GP, et al. The SAGES Guidelines Committee. Guidelines for surgical treatment of gastroesophageal reflux disease. *Surg Endosc* 2010; 24:2647–69. doi 10.1007/s00464-010-1267-8

Literature for ingestion of caustics

1 Cabral C, Chirica M, de Chaisemartin C, et al. Caustic injuries of the upper digestive tract: a population observational study. *Surg Endosc* 2012 Jan; 26(1):214–21. doi: 10.1007/s00464-011-1857-0

2 Atiq M, Kibria RE, Dang S, et al. Corrosive injury to the GI tract in adults: a practical approach. *Expert Rev Gastroenterol Hepatol* 2009 Dec; 3(6):701–9. doi: 10.1586/egh.09.56.

3 Tohda G, Sugawa C, Gayer C, et al. Clinical evaluation and management of caustic injury in the upper gastrointestinal tract in 95 adult patients in an urban medical center. *Surg Endosc* 2008 Apr; 22(4):1119–25.

4 Cheng HT, Cheng CL, Lin CH, et al. Caustic ingestion in adults:

the role of endoscopic classification in predicting outcome. *BMC Gastroenterol* 2008; 8:31.

5   Corrosive injury, Chapter 36, p. 515. in Pearson et al., *Esophageal Surgery*, 2nd edn., Churchill Livingstone, 2002.

Literature for hiatal hernias

1   Oelschlager BK, Petersen RP, Brunt LM, et al. Laparoscopic paraesophageal hernia repair: defining long term clinical and anatomic outcomes. *J Gastrointest Surg* 2012 Mar; 16(3):453–9.

2   Oelschlager BK, Pellegrini CA, Hunter JG, et al. Biologic prosthesis to prevent recurrence after laparoscopic paraesophageal hernia: long-term follow-up from a multicenter, prospective, randomized trial. *J Am Coll Surg* 2011 Oct; 213(4):461–8.

3   Mattar SG, Bowers SP, Galloway KD, et al. Long-term outcome of laparoscpic repair of paraesophageal hernia. *Surg Endosc* 2002 May; 16(5):745–9.

4   Soper NJ, Swanstrom LL, Eubanks WS. *Mastery of Endoscopic and Laparoscopic Surgery*, 2nd edn. Lippincott William and Wilkins, 2005.

Literature for diverticuli

1   Payne WS. The treatment of pharyngoesophageal diverticulum: the simple and complex. *Hepatogastroenterology* 1992; 39(2):109.

2   Chang CY, Payyapilli RJ, Scher RL. Endoscopic staple diverticulostomy for Zenker's diverticulum: review of literature and experience in 159 consecutive cases. *Laryngoscope* 2003; 113(6):957.

3   Zaninotto G, Portale G, Costantini M, et al. Therapeutic strategies for epiphrenic diverticula: systematic review. *World J Surg* 2011 Jul; 35(7):1447–53. doi: 10.1007/ s00268-011–1065-z.

4   Kilic A, Schuchert MJ, Awais O, et al. Surgical management of epiphrenic diverticula in the minimally invasive era. *JSLS* 2009 Apr–Jun; 13(2):160–4. Review.

5   Hudspeth DA, Thorne MT, Conroy R, Pennell TC. Management of epiphrenic esophageal diverticula: a fifteen- year experience. *Am Surg* 1993 Jan; 59(1):40–2.

6   Esophageal diverticula, Chapter 31, p. 515 in Pearson et al., *Esophageal Surgery*, 2nd edn. Churchill Livingstone, 2002.

Literature for motility disorders

1   Richter JE. Oesophageal motility disorders. *Lancet* 2001 Sep 8; 358(9284):823–8.

2   Herbella FA, Tineli AC, Wilson JL Jr, Del Grande JC. Surgical treatment of primary esophageal motility disorders. *J Gastrointest Surg* 2008 Mar; 12(3):604–8.

3   Patti MG, Gorodner MV, Galvani C, et al. Spectrum of esophageal motility disorders: implications for diagnosis and treatment. *Arch Surg* 2005 May; 140(5):442–8; discussion 448–9.

4   Primary esophageal motor disorders, Chapter 32, p. 515 in Pearson et al., *Esophageal Surgery*, 2nd edn., Churchill Livingstone, 2002.

5   Achalasia: thoracoscopic and laparoscopic myotomy, Chapter 35, p. 569 in Pearson et al., *Esophageal Surgery*, 2nd edn. Churchill Livingstone, 2002.

Esophageal cancer

Gail Darling

Chapter 24

Surgical anatomy

The esophagus begins at the level of the cricopharyngeus or upper esophageal sphincter (UES) and descends in the posterior mediastinum, through the esophageal hiatus at the level of T10, to join the stomach. In the absence of a hiatal hernia, the gastroesophageal junction lies 2–4 cm below the esophageal hiatus. Important relations of the esophagus anteriorly are the trachea from the level of the UES to the tracheal carina at T4, which is approximately 25 cm from the incisor teeth endoscopically, the left main bronchus. Below T4/5, the heart, specifically the left atrium, and inferior pulmonary veins lie anterior to the esophagus. Posteriorly lie the aorta and spine and laterally the lungs, the azygous vein, and thoracic duct. Understanding the anatomic relations is important in considering treatment because these structures may be invaded by an esophageal tumor or may be injured during esophagectomy.

The esophagus consists of a mucosal layer, a circular muscle layer, and a longitudinal muscle layer. It lacks a serosa. The lymphatics of the esophagus originate in the submucosal layer and have both indirect and direct connections to longitudinal lymphatic channels and the thoracic duct. The longitudinal lymphatic channels allow for extensive proximal and distal spread of cancer cells. This anatomic feature allows for extensive intramural spread of cancer as well as early dissemination of esophageal cancer once the tumor breaches the lamina propria and invades the submucosa. Because of potential intramural spread, proximal resection margins of 5–10 cm are required when performing an esophagectomy in order to achieve an R0 resection.

The esophagus is lined by squamous epithelium; however, it may acquire a columnar lining in response to chronic severe gastroesophageal reflux. This metaplastic epithelium, Barrett's esophagus, may develop dysplastic changes, which then progress to adenocarcinoma. Thus there are two dominant histologies in esophageal cancer: squamous cell carcinoma and adenocarcinoma. However, other malignancies may also occur as primary tumors in the esophagus, including small cell carcinoma, melanoma, carcinosarcoma, leiomyosarcoma, angiosarcoma, granular cell tumor, and lymphoma.

Epidemiology/etiology

Esophageal cancer is the eighth most common cancer. Although squamous cell carcinoma is the dominant histology worldwide, adenocarcinoma has been increasing in frequency since the 1980s and is now the dominant histology in North America and Western Europe. Risk factors for adenocarcinoma include obesity, gastroesophageal reflux, smoking, and possibly dietary factors. Risk factors for squamous cell carcinoma include smoking, alcohol, chronic inflammation or irritation related to caustic ingestion, achalasia, thermal injury (e.g. drinking very hot tea), and chewing Betel nut. Certain geographic regions (Iraq, Iran, India, China) have a higher incidence of esophageal cancer, which may be related to genetic factors because populations in these regions have some common ancestry (Turkman and Mongolian) or dietary factors.

Clinical presentation

Most patients with esophageal cancer present with dysphagia. The term "progressive mechanical dysphagia" is used to describe the progression of dysphagia for solid foods, which progresses until the patient cannot even swallow liquids, including their own

Core Topics in Thoracic Surgery, ed. Marco Scarci, Aman Coonar, Tom Routledge and Francis Wells. Published by Cambridge University Press. © Cambridge University Press 2016

saliva. Weight loss is common, while odynophagia is less frequent. Constant pain located in the chest, back, or epigastrium is an ominous symptom that suggests invasion of local structures including splanchnic nerves. Distant metastatic disease most often is suggested by poor performance status.

Investigations

Initial investigations include esophagogastroscopy with biopsy for diagnosis, and staging with endoscopic ultrasound (EUS), CT scan of the chest and abdomen, and PET-CT. A contrast swallow may be the initial diagnostic test but may be omitted if prompt endoscopy is performed. Staging laparoscopy is not commonly performed for esophageal tumors but should be considered for tumors of the gastric cardia that involve the gastroesophageal junction, especially if the tumor is T3 or T4. Tumors that appear to be T1 on EUS may be further evaluated by endomucoscal resection (EMR) to differentiate T1a versus T1b.

In addition to routine histology, tumor samples should be evaluated by immunohistochemistry to precisely determine the tumor type. Descriptions such as undifferentiated carcinoma should prompt further evaluation because these often turn out to be unusual tumors such as small cell or sarcoma.

Testing for HER2 status is now standard for esophageal adenocarcinomas because up to 33% of these tumors overexpress HER2. In the setting of advanced disease, trastuzumab has been shown to be useful for such patients.

Staging

Staging evaluation includes CT scan, PET-CT, and EUS (Table 24.1). PET-CT has been demonstrated to be superior to CT alone for detection of distant metastatic disease. The use of PET-CT in T1 cancers is controversial and is considered by many to be unnecessary. Contrast-enhanced CT using an esophageal or gastric protocol provides morphologic detail, which is useful in considering resectability. Lymph nodes may be identified on CT, but the absence of visible lymph nodes does not rule out lymph node involvement. While PET-CT may identify metastatic lymph nodes regardless of their location, it has a lower sensitivity for locoregional nodal disease because this may be overshadowed by high uptake in the primary tumor or may not be visible if the burden of disease is limited.

Table 24.1 Union for International Cancer Control (UICC) staging of cancer of the esophagus and esophagogastric junction 7. (www. uicc.org)

Tumor

Tis: carcinoma in situ, high-grade dysplasia
T1a: tumor limited to mucosa, does not invade lamina propria/muscularis mucosa
T1b: tumor invades beyond the lamina propria or muscularis mucosa into submucosa
T2 : tumor invades muscularis propria
T3: tumor invades adventitia
T4a: tumor invades pleura, pericardium, peritoneum, diaphragm
T4b: tumor invades other adjacent structures (aorta, vertebra, trachea)

Nodes

N0: no regional lymph node metastases
N1: 1–2 nodes regional lymph nodes
N2: 3–6 nodes
N3: > 6 nodes

Metastases

M0: no distant metastases
M1: distant metastases

Stage groupings			
IA	T1	N0	M0
IB	T2	N0	M0
IIA	T3	N0	M0
IIB	T1/T2	N1	M0
IIIA	T4a	N0	M0
	T3	N1	M0
	T1/T2	N2	M0
IIIB	T3	N2	M0
IIIC	T4a	N1/N2	M0
	T4b	any N	M0
	any T	N3	M0
IV	any T	any N	M1

Endoscopic ultrasound is used for determining T and N stage. However, EUS is limited in its ability to distinguish T1a versus T1b. This distinction is becoming increasingly important because more patients with T1a disease are being treated with EMR rather than esophagectomy. When a T1 tumor is identified by EUS, EMR may be used to provide more precise staging and distinguish T1a from T1b. EMR may also be therapeutic if the tumor is T1a. Endoscopic submucosal dissection (ESD) also has the ability to resect mucosal lesions but permits larger resections.

Thus EMR and ESD are increasingly used as both a staging and a therapeutic tool for early tumors.

Treatment

Treatment depends on the stage of the cancer and the patient's functional status. Esophagectomy has been the mainstay of treatment except for stage IV disease. However, recently, EMR has been used for patients with T1a tumors and patients with high-grade dysplasia. Standard therapy for these patients has been esophagectomy, but less invasive therapies such as EMR or ESD are now considered acceptable alternatives for T1a cancers.

The primary goal of therapy for patients with stage IV disease is relief of dysphagia. Options include brachytherapy, esophageal stent, external beam radiation, laser, or chemotherapy. The choice of treatment depends further on the patient's functional status and estimated survival. For patients with stage IV disease, estimated survival is measured in months, so prompt palliation of dysphagia is important. However, minimizing the number of interventions required to achieve relief of dysphagia is also desirable. For patients with limited survival, self-expanding metal stents (SEMS) provide the most immediate relief of dysphagia; however, these have their own potential complications, such as perforation, hemorrhage, food impaction, tumor overgrowth, and erosion. Laser or cryotherapy provides immediate but short duration of palliation.

External beam radiation is useful in providing more durable palliation of dysphagia, but the onset of dysphagia relief is not immediate and may take several weeks. Depending on the patient's duration of survival, tumor regrowth may occur, leading to recurrent dysphagia. External beam radiation may be repeated depending on the total dose of radiation given initially. Alternatively, brachytherapy may be used either alone or in conjunction with external beam radiation. Brachytherapy provides more immediate relief of dysphagia than external beam, may be repeated, and provides minimal radiation to surrounding tissues; hence it may be used in a patient who has had previous external beam radiation (depending on total dose) and may be given in a single fraction in one treatment or as two to three treatments given 1 week apart. For patients with adequate functional status, systemic chemotherapy may be appropriate and can relieve dysphagia. Chemotherapy may be repeated, treats systemic disease as well as local disease, and does not preclude other treatments for dysphagia.

Although SEMS are probably used most often for dysphagia relief, a randomized trial comparing SEMS and brachytherapy reported more prompt relief of dysphagia with esophageal stents but more prolonged relief of dysphagia and better quality of life with brachytherapy.

For stage I cancer, surgery alone is the standard of care. However, recently EMR or ESD has been used for patients with T1a disease. Although initially utilized in patients who were at high risk for surgery, these techniques have been used increasingly even for standard-risk patients, thus avoiding esophagectomy. Chemoradiation and even radiation alone are alternatives to surgery, particularly for squamous cell cancer.

The management of clinical T2N0M0 remains controversial. True T2N0M0 tumors are rare. It has been clearly demonstrated that clinical staging of T2N0M0 is inaccurate, and most patients are either up or down staged. Based on T status alone, the likelihood of nodal involvement for T2 is 50–60%, suggesting that such patients may benefit from combined-modality therapy. However, if the tumor is really T2N0 or T1N0, surgery alone is appropriate. Similar to stage I, chemoradiation would be an alternative to surgery. Ongoing research is trying to address this controversy.

For patients with locally advanced disease, T3, T4a, or N1-3M0, surgery alone may provide relief of dysphagia, but combined-modality therapy including preoperative chemoradiation offers improved survival and improved locoregional control. Combined-modality therapy has become the standard of care in many centers for locally advanced disease.

Although clinical staging is inherently inaccurate, it is clear that the risk of lymph node metastases increases with increasing T stage such that patients with T3 tumors have a 75–80% chance of having lymph node metastases. Similarly, the more lymph nodes involved, the higher is the chance of systemic disease. When eight or more lymph nodes are involved, the likelihood of systemic disease approaches 100%.

Because of the likelihood of systemic disease, it is reasonable to add chemotherapy to the therapeutic regimen. Whether radiation is also required is considered controversial by some, but the data are clear that the use of radiation increases the likelihood of an R0 resection. Given the anatomy of the esophagus in that it lacks a serosa and lies in intimate association with vital structures such as the tracheobronchial tree,

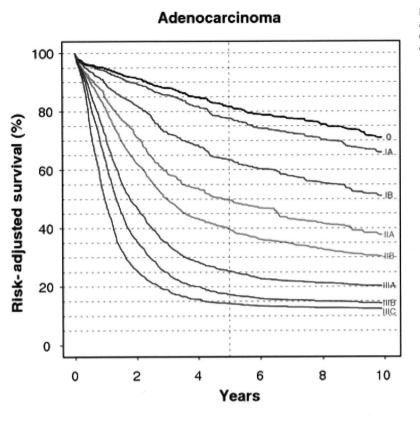

Adenocarcinoma

Figure 24.1 Risk-adjusted survival for adenocarcinoma according to the 7th edition of the American Joint Committee on Cancer (AJCC)/UICC staging system.

the heart, the aorta, and the spine, it is difficult to achieve an R0 resection with surgery alone for locally advanced tumors. The role of chemotherapy is twofold: to treat the systemic disease but also as a radiosensitizer.

Many clinical trials and meta-analyses of preoperative chemoradiation plus surgery for esophageal cancer have been completed. Until recently, only two trials were positive, but one was flawed by imbalance of stage in the two treatment arms and the other was very small. The meta-analyses have reported a significant survival benefit with combined-modality therapy, but the variability of the trials included weakens the conclusions. However, in 2010, the Cross group presented the results of the largest randomized trial of surgery alone versus chemoradiation followed by surgery. In this trial of 368 patients, 75% of whom had adenocarcinoma, median survival was 49.4 months in the trimodality arm compared to 24 months in the surgery-alone arm (HR = 0.0657; 95% CI 0.495–0.871, p = 0.003) (Figure 24.1). Although patients with squamous cancer had the best results with 49% complete pathological response, survival benefit was found for

both squamous cell cancers and adenocarcinoma (Figure 24.2).

It is increasingly recognized that the quality of surgery is important in achieving good outcomes. Surgeons reporting single-center experience with en bloc or modified en bloc esophagectomy report 5-year survivals similar to those achieved in the Cross trial. Although some have argued that good surgery obviates the need for preoperative chemoradiation, the evidence doesn't support this. Nonetheless, it is incumbent on the surgeon to provide the highest-quality resection possible. This mandates an adequate lymphadenectomy, adequate margins, R0 resection, and reliable and functional reconstruction performed with the least morbidity and mortality.

Surgery has been the mainstay of treatment for those with locoregional disease who are fit enough from a cardiorespiratory perspective. There are a number of surgical approaches. The principles of cancer surgery should be considered when deciding on the operative approach as well as the patient's comorbidities. The standard approaches by open surgery include Ivor Lewis (laparotomy and right

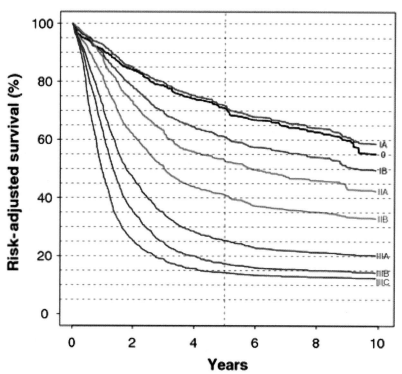

Figure 24.2 Risk-adjusted survival for squamous cell carcinoma according to the 7th edition of the AJCC/UICC staging system.

thoracotomy), McKeown (right thoracotomy, laparotomy and left cervicotomy), transhiatal (laparotomy and left cervicotomy), left thoracoabdominal with or without left cervicotomy, and left transdiaphragmatic with or without left cervicotomy. More recently, minimally invasive approaches have developed including either hybrid or fully minimally invasive equivalents of the Ivor Lewis or McKeown approaches.

The choice of operative approach depends on the location of the tumor, patient comorbidities, and surgeon experience. The best surgery is the one that provides the best cancer operation with the lowest morbidity and mortality.

An adequate cancer operation requires an R0 resection: microscopically negative margins. Distally, a margin of 5 cm is appropriate, while the proximal margin should be 7–10 cm in situ. Although a microscopically negative radial margin is desirable, it may be difficult to achieve because of the anatomic relations of the esophagus. Preoperative radiation has been shown to improve the likelihood of a negative radial margin.

An adequate lymph node dissection is essential for both staging and prognosis. It appears that the number of lymph nodes required depends on the T stage. For T1 tumors, 10–16 nodes are required, while for T3 or T4 tumors, 20 or more nodes must be resected. These data are based on patients who were not treated with neoadjuvant therapy. There is no data regarding the number of nodes required for an adequate resection after neoadjuvant therapy.

Tumors of the middle or upper esophagus are best approached using the McKeown approach either open or minimally invasive equivalent. Tumors of the distal third of the esophagus are best approached using Ivor Lewis, thoracoabdominal, McKeown, or minimally invasive equivalent. Tumors of the gastroesophageal junction may be approached by any of the aforementioned approaches as well as the transhiatal approach.

Minimally invasive esophagectomy or transhiatal esophagectomy has both been shown to be associated with reduced pulmonary morbidity. For patients with limited pulmonary reserve, these operative approaches should be considered. For patients with cardiac comorbidity, a transhiatal approach is less desirable.

Although there is some suggestion that transthoracic approaches may offer a survival benefit over transhiatal esophagectomy, both approaches are considered acceptable. Minimally invasive esophagectomy appears to be equivalent to open approaches at least in terms of short-term outcomes and lymph node harvest and is associated with reduced pulmonary morbidity.

Finally, surgeon experience is important. Esophagectomy is one of the complex operative procedures wherein surgeon experience has been shown to have an impact on outcome. The exact operative approach is probably less important.

Outcomes

Esophageal cancer has the second highest case fatality ratio of any solid tumor, second only to pancreas. This is related to esophageal anatomy, wherein lymphatic and systemic dissemination occur at an early stage, as well as its silent nature until locally advanced.

Five-year survival is stage dependent, as for any other tumor, but also depends on histology, grade, and features such as lymphovascular invasion. Surgical approach also contributes. For patients treated with surgery alone, 5-year survival for transhiatal esophagectomy is approximately 25%; with en bloc esophagectomy, 5-year survival up to 54% is seen for stage III patients.

Operative mortality in high-volume centers with high-volume surgeons ranges from 2–5%. Mortality in low-volume centers is significantly higher, up to 20%. Morbidity of esophagectomy is high regardless of approach or center volume, with 50% of patients experiencing one or more postoperative complications. Pneumonia (10–20%) has been a major source of morbidity, and 50% of operative mortality has been attributed to pneumonia. Minimally invasive esophagectomy and transhiatal esophagectomy have lower rates of pneumonia compared to transthoracic open esophagectomy. Atrial fibrillation is reported in approximately 15% of patients. Importantly, atrial fibrillation should be considered as a sign of other complications, including pulmonary embolus, myocardial infarction, pneumonia, anastomotic leak, and gastric conduit necrosis. Gastric conduit necrosis is rare (1%) but catastrophic, requiring immediate reoperation and resection of the conduit. Anastomotic leak rates (<5–24%) vary depending on technique and location. Cervical anastomoses have a higher rate of leak. Stapled anastomoses have a lower rate of leak.

Functional outcomes depend on an adequate anastomotic lumen, a straight, nonredundant, and not twisted conduit. Use of a gastric emptying procedure and feeding jejunostomy is generally recommended.

Essentials of postoperative care are careful fluid balance avoiding volume overload, which contributes to congestion of the conduit and ischemia; attention to electrolytes, particularly phosphate, which may drop when feeding is initiated if the patient had poor nutrition preoperatively; supplementation with magnesium to keep serum levels in the normal range; pulmonary toilet; and nutrition. DVT prophylaxis in hospital is essential, and some consider continuing this after discharge for 4–8 weeks.

References

1 Li Z, Rice TW. Diagnosis and staging of cancer of the esophagus and esophagogastric junction [review]. *Surg Clin North Am* 2012 Oct; 92(5):1105–26.

2 Van Hagen P, Hulshof MCCM, van Lanschot JJB, et al. Preoperative chemoradiotherapy for esophageal or junctional cancer. *N Engl J Med* 2012; 366:2074–84.

3 Biere SS, van Berge Henegouwen MI, Maas KW, et al. Minimally invasive versus open oesophagectomy for patients with oesophageal cancer: a multicentre, open-label, randomized, controlled trial. *Lancet* 2012; 379: 1887–92.

4 Rizk NP, Ishwaran H, Rice TW, et al. Optimum lymphadenectomy for esophageal cancer. *Ann Surg* 2010; 251:46–50.

5 Zehetner J, DeMeester SR, Hagen JA, et al. Endoscopic resection and ablation versus esophagectomy for high-grade dysplasia and intramucosal adenocarcinoma. *J Thorac Cardiovasc Surg* 2011; 141:39–47.

Chapter 25

Esophageal perforation

Michael J. Shackcloth and George John

Introduction

Oesophageal perforation is a potentially life-threatening condition that presents a diagnostic and therapeutic challenge. It is a surgical emergency associated with high mortality and morbidity, especially if the diagnosis is delayed. Presentation is often ambiguous or atypical, making diagnosis challenging, and management remains controversial. Evidence for treatment is mainly based on case series and fraught with bias.

The first case of spontaneous perforation of the oesophagus was described by Boerhaave in 1723[1]. The first successful repair of a spontaneous perforation of the oesophagus were reported by Barrett[2] and Olsen[3] in 1947. Although spontaneous perforation of the oesophagus is a relatively uncommon condition, the dramatic increase in the use of endoscopy for the diagnosis and treatment of gastrointestinal diseases has led to a significant increase in incidence of oesophageal perforation.

Etiology and pathophysiology

In order to understand the aetiology and pathophysiology better, one should have a good anatomical knowledge of the oesophagus. The oesophagus is a muscular tube approximately 25 cm in length, starting from the lower border of the cricoid cartilage and ending at the gastro-oesophageal junction, where it joins the stomach. There are three anatomical points of narrowing: the cricopharyngeus muscle, broncho-aortic constriction and the gastro-oesophageal junction. Perforation can occur anywhere as the oesophagus lacks a serosal layer which provides stability through elastin and collagen fibres, but these anatomical narrowings are more prone to rupture.

Perforation of the oesophagus leads to leakage of oesophageal and gastric contents, saliva, bile, digestive enzymes and other substances into the mediastinum, causing soiling and leading to mediastinitis. The mediastinal collection often ruptures into the pleural cavity leading to pleural effusion, empyema or hydropneumothorax.

The degree of inflammation depends upon the time interval between the actual perforation and the clinical presentation and the amount of contamination. The presence of bacteria in saliva and the digestive enzymes in the stomach lead to a mixed necrotizing infection. Left untreated, it rapidly progresses to sepsis and multi-organ failure.

Etiology

Oesophageal perforations can broadly be divided into intraluminal and extraluminal causes (Table 25.1).

Intraluminal causes
Iatrogenic/instrumental injuries

With the increased use of endoscopy and endoluminal therapies, this has become the leading cause of oesophageal perforation. Up to 70% of oesophageal injuries are caused by instrumentation[4-9]. In 1974, the Society of American Gastrointestinal Endoscopic Survey looked at 211,410 endoscopic procedures to reveal a perforation rate of 0.03% in all simple upper endoscopies and 0.25% of procedures involving bougienage[10].

The most vulnerable area for perforation is in the region of Killian's dehiscence. This is a triangular area in the wall of the pharynx between the thyropharyngeus part of the inferior constrictor muscle, cricopharyngeus muscle and inferior constrictor muscle

Core Topics in Thoracic Surgery, ed. Marco Scarci, Aman Coonar, Tom Routledge and Francis Wells. Published by Cambridge University Press. © Cambridge University Press 2016

Table 25.1 Atiology of oesophageal perforations

Intraluminal	Extraluminal
A) Instrumentation/ iatrogenic	**A) Trauma**
1. Oesophagoscopy – diagnostic or therapeutic	1. Penetrating – stab or gunshot
2. Bougienage	2. Blunt – motor vehicle accident
3. Pneumatic dilatation and photodynamic therapy	
4. Oesophageal varices, banding and sclerotherapy	
5. Placement of intra-oesophageal tubes like Sengstaken-Blakemore or Minnesota tube for varices, nasogastric or nasojejunal, prostheses and others	
6. Endotracheal intubations	**B) Operative injuries**
7. Trans-oesophageal echocardiography	1. Mediastinoscopy
8. Mini-tracheostomy	2. Thyroid surgery
	3. Anterior spinal surgery
B) Foreign bodies	4. Laparoscopic Nissen fundoplication
	5. Pneumonectomy
Fish bones, coins, impacted food or pills, dentures	6. Vagotomy
C) Caustic agents like acid and alkali	
D) Spontaneous/barotrauma	
1. Boerhaave's syndrome	
2. Heimlich maneuver	
3. Mallory-Weiss tears	
E) Severe reflux and Barrett's oesophagitis	
F) Infections	
1. Human immunodeficiency virus (HIV)	
2. Herpes simplex virus (HSV)	

3. *Candida* species

4. Tuberculosis

5. Syphilis

G) Malignancy

1. Oesophageal

2. Lung

3. Other mediastinal structures

of the pharynx. It is situated at the level of C5 and C6 vertebrae. The posterior oesophageal mucosa is covered only by fascia in this area, thus making the risk of perforation high. The risk is further increased with hyperextension of the neck. Jackson in 1957 named this area the 'pass of Bal-el-mandeb' or the 'gate of tears'[11].

Other causes of intraluminal oesophageal instrumentation injuries are during sclerotherapy and banding for oesophageal varices (1–6%)[9], endoscopic stenting of advanced oesophageal cancers[12], endoscopic laser therapy, photodynamic therapy and during biopsies. Placement of intra-oesophageal tubes such as nasogastric tube[13–15], Sengstaken-Blakemore or Minnesota[16] may cause oesophageal perforation. There are a few cases of oesophageal perforation after traumatic endotracheal intubation[17;18], although the risk is very low. It has also been reported after insertion of mini-tracheostomy[19,20].

The use of trans-oesophageal echocardiography is increasing, especially in evaluating patients with valvular dysfunction intra-operatively, in ensuring there is no paravalvular leak after valve repair or in excluding tamponade after cardiac surgery. Kallmeyer et al. in 2001 reported a case series looking at 7,200 cardiac surgical patients to find a perforation rate of 0.01%[21]. Trans-oesophageal echocardiography may cause injury via direct tissue trauma or by the thermal energy from the probe[22].

Foreign bodies

Foreign-body ingestion causes about 12% of all oesophageal perforations[9]. Children below the age of 5 years are most likely to swallow and lodge a foreign body in their oesophagus. A study done by Little et al. in 2006 looked at 500 paediatric patients over a 16-year period and concluded that 88% of the objects swallowed were coins and 73% were lodged in the superior oesophagus. The mean age was 3.24 years[23]. Perforation is more likely to occur if the foreign body has been lodged for greater than 4 hours[24]. Other objects swallowed include batteries, buttons, pins and dentures in the elderly[25]. Fish bones can get lodged into the oesophageal mucosa causing delayed tissue necrosis, which ultimately causes local perforation. Oesophageal perforation is a potential occupational hazard for sword swallowers, with two cases reported in the literature[26–28]. The incidence may be higher than previously thought as some cases are probably self-treated[29].

Spontaneous

Spontaneous perforation is becoming more frequent as it is recognized earlier as compared to the past when this condition was often missed altogether. Evidence is limited, but a study from Iceland showed an age-standardized incidence of 3.1/1,000,000 per study year[30]. According to hospital episode statistics, there were 340 admissions for oesophageal rupture during 2005–6 in England[31]. Hermann Boerhaave, a Dutch botanist, humanist and physician of European fame, first described this phenomenon in 1724 after the oesophageal rupture suffered by the High Admiral of the Dutch Navy, Baron Van Jon Wassenaer, who died after a gluttonous meal with alcohol and subsequent vomiting. Post mortem revealed an oesophageal rupture[1]. Spontaneous perforation accounts for 33% of all causes of perforations[32]. They result from a sudden rapid increase in intra-oesophageal pressure with incoordination of the upper oesophageal sphincter. Perforation usually occurs on the left posterolateral side of the lower oesophagus, about 2–3 cm from the gastro-oesophageal junction, and extends into the pleural cavity in 80% of cases.

Caustic injuries, reflux oesophagitis and Barrett's oesophagus

Caustic injuries due to ingestion of insecticides and pesticides are seen in developing countries like India as a mean for suicide, whereas alkaline materials are more common in developed countries. These are more likely to cause perforation of the intrathoracic oesophagus.

Reflux oesophagitis and Barrett's oesophagus are becoming less common now with the wide usage of proton pump inhibitors; hence the incidence of perforation is also very low.

Infections and malignancy

Various infections, as mentioned in Table 25.1, are also reported to cause perforations, but with appropriate treatment available in this current era, the risk is much reduced. Oesophageal cancer in its advanced stage can erode through the oesophageal wall, leading to perforation and sepsis. Other reported cases are lung and mediastinal tumours with oesophageal involvement, generally carrying a poor prognosis.

Extraluminal causes

Trauma

Perforations from either blunt or penetrating trauma are usually in the cervical oesophagus. Penetrating injuries to the chest only rarely cause oesophageal perforation[33]. Blunt trauma to the oesophagus is rare. It is most commonly seen after motor vehicle accidents where the oesophagus is crushed between sternum and the spine[34], although it has been reported after a Heimlich maneuver[35].

Operative injuries

There are certain non-oesophageal surgeries that can inadvertently cause trauma to the oesophagus leading to perforation. The reported cases are during mediastinoscopy[36], thyroid surgery[37,38], laparoscopic Nissen fundoplication[26,39], spinal surgery[40,41] and vagotomy[42,43]. Radiofrequency ablation of the atrial appendage during cardiac surgery[44] and pneumonectomy[45] are also at risk of oesophageal perforation.

Clinical features

The clinical features of a patient with oesophageal perforation will depend on the aetiology of the perforation, the site of the perforation, the degree of contamination and the time from injury. Possible signs and symptoms of oesophageal perforation are listed in Table 25.2.

Perforation of the cervical oesophagus is usually less severe and presents with a sore throat, odynophagia, neck tenderness and surgical emphysema. Perforation of the thoracic oesophagus will present with chest pain, dysphagia and surgical emphysema. Abdominal oesophageal perforation usually presents with abdominal pain and signs of peritonitis.

Later manifestations are those of infection and septic shock, which include pyrexia, sweating, tachypnoea, tachycardia, hypotension and oliguria.

Table 25.2 Symptoms and signs of oesophageal perforation

Symptoms	Signs
Chest pain	Surgical emphysema
Dysphagia	Tachypnoea
Odynodysphagia	Tachycardia
Sore throat	Hypotension
Abdominal pain	Pyrexia
Neck pain	Sweating
	Oliguria
	Peritonitis

The differential diagnosis of oesophageal perforation is wide, often leading to delays in the diagnosis. Possible differential diagnoses include pneumonia, pulmonary embolism, gastroenteritis, myocardial infarction, peptic ulcer disease, acute pancreatitis and acute aortic dissection. In one study the initial diagnosis was correct in only 17 of 51 cases[46].

Investigations
Chest X-ray

In the early stages of an oesophageal perforation with minimal contamination, chest X-ray signs can be very subtle. Chest X-ray abnormalities may include surgical emphysema, pneumomediastinum, pleural effusion, pneumothorax and hydropneumothorax (Figure 25.1).

Contrast swallow

This remains the most accepted method for the diagnosis of a perforated oesophagus. A positive result clearly indicates the level of perforation as well as the site, side and extent of contamination of the pleural space, enabling planning of any treatment. A normal contrast study does not completely exclude a small perforation. There is a false-negative rate of between 10 and 20%[47]. Non-ionic contrast medium such as gastrografin or gastromyelin is the agent of choice as it is less harmful to the mediastinum. If aspirated, gastrografin can cause a severe necrotizing pneumonitis due to its hypertonicity[47]. It should therefore be avoided in patients at risk of aspiration or with a suspected trache-oesophageal fistula. A contrast swallow has its limitations and is not possible in a ventilated patient.

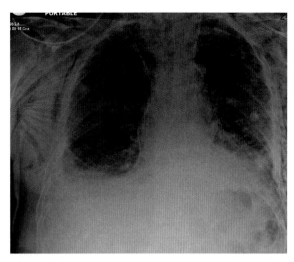

Figure 25.1 Chest x-ray of a man following a spontaneous perforation of the oesophagus. The left hydropneumothorax has been drained. Surgical emphysema is present and a slight pneumomediastinum can be made out on the right heart border.

Computed tomography

This is the method of choice for assessing a perforated oesophagus in the ventilated patient. Computed tomography (CT) is good at assessing the degree of contamination and localizing pleural and mediastinal collections. It also identifies any underlying pathology and eliminates any other serious conditions that may have been in the differential diagnosis (Figures 25.2A, 25.2B, and 25.3).

Endoscopy

In experienced hands, flexible endoscopy provides direct visualization of the perforation and provides details to determine the aetiology of the perforation. Figure 25.4 shows the endoscopic finding in a gentleman suspected of having a spontaneous perforation of the oesophagus. In the emergency setting of assessing a perforated oesophagus secondary to penetrating trauma, it is associated with 100% sensitivity and a specificity of 83%[48]. The role of endoscopy remains controversial due to the worry of further damaging the oesophagus and causing an increase in pneumomediastinum or pneumothorax. Endoscopy does, however, allow for the assessment of any associated pathology in the oesophagus or stomach. It also allows for the assessment as to whether any endoscopic treatment options would be possible.

243

(a)

(b)

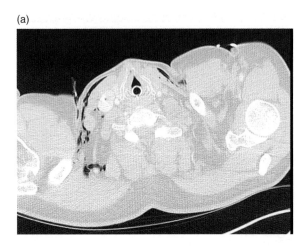
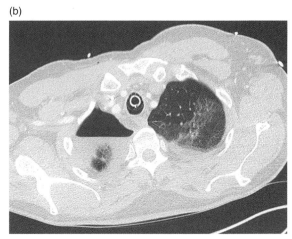

Figure 25.2 CT scan following a perorated oesophagus. **(A)** surgical emphysema. **(B)** hydropneumothorax.

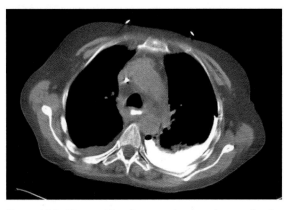

Figure 25.3 CT scan with oral contrast showing a large perforation of the oesophagus into the left chest.

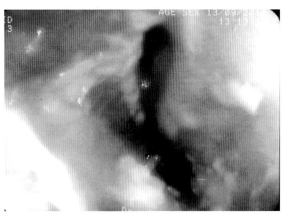

Figure 25.4 Endoscopy view showing a tear in the left lateral wall of the oesophagus just above the gastro-oesophageal junction following a spontaneous perforation.

Treatment

Oesophageal perforations represent a heterogeneous group, ranging from an iatrogenic perforation on a normal oesophagus to spontaneous perforations. The location, aetiology of the perforation, degree of mediastinal contamination and time to diagnosis are the most important factors on which to base treatment[4,7,8,49,50].

Cervical oesophageal perforations, because of the containment of the contents within the fascial planes of the neck, tend to incite less of a systemic inflammatory response than thoracic and abdominal perforations. Perforations occurring in these lower areas are not as well contained and thus elicit more of both a local and systemic inflammatory response leading to a compromise in many organ systems, particularly respiratory function, and lead to a higher mortality and morbidity[51].

Perforation of the oesophagus into the thoracic cavity is a potential life-threatening condition and still remains a true surgical emergency.

Initial management

Patients presenting with a perforated oesophagus are often in septic shock, and therefore, initial treatment involves keeping the patient nil by mouth, intravenous antibiotics, anti-fungal agents, reduction of gastric acid production with proton pump inhibitors and fluid resuscitation. If there is a large pleural collection or pneumothorax, then a large-bore chest drain should be inserted. Organ support may be necessary in intensive care.

Non-operative

Most instrumental perforations are small and, if identified early, respond to conservative measures as described earlier. If a decision is made to treat a patient non-operatively, then one has to monitor the patient's clinical condition closely and be prepared to change the management strategy.

Strict criteria for the non-operative management of oesophageal perforations have been proposed[4,52,53]. Even with these strict criteria for non-operative treatment, 20–54% of patients will develop multiple complications and require operative intervention[4,52].

Operative

Cervical perforations

Due to the reasons described earlier, these perforations are often small and well contained and can be managed by drainage alone.

Intrathoracic and abdominal

The treatment of choice is primary closure. To achieve this, the tissues of the oesophageal wall need to be fairly healthy. The longer the time interval before diagnosis, the less likely this is to be the case. Where possible, the patient should undergo single lung ventilation. A posterolateral thoracotomy is performed. The side and level of the posterolateral thoracotomy will be determined by the information gained from the contrast study. The lung is fully mobilized, and any pleural debris and fluid are removed. The mediastinal pleura is opened. The tear in the oesophagus may not always be obvious. The careful placement of a Maloney bougie preoperatively may help the identification of it. The upper and lower limits of the tear are identified. The mucosal tear is often longer than the tear in the muscular layer; therefore, one has to open the muscle layer to fully demarcate the upper and lower margins. The mucosa is then approximated using interrupted sutures such as 3-0 Monocryl. The muscle layer is then closed in a similar fashion. Sometimes if the edges of the tear are necrotic, excision is necessary. Also, a single-layer closure may sometimes be possible.

After primary closure, the repair should be buttressed using vascularized tissue. The author's first choice is a pedicled intercostal muscle flap, which can be harvested at the beginning of the procedure. Other options include diaphragm or pericardium.

An NG tube is passed into the stomach with careful guidance past the repair. Two large-bore 32F drains are inserted, one basal and one adjacent to the repair.

One then has to consider how the patient will be fed; options include total parental nutrition (TPN) or performing a mini-laparotomy and insertion of a feeding jejunostomy.

Post-operative care includes intravenous antibiotics, free drainage and 4-hourly aspirations of NG tube and proton pump inhibitors. Consideration should be given to putting the patient on anti-fungal agents such as fluconazole. The patient is kept nil by mouth (NBM) for 5–7 days when a contrast swallow is performed.

Oesophagectomy

Performing an oesophagectomy for an oesophageal perforation is controversial[51]. If the perforation is an instrumental perforation due to a benign or malignant stricture, then resection may be the treatment of choice. The approach and extent of resection will depend on the site of the pathology.

Saarnio et al. have recently advocated a two-staged repair of oesophageal perforations, with initial oesophageal resection and cervical oesophagostomy and gastrostomy in cases of severe mediastinal sepsis[54]. At a later date, continuity of the upper gastrointestinal tract is restored with a second operation. Altorjay et al. have presented a series of 27 cases of oesophageal resection with a mortality rate of 3.7%[5]. Proponents of performing an oesophagectomy argue that it provides the best option for controlling the sepsis as there will be no chance of a residual leak. The disadvantages are the need for a second major operation to restore continuity of the gastrointestinal tract and the long-term complications of a stomach tube or colonic interposition.

Thoracoscopy

The use of thoracoscopy in the management of oesophageal perforations is limited[9]. Although its use in the primary repair has been reported[55–58], it is more widely used to drain pleural and mediastinal collections.

Endoscopic therapies

Over the last decade, developments in the minimally invasive endoluminal approach in the management of oesophageal perforations include closure of the

(a)

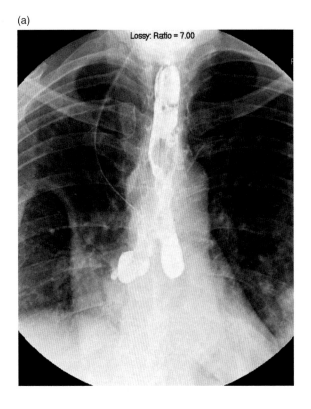

(b)

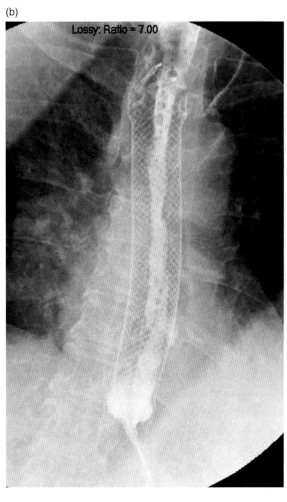

Figure 25.5 **(A)** Contrast swallow showing a large oesophageal perforation into the right chest. **(B)** Contrast swallow following placement of a covered stent showed no leak.

perforation with clips or sutures, covering the leaks with a covered stent and/or endoluminal drainage of the mediastinal infection.

Endoscopic clips are either deployed through the endoscope or over the scope (Over The Scope Clip [OTSC], Ovesco, Tubingen, Germany). In a systematic review of endoclip closure for oesophageal perforations in 17 patients, through the scope clip was used to close perforations from 3–25 mm. The OTSC is a 12-mm Nitonol clip that fits on the tip of the endoscope. It can be used to close perforations up to 30 mm in diameter. In a multicentre study, all five oesophageal perforations were closed successfully[59].

Stents can be used to close oesophageal perforations. Stents may be plastic, covered metal or covered biodegradable material[60]. Dai et al.[61]

reported a retrospective series of 41 oesophageal leaks (6 of which were for perforations) treated with covered stents. Complete healing was observed in six leaks with one death. Figures 25.5a and 25.5b show a large oesophageal perforation that was treated with a covered stent.

Possible complications of covered stents include stent migration or leakage around the stent. Patients treated with oesophageal stents therefore require close monitoring clinically for signs of sepsis and radiologically for signs of stent migration.

Vacuum-assisted closure is now routinely used to treat many different wounds. The principles behind it are the utilization of suction to remove bacterial contamination, secretions and oedema, thereby promotingthe development of granulation tissue and

(a)

(b)

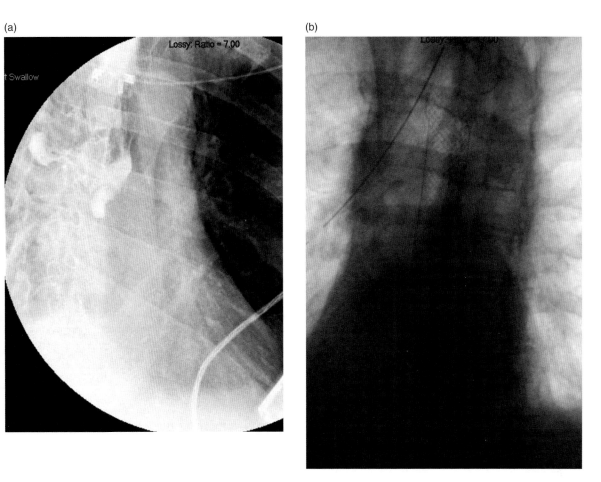

Figure 25.6
a) Contrast swallow showing a residual leak into the right chest following primary repair of a spontaneous oesophageal perforation into the right chest with intercostal muscle flap.
b) The residual leak was treated with a covered stent. Contrast swallow following placement of the stent showed no residual leak.

healing by secondary intention. Endoscopically placed vacuum-assisted therapy has been used to treat oesophageal perforations[62–64]. The device consists of a nasogastric tube with a sponge attached, which is placed endoscopically through the oesophageal defect into the mediastinal cavity. Once the sponge is in the desired position, suction of 75–125 mmHg is applied to the NG tube. The sponge is changed at regular intervals.

Results

In a review of the literature between 1990 and 2003, Brinster et al. found the overall mortality from oesophageal perforation to be 18%[9]. Various factors have been found to affect the mortality rate. These include reason for perforation, underlying pathology, time to diagnosis and method of treatment[4,50,65].

Brinster et al. reported a mortality rate of 36% for spontaneous perforations (range 0–70%), 19% for iatrogenic perforations (range 7–33%) and 7% for traumatic perforations (range 0–33%)[9]. Spontaneous perforations probably have the highest mortality rate due to the high degree of mediastinal contamination and frequent delay in diagnosis. Iatrogenic perforations usually occur following endoscopy and are therefore more easily recognized. The patient usually is starved prior to the procedure, leading to less contamination. Traumatic perforations are often confined to the cervical oesophagus with limited contamination of the mediastinum.

In the same study, cervical oesophageal perforations were associated with a 6% mortality (range 0–16%), thoracic perforations a 27% mortality (range 0 to 44%) and intra-abdominal perforations with a 21% mortality (range 0–43%)[9]. As mentioned previously, cervical leaks are often contained in the neck with limited contamination.

The time interval between perforation and treatment affects mortality and morbidity[7,49,50,66–68]. In their review, Brinster et al. found that a delay in treatment of more than 24 hours was associated with a doubling of mortality[9]. In the past, the first 24 hours have been described as the 'golden 24 hours'. It was suggested that primary repair should only be performed if less than 24 hours after presentation; after 24 hours, treatment should be more conservative with drainage of pleural collections. However, there are many case series of primary repairs performed after 24 hours with excellent results[7,66–73].

Factors shown to be associated with a poor prognosis include pre-operative respiratory failure requiring mechanical ventilation, malignant perforation, a Charlson co-morbidity index of 7.1 or greater, the presence of a pulmonary co-morbidity and sepsis[51].

The type of treatment of the oesophageal perforation seems to be an important determinant of survival. In their review of the literature containing 726 patients, Brinster et al. found that primary repair had a mortality rate of 12% (range 0–31%), compared with 36% (range 0–40%) for drainage and 17% (range 0–33%) for non-operative management[9]. Careful interpretation of these results is vital, as they are based on case series where significant selection bias would have occurred and the management strategy was individualized for every patient.

After primary repair of intrathoracic perforations, 25–50% of patients have been reported to have a residual leak[51,68,71,73,74]. The majority of these can be managed conservatively, although the author tends to consider placement of a covered stent at 2 weeks post-operatively if there is still a residual leak. Patients treated late are at increased risk of having residual leaks[68].

Although limited data are available on the long-term follow-up of patients who have successfully survived an oesophageal perforation, the outlook is generally good. Three case series provide data on medium- to long-term survival with an average of 3[67], 3.7[75] and 12.5[6] years with survival rates of 90, 88 and 64%, respectively.

Summary

Oesophageal perforation is a surgical emergency that carries a significant mortality and morbidity. Prompt and accurate diagnosis is essential. The management has to be tailored to the individual patient.

References

1 Barrett NR. Spontaneous perforation of the oesophagus; review of the literature and report of three new cases. *Thorax* 1946 Mar; 1:48–70.

2 Barrett NR. Report of a case of spontaneous perforation of the oesophagus successfully treated by operation. *Bri J S* 1947 Oct; 35(138):216–8.

3 Olsen AM, Clagett OT. Spontaneous rupture of the esophagus; report of a case with immediate diagnosis and successful surgical repair. *Postgrad Med* 1947 Dec; 2(6):417–21.

4 Altorjay A, Kiss J, Voros A, Bohak A. Nonoperative management of esophageal perforations: is it justified? *Ann Surg* 1997 Apr; 225(4):415–21.

5 Altorjay A, Kiss J, Voros A, Sziranyi E. The role of esophagectomy in the management of esophageal perforations. *Ann Thorac Surg* 1998 May; 65(5):1433–6.

6 Iannettoni MD, Vlessis AA, Whyte RI, Orringer MB. Functional outcome after surgical treatment of esophageal perforation. *Ann Thorac Surg* 1609 Oct; 64(6):1606–9.

7 Salo JA, Isolauri JO, Heikkila LJ, et al. Management of delayed esophageal perforation with mediastinal sepsis: esophagectomy or primary repair? *J Thorac Cardiovasc Surg* 1993 Dec; 106(6):1088–91.

8 Tilanus HW, Bossuyt P, Schattenkerk ME, Obertop H. Treatment of oesophageal perforation: a multivariate analysis. *Br J Surg* 1991 May; 78(5):582–5.

9 Brinster CJ, Singhal S, Lee L, et al. Evolving options in the management of esophageal perforation [review] [95 refs]. *Ann Thorac Surg* 2004 Apr; 77(4):1475–83.

10 Silvis SE, Nebel O, Rogers G, et al. Endoscopic complications: results of the 1974 American Society for Gastrointestinal Endoscopy Survey. *JAMA* 1976 Mar 1; 235(9):928–30.

11 Jackson CL. Foreign bodies in the esophagus. *Am J Surg* 1957 Feb; 93(2):308–12.

12 Kinsman KJ, DeGregorio BT, Katon RM, et al. Prior radiation and chemotherapy increase the risk of life-threatening complications after insertion of metallic stents for esophagogastric malignancy. *Gastrointest Endosc* 1996 Mar; 43(3):196–203.

13 Robinson P, Thomas NB. Intra-abdominal oesophageal perforation following naso-gastric tube insertion. *Eur Radiol* 1999; 9(8):1697–8.

14 Gruen R, Cade R, Vellar D. Perforation during nasogastric and orogastric tube insertion. *Aust NZ J Surg* 1998 Nov; 68(11):809–11.

15 de DF, Rekik R, Merlusca G, et al. [Esophageal perforation during nasogastric tube insertion in a patient with right-sided aortic arch and thoracic aorta. Pathophysiology and surgical implications] [French]. *J Chir* 2009 Aug; 146(4):419–22.

16 Lee JG, Lieberman DA. Complications related to endoscopic hemostasis techniques [review] [82 refs]. *Gastrointest Endosc Clin North Am* 1996 Apr; 6(2):305–21.

17 Ku PK, Tong MC, Ho KM, et al. Traumatic esophageal perforation resulting from endotracheal intubation. *Anesth Analge* 1998 Sep; 87(3):730–1.

18 Jougon J, Cantini O, Delcambre F, et al. Esophageal perforation: life threatening complication of endotracheal intubation. *Eur Cardio thorac Surg* 2001 Jan 10; 20(1):7–10.

19 Allen PW, Thornton M. Oesophageal perforation with minitracheostomy. *Intensive Care Med* 1989; 15(8):543.

20 Claffey LP, Phelan DM. A complication of cricothyroid "minitracheostomy"–oesophageal perforation. *Intensive Care Med* 1989; 15(2):140–1.

21 Kallmeyer IJ, Collard CD, Fox JA, et al. The safety of intraoperative transesophageal echocardiography: a case series of 7,200 cardiac surgical patients. *Anesthes Analge* 2001 May; 92(5):1126–30.

22 Elsayed H, Page R, Agarwal S, Chalmers J. Oesophageal perforation complicating intraoperative transoesophageal echocardiography: suspicion can save lives. *Interact Cardiovasc Thorac Surg* 2010 Sep; 11(3):380–2.

23 Little DC, Shah SR, St Peter SD, et al. Esophageal foreign bodies in the pediatric population: our first 500 cases. *J Pediatr Surg* 2006 May; 41(5):914–8.

24 Chaikhouni A, Kratz JM, Crawford FA. Foreign bodies of the esophagus. *Am Surg* 1985 Apr; 51(4):173–9.

25 Delince P, Amiri-Lamraski MH. [Perforating injury of the thoracic esophagus caused by a dental prosthesis] [French]. *Acta Chir Belg* 1984 Jan; 84(1):13–7.

26 Flum DR, Bass RC. The accuracy of gastric insufflation in testing for gastroesophageal perforations during laparoscopic Nissen fundoplication. *J Soc Laparoendosc Surg* 1999 Oct; 3(4):267–71.

27 Martin M, Steele S, Mullenix P, et al. Management of esophageal perforation in a sword swallower: a case report and review of the literature [review] [30 refs]. *J Trauma Injury Infect Crit Care* 2005 Jul; 59(1):233–5.

28 Scheinin SA, Wells PR. Esophageal perforation in a sword swallower. *Texas Heart Inst J* 2001; 28(1):65–8.

29 Witcombe B, Meyer D. Sword swallowing and its side effects. *BMJ* 2006 Dec 23; 333(7582):1285–7.

30 Vidarsdottir H, Blondal S, Alfredsson H, et al. Oesophageal perforations in Iceland: a whole population study on incidence, aetiology and surgical outcome. *Thorac Cardiovasc Surg* 2010 Dec; 58(8):476–80.

31 Blencowe NS, Strong S, Hollowood AD. Spontaneous oesophageal rupture [review]. *BMJ* 2013; 346:f3095.

32 Soreide JA, Viste A. Esophageal perforation: diagnostic work-up and clinical decision-making in the first 24 hours [review]. *Scand J Trauma Resuscitation Emergency Med* 2011; 19:66.

33 Oparah SS, Mandal AK. Operative management of penetrating wounds of the chest in civilian practice: review of indications in 125 consecutive patients. *J Thorac Cardiovasc Surg* 1979 Feb; 77(2):162–8.

34 Beal SL, Pottmeyer EW, Spisso JM. Esophageal perforation following external blunt trauma. *J Trauma Injury Infect Crit Care* 1988 Oct; 28(10):1425–32.

35 Cumberbatch GL, Reichl M. Oesophageal perforation: a rare complication of minor blunt trauma. *J Accident Emerg Med* 1996 Jul; 13(4):295–6.

36 Dernevik L, Larsson S, Pettersson G. Esophageal perforation during mediastinoscopy: the successful management of two complicated cases. *Thorac Cardiovasc Surg* 1985 Jun; 33(3):179–80.

37 Akbulut G, Gunay S, Aren A, Bilge O. A rare complication after thyroidectomy: esophageal perforation. *Ulusal Travma Dergisi* 2002 Oct; 8(4):250–2.

38 Ozer MT, Demirbas S, Harlak A, et al. A rare complication after thyroidectomy: perforation of the oesophagus: a case report. *Acta Chir Belg* 2009 Jul; 109(4):527–30.

39 Schauer PR, Meyers WC, Eubanks S, et al. Mechanisms of

249

gastric and esophageal perforations during laparoscopic Nissen fundoplication. *Ann Surg* 1996 Jan; 223(1):43–52.

40 Rueth N, Shaw D, Groth S, et al. Management of cervical esophageal injury after spinal surgery. *Ann Thoracic Surg* 2010 Oct; 90(4):1128–33.

41 Zairi F, Tetard MC, Thines L, Assaker R. Management of delayed oesophagus perforation and osteomyelitis after cervical spine surgery: review of the literature [review]. *Br J Neurosurg* 2012 Apr; 26(2):185–8.

42 Sapounov S. [Esophageal perforations after vagotomy] [German]. *Rofo: Fortschritte auf dem Gebiete der Rontgenstrahlen und der Nuklearmedizin* 1982 Sep; 137(3):321–4.

43 Vinz H, Reisig J, Machura R. [Complications of vagotomy (author's transl)] [German]. *Zentralblatt fur Chirurgie* 1980; 105(9):605–10.

44 Doll N, Borger MA, Fabricius A, et al. Esophageal perforation during left atrial radiofrequency ablation: Is the risk too high? *J Thorac Cardiovasc Surg* 2003 Apr; 125(4):836–42.

45 Venuta F, Rendina EA, De GT, et al. Esophageal perforation after sequential double-lung transplantation. *Chest* 2000 Jan; 117(1):285–7.

46 Griffin SM, Lamb PJ, Shenfine J, et al. Spontaneous rupture of the oesophagus. *Br J Surg* 2008 Sep; 95(9):1115–20.

47 Foley MJ, Ghahremani GG, Rogers LF. Reappraisal of contrast media used to detect upper gastrointestinal perforations: comparison of ionic water-soluble media with barium sulfate. *Radiology* 1982 Jul; 144(2):231–7.

48 Horwitz B, Krevsky B, Buckman RF Jr, et al. Endoscopic evaluation of penetrating esophageal injuries.

Am J Gastroenterol 1993 Aug; 88(8):1249–53.

49 Attar S, Hankins JR, Suter CM, et al. Esophageal perforation: a therapeutic challenge. *Ann Thorac Surg* 1950 Jan; 50(1):45–9.

50 White RK, Morris DM. Diagnosis and management of esophageal perforations. *Am Surg* 1992 Feb; 58(2):112–9.

51 Bhatia P, Fortin D, Inculet RI, Malthaner RA. Current concepts in the management of esophageal perforations: a twenty-seven year Canadian experience. *Ann Thorac Surg* 2011 Jul; 92(1):209–15.

52 Minnich DJ, Yu P, Bryant AS, et al. Management of thoracic esophageal perforations. *Eur J Cardio thorac Surg* 2011 Oct; 40(4):931–7.

53 Cameron JL, Kieffer RF, Hendrix TR, et al. Selective nonoperative management of contained intrathoracic esophageal disruptions. *Ann Thorac Surg* 1979 May; 27(5):404–8.

54 Saarnio J, Wiik H, Koivukangas V, et al. A novel two-stage repair technique for the management of esophageal perforation. *J Thorac Cardiovasc Surg* 2007 Mar; 133(3):840–1.

55 Ikeda Y, Niimi M, Sasaki Y, et al. Thoracoscopic repair of a spontaneous perforation of the esophagus with the endoscopic suturing device. *J Thorac Cardiovasc Surg* 2001 Jan; 121(1):178–9.

56 Kiel T, Ferzli G, McGinn J. The use of thoracoscopy in the treatment of iatrogenic esophageal perforations. *Chest* 1993 Jun; 103(6):1905–6.

57 Nathanson LK, Gotley D, Smithers M, Branicki F. Videothoracoscopic primary repair of early distal oesophageal perforation. *Aust NZ J Surg* 1993 May; 63(5):399–403.

58 Cho JS, Kim YD, Kim JW, HS I, Kim MS. Thoracoscopic primary

esophageal repair in patients with Boerhaave's syndrome. *Ann Thorac Surg* 2011 May; 91(5):1552–5.

59 Voermans RP, Le MO, von RD, et al. Efficacy of endoscopic closure of acute perforations of the gastrointestinal tract. *Clin Gastroenterol & Hepatol* 2012 Jun; 10(6):603–8.

60 Cerna M, Kocher M, Valek V, et al. Covered biodegradable stent: new therapeutic option for the management of esophageal perforation or anastomotic leak. *Cardiovasc Intervent Radiol* 2011 Dec; 34(6):1267–71.

61 Dai Y, Chopra SS, Kneif S, Hunerbein M. Management of esophageal anastomotic leaks, perforations, and fistulae with self-expanding plastic stents. *J Thorac Cardiovasc Surg* 2011 May; 141(5):1213–7.

62 Ahrens M, Schulte T, Egberts J, et al. Drainage of esophageal leakage using endoscopic vacuum therapy: a prospective pilot study. *Endoscopy* 2010 Sep; 42(9):693–8.

63 Kuehn F, Schiffmann L, Rau BM, Klar E. Surgical endoscopic vacuum therapy for anastomotic leakage and perforation of the upper gastrointestinal tract. *J Gastrointest Surg* 2012 Nov; 16(11):2145–50.

64 Schorsch T, Muller C, Loske G. Endoscopic vacuum therapy of anastomotic leakage and iatrogenic perforation in the esophagus. *Surg Endosc* 2013 Jun; 27(6):2040–5.

65 Bufkin BL, Miller JI Jr, Mansour KA. Esophageal perforation: emphasis on management. *Ann Thorac Surg* 1996 May; 61(5):1447–51.

66 Muir AD, White J, McGuigan JA, et al. Treatment and outcomes of oesophageal perforation in a tertiary referral centre. *Eur J Cardio thorac Surg* 2003 May; 23(5):799–804.

67 Shaker H, Elsayed H, Whittle I, et al. The influence of the 'golden 24-h rule' on the prognosis of oesophageal perforation in the modern era. *Eur J Cardio thorac Surg* 2010 Aug; 38(2):216–22.

68 Wright CD, Mathisen DJ, Wain JC, et al. Reinforced primary repair of thoracic esophageal perforation. *Ann Thorac Surg* 1995 Aug; 60(2):245–8.

69 Jougon J, Mc BT, Delcambre F, et al. Primary esophageal repair for Boerhaave's syndrome whatever the free interval between perforation and treatment. *Eur J Cardio thoracic Surg* 2004 Apr; 25(4):475–9.

70 Lawrence DR, Moxon RE, Fountain SW, et al. Iatrogenic oesophageal perforations: a clinical review. *Ann R Colle Surg Engl* 1998 Mar; 80(2):115–8.

71 Ohri SK, Liakakos TA, Pathi V, et al. Primary repair of iatrogenic thoracic esophageal perforation and Boerhaave's syndrome. *Ann Thorac Surg* 1993 Mar; 55(3):603–6.

72 Port JL, Kent MS, Korst RJ, et al. Thoracic esophageal perforations: a decade of experience. *Ann Thorac Surg* 2003 Apr; 75(4):1071–4.

73 Wang N, Razzouk AJ, Safavi A, et al. Delayed primary repair of intrathoracic esophageal perforation: is it safe? *J Thorac Cardiovasc Surg* 1996; 111(1):114–21.

74 Kiev J, Amendola M, Bouhaidar D, et al. A management algorithm for esophageal perforation. *Am J Surg* 2007 Jul; 194(1):103–6.

75 Kumar P, Sarkar PK. Late results of primary esophageal repair for spontaneous rupture of the esophagus (Boerhaave's syndrome). *Int Surg* 2004 Jan; 89(1):15–20.

Thoracic trauma

26

Gregor J. Kocher and Ralph A. Schmid

Introduction

Thoracic trauma, whether blunt or penetrating, is the leading cause of death in trauma victims in Europe and North America after injuries to the head and spinal cord. The proportion of penetrating trauma varies geographically. In Europe, the incidence of penetrating trauma is generally lower (about 10%) than in the United States (about 20%). While blunt trauma frequently leads to respiratory compromise with hypoxia, hypercarbia and acidosis, penetrating forces often result in a certain degree of blood loss and occasionally in life-threatening, exsanguinating injuries to the heart and great vessels. The majority of traumatic chest injuries can be managed by airway control and placement of a chest tube.

After elucidating some general aspects of blunt and penetrating injuries to the chest, the diagnosis and management of specific injuries are discussed.

Blunt chest trauma

Blunt injury to the thorax directly accounts for approximately 25% of trauma-related mortality and is a major contributor in another more than 25% of deaths, as it is often associated with trauma to the abdomen and particularly the head. In-hospital mortality rates for isolated blunt chest injuries are in the range of 1–2%. The most important causes of blunt chest trauma in Europe and Northern America include traffic accidents, followed by violence. Fortunately, approximately 90% of blunt chest injuries can be managed non-operatively by appropriate analgesia, tube thoracostomy and aggressive respiratory therapy, eventually including endotracheal intubation and mechanical ventilation. Emergency thoracotomy is rarely required (in about 2%) in blunt thoracic

trauma victims and is generally only indicated in patients suffering from cardiac arrest due to pericardial tamponade and in situations of a witnessed cardiac arrest in the emergency department.

Important details, which should be obtained in the patient's clinical history in order to raise suspicion of specific injuries, are the mechanism (fall/car crash, height/velocity) and time of injury as well as cardiopulmonary co-morbidities. As direct impacts over the thorax may lead to rib fractures (including flail chest), pulmonary and cardiac contusions, high-velocity impacts with simultaneous presence of a closed glottis may even cause bronchial disruption. In addition, impacts on the abdomen lead to associated injuries of abdominal organs and may cause diaphragmatic rupture due to a sudden rise in intra-abdominal pressure. Rapid deceleration (fall from height, car crash) can lead to aortic rupture as well as tracheobronchial injuries as a result of antero-posterior compression of the chest.

Penetrating chest trauma

In general, in-hospital mortality from isolated penetrating chest injury is higher, in the range of 8–14%, compared to blunt thoracic trauma (1–2%) and often related to shock as a result of vascular or cardiac injury. Stab wounds and gunshot wounds comprise the vast majority of penetrating injuries, whereas industrial accidents or high-velocity motor vehicle accidents can lead to open or penetrating chest injuries. In patients who reach the hospital alive, rapid assessment and interventions, such as tube thoracostomy and airway control, are of capital importance, and detailed imaging studies are reserved for haemodynamically stable patients. About 10–30% of penetrating trauma patients will require emergency or at

Core Topics in Thoracic Surgery, ed. Marco Scarci, Aman Coonar, Tom Routledge and Francis Wells. Published by Cambridge University Press. © Cambridge University Press 2016

least prompt thoracotomy. Especially concomitant abdominal injuries as well as a low systolic blood pressure on presentation in the emergency room are risk factors for higher mortality rates.

Low-energy trauma (i.e. stab wound, impalement, car accidents) can be separated from injuries caused by low- (<250 m/s; i.e. small handguns), medium- (250–750 m/s; i.e. most handguns and hunting rifles) and high-velocity missiles (750–1,000 m/s; i.e. machine guns, military rifles). This is important in the light that the degree of injury is directly related to the kinetic energy of the projectile, which grows proportionally to its velocity squared (kinetic energy = 0.5 × mass × velocity²). Hence, among the worst injuries can be caused by fragments with extremely high velocity (>1,000 m/s) originating not only from military mines and grenades but also from improvised explosive devices. In addition to multiple penetrating wounds with unpredicted fragment paths, they also produce severe burn and blast injuries. While knifes and low-energy missiles usually 'only' lacerate the tissues they penetrate (i.e. they lead to a permanent cavity), higher missile velocities result in even more collateral tissue damage as tissue particles are driven away from the bullet tract, causing an increasing effect of cavitation (i.e. they cause an additional 'temporary' cavity). Furthermore bullets often cause secondary missiles, such as rib fragments, when hitting the chest wall, at the same time possibly leading to an altered trajectory of the missile.

Initial assessment and management

Initial evaluation

After obtaining a clinical history and details about the time and mechanism of injury, initial evaluation of the patient should be performed according to the *Advanced Trauma Life Support (ATLS) Guidelines*. First of all, rapid recognition and treatment of immediately life-threatening injuries is done during the *primary survey*, including assessment of airway (A), breathing (B) and circulation (C). After a rapid neurologic evaluation (D – disability), the patient will be shortly undressed and thoroughly examined (E – exposure). Body temperature control (E – environmental control) must not be underestimated, since hypothermia aggravates coagulopathy and acidosis.

Subsequently, the *secondary survey* allows patient evaluation for other potentially life-threatening injuries in a systematic manner.

Imaging studies

The **chest radiograph** is an important adjunct to the *primary survey* and can be helpful in evaluating breathing difficulties ('B-problems'), as well as the position and effect of an inserted chest tube. It mainly shows pneumothorax, hemothorax and mediastinal abnormalities and severely displaced rib fractures (Figure 26.1). Due to the limited sensitivity of the chest radiograph, **computed tomography** is frequently performed, during the *secondary survey* for further evaluation of the hemodynamically stable trauma victim.

Focused assessment with **sonography** for trauma (FAST) is another important adjunct to the *primary survey* in the patient with a 'C-problem'. Besides the evaluation for associated abdominal injuries, it is useful to detect pericardial effusion or tamponade in the thoracic trauma patient. Furthermore, thoracic ultrasound not only has the potential to detect intrapericardial bleeding, but in the hands of an experienced investigator it may also allow recognition of hemothoraces and assessment of the heart and its function.

Airways

Consider that airway obstruction may be caused by blood, secretions and foreign objects (e.g. tooth), as well as by injuries of the airway itself or compression from the outside.

Laryngotracheal injury

Despite its protected position between mandible and sternum, the larynx and cervical trachea can be

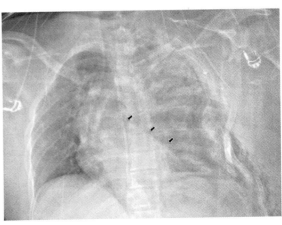

Figure 26.1 Severe blunt chest trauma with mediastinal shift to the right (arrows) due to left tension hemopneumothorax.

injured by blunt trauma (e.g. hyperextended neck against dashboard in unrestrained passengers, direct blows, strangulation by seatbelt/rope/manually) as well as by penetrating forces (e.g. knife, projectile). Patients may present with stridor, hemoptysis, hoarseness (due to vocal cord injury/displacement or recurrent laryngeal nerve injury, often associated with lesions to the cricotracheal junction) and neck pain. Besides concomitant soft tissue injury (erosion, haematoma), cervicomediastinal emphysema can be present. In stable patients, thorough examination by CT scan and flexible endoscopy allows systematic assessment of the injury, including potentially associated lesions of the esophagus. In patients with severe respiratory distress, oro- or nasotracheal intubation past the area of trauma is advised. Wherever applicable, this is best performed by guidance of a flexible bronchoscope, in order to avoid additional tissue damage with the risk of complete airway disruption. In cases of unsuccessful intubation due to severe edema or concomitant maxillofacial injury, emergency tracheostomy may be required.

Early surgical exploration with definitive reconstruction through a collar incision is recommended. In cases of laryngotracheal lesions with possible bilateral vocal cord and/or recurrent laryngeal nerve injury, consider the placement of a tracheostomy cannula at the end of the procedure.

Tracheal compression by sternoclavicular dislocation

Trauma to the upper chest can result in posterior sternoclavicular joint dislocation or sternoclavicular fracture dislocations, in which the medial end of the clavicle may come to rest on the trachea and cause upper airway obstruction. Amongst inspiratory stridor and a palpable defect in the region of the sternoclavicular joint, patients may also present with signs of vascular compression of the ipsilateral extremity. Treatment consists of immediate reduction of the medial end of the clavicula, best achieved by pulling both shoulders backwards, eventually with the help of a cushion positioned between the shoulder blades, and by additionally pulling at the medial end of the clavicula with a pointed clamp. Once reduction is achieved it is usually stable, and if so, conservative treatment (shoulder immobilization for 3 weeks) is sufficient. In contrast, anterior sternoclavicular dislocations are more common, and reduction is easier, but reduction is rarely stable, and operative fixation is often necessary.

Intrathoracic trachea

Based on the firm constitution of the trachea, especially in its cartilaginous anterior part, rupture is a very uncommon finding. However, if it does happen, it usually occurs due to a sudden increase in intratracheal pressure against the closed glottis, which mainly leads to vertical tears in the posterior, membranous part. These tracheal lesions can also result from forceful intubations. Patients present with haemoptysis, mediastinal emphysema and eventually pneumothorax (uni- or bilaterally), which are generally characterized by large air leaks through an indwelling chest tube. After establishing diagnosis by bronchoscopy and securing the airway by orotracheal intubation, prompt primary repair is advised. Access to the trachea is gained either through a collar incision for cranial lesions with possible extension into an upper partial sternal split or through a right thoracotomy, allowing better exposure of the lower and especially dorsal part of the trachea.

Bronchial rupture

Most bronchial ruptures occur due to shearing forces and forceful antero-posterior compression of the chest, as seen in most car accidents, leading to distracting forces of the laterally displaced lungs at the relatively fixed carina. Most tears occur within 2.5 cm of the carina and are usually found on the right, due to the shorter length and relatively unprotected position of the right mainstem bronchus. Patients may present with only subtle symptoms such as haemoptysis and discrete emphysema if the tear is covered. In tears communicating with the pleural space, pneumothorax with large air leaks through the chest drains may occur and suction on the chest drain may even worse dyspnea. The typical radiological sign is that of a collapsed lung at the bottom of the hemithorax (as opposed to a lung collapse around the hilum seen in 'conventional' pneumothorax); therefore it is also referred to as 'dropped lung' sign. Again, bronchoscopy establishes the diagnosis, and prompt direct repair through thoracotomy under single-lumen ventilation should be preferred to resectional procedures. Asymptomatic, minor bronchial tears can be managed conservatively in the presence of a fully expanded lung with no air leak being present. In those patients, bronchoscopic examinations should be performed on a regular basis for early recognition of strictures or bronchiectasis, which may develop at a later time in the course of recovery.

Lungs

Pneumothorax

The most common injury resulting from thoracic trauma is a **simple pneumothorax**. It is either caused by laceration of the visceral pleura by a sharp object (e.g. fractured rib, knife, bullet) or due to rupture of the visceral pleura caused by deceleration or barotrauma. While small pneumothoraces (up to 2 cm) in stable blunt chest trauma victims can be managed conservatively, all patients with pneumothorax and penetrating injury, unstable respiratory situation or otherwise intended intubation and mechanical ventilation need tube thoracostomy. Chest tubes may be removed when the lung is fully expanded (no persistent blood or air in the thoracic cavity), if the air leak has completely resolved and if fluid drainage is less than about 200 ml/24 hours.

The deadliest form of pneumothorax is **tension pneumothorax**, which develops when a one-way valve-like air leak occurs from the lung. The increasing accumulation of air in the thoracic cavity leads to a complete collapse of the affected lung and a mediastinal shift to the contralateral side with compression of the contralateral lung and venae cavae. The result is a rapidly increasing hemodynamic instability due to decreased venous return, followed by rhythm disturbances (tachyarrhythmia). Patients correspondingly present with chest pain, respiratory distress, tachycardia, hypotension, distended neck veins and a unilateral absence of breath sounds with hyper-resonance to percussion. Sometimes clinical diagnosis can be difficult, since associated hemothorax, lung contusions and hypovolaemia can mask the typical aforementioned clinical signs (Figure 26.1). Radiological confirmation of diagnosis is usually obsolete, and immediate decompression is mandatory by inserting a large-calibre needle through the second intercostal space in the mid-clavicular line. Definitive management consists of insertion of a chest tube in the fifth intercostal space in the anterior axillary line.

Also **open pneumothorax** can lead to a certain amount of tension in the thoracic cavity if there is a one-way-valve-like tissue flap (or inappropriately placed wound dressing!) that allows air to enter

through the opening in the chest with every breath. Management includes coverage of the open chest wound with a three-way occlusive dressing that allows air to go out and at the same time prevents air from entering the thoracic cavity. Then a tube thoracostomy is performed remote from the wound until operative debridement and closure of the defect are possible. Local muscle or myocutaneous flaps should be preferred over prosthetic material (e.g. polypropylene mesh) in the reconstruction process, since wound contamination usually has to be expected.

Hemothorax

Hemothorax can compromise respiration itself on the one hand, and on the other hand, hypotension due to blood loss contributes even more to poor tissue oxygenation. Hemothorax can occur from bleeding due to lung laceration, vessel laceration (usually intercostal or internal mammary vessels) or from fractured ribs, sternum or spine. Small bleeds are self-limiting, and patients with major bleeds, for example, due to hilar vessel injury, heart injury (chamber rupture) or aortic dissection, rarely even reach the hospital alive. Hemothoraces are evacuated using a large-caliber chest tube and the application of autologous blood salvage systems (e.g. Hemovac, Cell Saver) can be helpful in cases of expected large volumes. Operative exploration should be considered if the initial amount of blood output is more than 1,500 ml and/or chest tube output is 200 ml or more for 2–4 hours, also taking into account the patient's condition. In uncertain situations or if the bleeding source is well localized (e.g. by CT angiography), a videothoracoscopic approach (VATS) can be chosen in hemodynamically stable patients. VATS also is applicable in the post-primary evacuation of large, clotted hemothoraces in order to allow lung re-expansion and prevent the formation of empyema and late fibrothorax.

Lung laceration

Pulmonary lacerations are seen in penetrating as well as blunt thoracic trauma victims and usually result in a combination of bleeding and air leak (i.e. hemopneumothorax). Minor lacerations can be treated by simple insertion of a chest tube. For larger, more centrally located lung injuries (Figure 26.2), characterized by large air leak or persistent blood loss (continuous blood loss of >200 ml per hour), consider

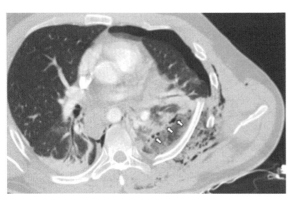

Figure 26.2 Blunt trauma victim with a large tear across the whole lower lobe (arrows), dislocated rib fractures and pneumothorax.

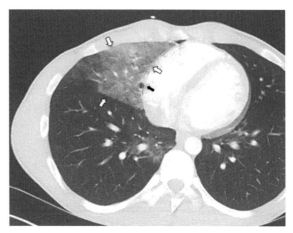

Figure 26.3 Lung contusion (white arrows) of the middle lobe with small pneumatocele (black arrow).

thoracotomy. Depending on the degree of injuries, either resectional procedures or, more desirable if applicable, parenchyma-saving techniques, such as pulmonary tractotomy, may be used. This technique initially was developed to avoid larger resectional procedures (i.e. lobectomy, pneumonectomy) in gunshot victims. The basic idea is to open the wound tract by dividing the healthy parenchymal bridge above it between two clamps (or by means of a stapling device), and subsequently bleeding vessels and small, leaking bronchi at the base of the tract can be ligated and oversewn, respectively.

Lung contusion

Direct lacerations of the lung, as well as the transmitted, indirect forces associated with blunt thoracic trauma, lead to diffuse bleeding and edema in the underlying lung parenchyma (Figure 26.3), resulting in pulmonary shunting (ventilation/perfusion mismatch).

The degree of respiratory impairment often varies with concomitant injuries (e.g. flail chest, pneumothorax, hemothorax) and pre-existing disabilities (lung emphysema); patients should be closely observed because the full impact on oxygen exchange emerges only hours after the initial trauma. Generally, blood gases deteriorate before radiological signs of lung edema appear; furthermore, these radiological signs might only be minimal if there is a short interval between the triggering injury and radiographical studies, which leads to a high degree of under-estimation in these patients. Therapy includes administration of humidified oxygen, carefully controlled administration of crystalloids (to prevent fluid overload) and close

patient observation in order to initiate, if necessary, endotracheal intubation and mechanical ventilation. Haematoma formation can be observed in 5–10% of patients with pulmonary contusions. Symptoms of haemoptysis and occasionally fever usually abate within 1 week, but haematoma resolution on chest radiographs takes about 1 month.

The most severe complication from lung contusion is acute respiratory distress syndrome (ARDS), whereas the risk for ARDS increases with the severity of injuries. Not only the injury to the lung itself but also its combination with associated injuries and the eventual need for endotracheal intubation and ventilation with its risk of ventilator-associated pneumonia finally may result in ARDS.

Chest wall

The thoracic wall protects the vital organs of the chest, notably the heart and lungs, but it also covers the well-perfused and fragile parenchymal abdominal organs of the abdomen such as the liver, spleen and kidneys. Every thoracic injury, whether blunt or penetrating, leaves certain damage to the chest wall. While in children the ribs are more elastic, stronger forces are needed to cause rib fractures, and thus, severe intrathoracic injuries in blunt trauma can occur without signs of broken ribs. Consider that rib fractures in toddlers up to 3 years occasionally result from child abuse. In contrast, in the elderly, simple coughing or a fall from a standing position can result in multiply fractured osteoporotic ribs without severe damage to intrathoracic organs.

Rib fractures

Rib fractures are the main finding in blunt thoracic trauma. Beside pain with the consequence of shallow breathing and atelectasis of the lung, significant respiratory impairment is mostly due to accompanying lung contusions and/or associated head injuries as well as pre-existing co-morbidities (i.e. poor pulmonary reserve). The direct impact on respiratory function as well as the pattern of associated injuries depends on the location (upper/lower ribs, single fracture/fracture in several places) and the number of broken ribs. Since the **upper ribs (1,2)** are well protected by the clavicles and the whole shoulder girdle, fractures of these ribs result only from strong forces, which should raise suspicion for particular associated injuries such as aortic rupture or tracheo-bronchial injury.

Fractures of the **middle ribs (3–8)** are the most common and may result from direct blows to the chest, as well as from indirect lateral fractures following forceful antero-posterior compression of the chest. Furthermore, trauma to the upper extremity often leads to a fracture of the clavicle first, then driving the scapula into the nearby chest, typically causing lateral and posterior fractures of the middle ribs.

Fractures of the **lower ribs (9–12)**, like those of the upper ones, rarely have major influence on respiratory mechanics, but injuries to the liver, spleen and kidneys, as well as diaphragmatic rupture, are sometimes associated with these injuries (Figure 26.4).

The cornerstone of initial **treatment** is undoubtedly sufficient pain control to allow appropriate pulmonary toilet. Shallow breathing and the avoidance to cough due to poor pain control inevitably lead to sputum retention, atelectasis and pneumonia. The broad possibilities of pain control reach from oral analgesics, including morphine and its derivatives, over self-administered IV opioids, to epidural analgesia and should be carefully adapted to the patient situation. Operative stabilization of fractured ribs is rarely indicated without the presence of a severe instability of the chest wall due to a series (three or more) of multiply broken ribs, which is called 'flail chest'.

One of the **late sequelae** after rib fractures, which may need further treatment, is pseudarthrosis (painful instability at the fracture site 6 or more months after trauma). If local infiltration with long-lasting anaesthetics and corticosteroids does not lead to pain relief and painful instability is one of the main clinical findings, operative measures, such as simple resection or debridement followed by plate osteosynthesis, have to be considered. One of the most difficult and also the most prevalent problems is chronic thoracic pain, which occurs in approximately 30% of patients, and therefore needs an interdisciplinary approach

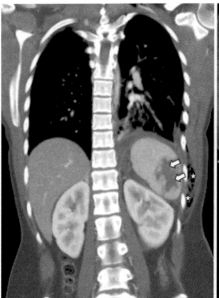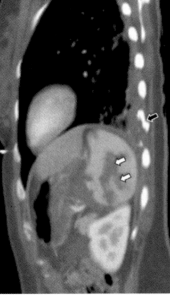

Figure 26.4 Fracture of lower ribs (black arrow) with associated second-degree splenic laceration (white arrows) and subcutaneus emphysema (stars).

between thoracic surgeons, anaesthetists and on occasion the help of a psychiatrist in the treatment of a post-traumatic stress disorder.

Flail chest

Flail chest is defined as a consecutive series of three or more rib fractures, which are broken in at least two different sites resulting in a free-floating chest wall segment. These patients are in the majority of cases referred after moderate to severe blunt trauma and suffer from respiratory-dependent pain and dyspnoea. In the spontaneously breathing patient, a paradoxical movement of the free-moving chest wall segment can be examined. But often, concomitant haematoma and/or emphysema of the chest wall soft tissue conceal these findings. The flail segment can be **anterior**, associated with contralateral anterior rib fractures, sternal fractures or separation of several ribs at their costochondral junction (invisible by plain radiographs and even difficult to detect by CT scan). In most cases, the floating segment is localized **laterally** due to direct impacts, antero-posterior compression or upper extremity trauma ('scapula against chest wall' effect). The least common variety lies **posterior** and often goes clinically unrecognized, since the chest wall in this region is well supported by the back muscles and the scapula.

As flail chest often results in respiratory insufficiency due to a combination of pain, increased work of breathing and, most important, associated pulmonary contusion; endotracheal intubation and ventilation sometimes are inevitable. As internal pneumatic stabilization by mechanical ventilation takes an average ventilation time of 10 days, the risk of ventilator-associated pneumonia as well as the high costs of ICU care are only some of the factors which may raise the question for early rib stabilization. Indications for rib stabilization include:

- Thoracotomy for another reason (e.g. haemorrhage or lung laceration)
- Severe chest wall instability with increasing respiratory insufficiency in patients with sufficient pain control and without the presence of major lung contusions

A relative indication for chest wall stabilization is an insufficient bronchial toilet due to inefficient coughing in flail chest patients. Roughly summarized, operative stabilization should aim at preventing intubation and prolonged mechanical ventilation. For rib stabilization, contourable reconstruction plates or anatomically precontoured titanium plates are available, which allow anatomical and physiological fracture reconstruction (Figure 26.5). Furthermore, intramedullary splints can be used with smaller incisions to reduce exposure and avoid further soft tissue damage. Implant removal is usually not required.

Sternal fractures

Sternal fractures are commonly caused by motor vehicle accidents, resulting from a direct impact on the steering wheel (without restraint) or forceful deceleration caused by the seat belt itself. Therefore, they are often associated with rib fractures and closed injuries of the head. Operative fixation is rarely needed but may be considered in patients with persisting painful instability (for 6 weeks or more) or severe fracture

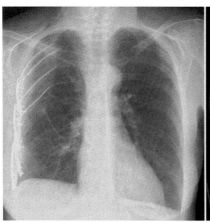
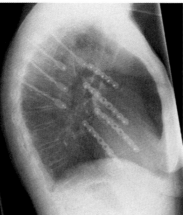

Figure 26.5 Result after stabilization of flail chest with osteosynthesis plates (lateral fracture line) and splints (latero-posterior fracture line).

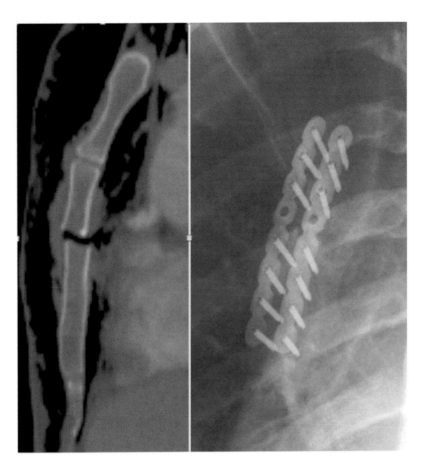

Figure 26.6 Instable sternal fracture 6 weeks after trauma, reduced and stabilized with two parallel angle-stable plates.

dislocation with high risk for non-union. Stabilization can be easily achieved by plate osteosynthesis, whereas two parallel plates offer the best results (Figure 26.6). It is important to be aware of associated cardiac injuries, especially cardiac contusions, which may lead to potentially life-threatening dysrhythmias.

Traumatic asphyxia

Severe crushing of the chest, for example, in passengers trapped inside or underneath a crashed vehicle, results, on the one hand, in immediate effects caused by the initial blow and, on the other hand, in subsequent effects caused by prolonged compression of the chest and thus increased venous pressure. The immediate effect consists of disruptions of the airways, while increased venous pressure levels eventually lead to swelling, cyanosis and petechiae of the head and neck, as well as subconjunctival hemorrhage. Furthermore, not only oedema of the head and neck but also cerebral oedema with subsequent loss of consciousness may occur. As neurological symptoms and the effects

of an impaired venous return are usually transient once the victim is rescued, associated injuries must be excluded during the work-up.

Chest wall defects

Large chest wall defects require prompt debridement and irrigation to avoid necrotizing wound infections. Once the patient's situation has stabilized and the local wound situation is under control (i.e. no signs of infection), reconstruction with or without prosthetic material (e.g. polypropylene mesh) is feasible, depending on the depth, localization and size of the defect. Especially in larger defects, myocutaneous rotation flaps (either from the latissimus dorsi or from the rectus abdominis muscle) have proven to be quite helpful in wound closure.

Associated skeletal injuries

Clavicle fractures are common in thoracic trauma patients and rarely need operative stabilization.

Absolute indications include open fractures and neurovascular injury requiring repair or exploration. Severe displacement is a relative indication for operative stabilization, which may prevent a high mal- and non-union rate in these patients.

Scapular fractures are associated with rib fractures and only need operative fixation in severely dislocated fractures of the coracoid, the acromion or the glenoid and in fractures of the humerus (mostly at its surgical neck), which are associated with lesions of the suprascapular nerve (innervation of the supraspinatus and infraspinatus muscles has to be evaluated by electromyography).

Sternoclavicular joint dislocations/fractures – see earlier section.

Esophagus

Esophageal injuries are uncommon in trauma, and when they appear, they are most commonly the result of a penetrating injury. On the other hand, severe blows to the abdomen can lead to an expulsion of gastric contents into the esophagus, which again can lead to linear tears of the lower esophagus (as seen in Boerhaave's syndrome). A high index of suspicion is needed for early diagnosis because symptoms often do not become apparent until the patient presents with signs of sepsis due to pleural empyema or sepsis. On occasion, gastric contents may be evacuated through an indwelling chest drain, which makes the diagnosis obvious. Esophagoscopy is the diagnostic tool of choice, followed by contrast (water-soluble) esophagogram. When both studies are combined and performed in sequence, over 95% of esophageal injuries are identified.

Prompt, direct repair with the use of well-vascularized reinforcement material (e.g. intercostal muscle, pleural or pericardial flap) is advised, since any delay in treatment increases morbidity and mortality (a delay of more than 24 hours has a 50% mortality). Only small lesions, which are usually attributable to mishaps of instrumentation (i.e. nasogastric tube insertion) rather than to the trauma itself, may be managed conservatively or eventually by esophageal stent placement. Tears of the lower third of the esophagus, as mostly seen in blunt trauma, are best approached through a left thoracotomy, while injuries to the middle or upper third need right thoracotomy for optimal exposure. In patients who are already in a septic state due to missed or delayed

diagnosis, a two-stage approach is often the only option. The first step consists of initial stapling of the distal esophageal end after insertion of a percutaneous catheter into the jejunum (feeding jejunostomy) and the creation of a cervical mucus fistula within the proximal esophageal end (cervical esophagostomy). Later on, tension-free reconstruction can be performed preferably using an autologous intestinal graft (stomach, small intestine or colon). Due to the injury mechanism in blunt trauma (forceful blow against the upper abdomen), associated injuries such as diaphragmatic rupture are sometimes seen.

Diaphragm

Diaphragmatic injuries must be suspected in patients who have sustained a forceful blow against the upper abdomen as a result of a high-speed motor vehicle accident or similar trauma. Patients may present with dyspnoea but also may suffer from hypovolemic shock due to associated injuries of the spleen or liver. Often the injury goes unrecognized until detected either by CT scan in haemodynamically stable patients or incidentally at the time of laparotomy or thoracotomy for hypovolemic shock. While blunt trauma causes diaphragmatic rupture in the range of 5% of cases and usually results in tears of 5–10 cm or more in the region of the tendinous part of the diaphragm, penetrating gunshot wounds lead to diaphragmatic injury in approximately 45% of cases, and injuries are generally (in 85% of cases) no longer than 2 cm. Large tears can immediately present by herniation of abdominal organs into the chest cavity (Figure 26.7), whereas smaller tears and those located on the right side may go unrecognized until the patient presents only months or sometimes years later (in 85% within 3 years) when visceral herniation occurs. Due to the high potential of visceral herniation into the chest, following the lower intrathoracic pressure, and eventually resulting in gangrene, prompt repair is warranted.

Large tears are best exposed through a low, lateral thoracotomy, which allows direct repair. But due to often-associated abdominal injuries, repair through a laparotomy approach might be more suitable in most cases. Peripheral injuries might require resuspension of the thoracic wall by encircling the ribs. Confronted with large defects, sometimes the additional use of a prosthetic mesh is useful. In uncertain situations, thoracoscopy or laparoscopy (depending on present

261

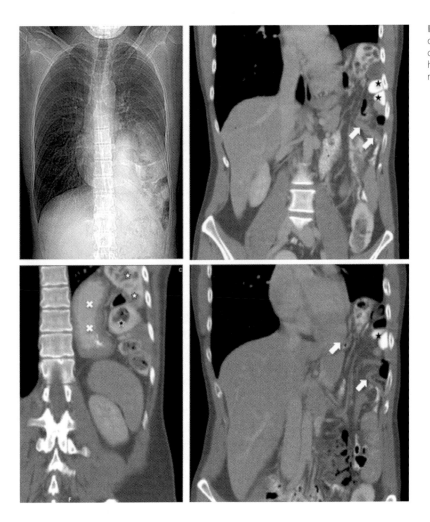

Figure 26.7 Large left-sided diaphragmatic tear with herniation of colon (stars) and gut (crosses) into the left hemithorax. The retracted diaphragm is marked with arrows.

or suspected associated injuries) may confirm a suspected diagnosis and allow direct repair of small lesions.

Missed lesions are best approached through thoracotomy since pulmonary adhesion formation is a common finding in those cases. Also, postero-lateral, right-sided tears are almost only accessible from the chest, since the liver interferes with an abdominal approach.

Thoracic duct/lymphatics

Injuries of the thoracic duct are rarely seen in trauma patients. They may be associated with blunt thoracic vertebral trauma, whereas the mechanism of injury often is a forceful hyper-extension or translation. Also, penetrating trauma can lead to thoracic duct injury. In both situations, diagnosis is generally made

incidentally after a few days, when the blood has cleared from the chest tubes, and the milky white appearance of the draining liquid due to its high triglyceride content actually confirms the diagnosis. Initial management is always non-operative, keeping the patient on total parenteral nutrition (nil by mouth) for about 7 days. If the conservative attempt fails, thoracic duct ligation can be achieved either thoracoscopically (for the experienced) or through a right-sided, low, lateral thoracotomy, ligating the thoracic duct just as it has traversed the diaphragm to enter the thoracic cavity. In selected cases (e.g. necessity of left thoracotomy for the treatment of associated injuries), an attempt to directly identify the leakage and ligate the leaking vessel may be justified in order to avoid a contralateral operation. The application of full-fat cream through a nasogastric tube, just half an hour before the operative procedure, may simplify direct visualization of the leak. A percu-taneous cannulation of the cysterna chyli with embo-lization of the thoracic duct has also been described by several authors and may be a valuable treatment option, if available, in these patients.

Thoracic great vessels

Over 90% of injuries of the thoracic great vessels are caused by penetrating trauma. In blunt trauma victims, aortic rupture is the second most common cause of death after head injury.

Aorta

It is estimated that only 25% of patients who sustain aortic injuries due to blunt thoracic trauma reach the hospital alive. In over 30% of these initial survivors, the aorta will rupture within 24 hours of trauma without initiation of therapy. Rapid deceleration is the main mechanism leading to aortic injury in blunt trauma victims, with traffic accidents and falls from heights the main underlying causes of trauma. Sudden deceleration leads to traction at the relatively immobile isthmus, where the ductus arteriosus forms a ligamentous attachment between the descending aorta and the pulmonary artery. Thus this region represents the transition zone between the relatively mobile arch and the relatively fixed descending aorta. Therefore, rupture most often occurs just below the isthmus (50–70%) followed by the ascending (18%) and descending (14%) aorta. Given that open vessel rupture leads to imminent death in the field, only patients with a contained rupture (containment by either adventitia or mediastinal pleura) may survive to reach the hospital. In these patients, only early diagnosis and rapid management may prevent cata-strophic rupture. Radiological signs of contained aortic rupture include a widened mediastinum (>8 cm), an indistinct ('blurred') aortic knob, depression of the left mainstem bronchus and deviation of the trachea and esophagus (nasogastric tube) to the right. A first rib fracture and a small apical hemothorax ('apical cap') may also be seen on occasion. Massive left haemothorax and profound hypotension are signs of an imminent rupture, thus calling for imme-diate surgery. Often, definitive diagnosis is made by contrast-enhanced CT scans in stable patients, and aortography is reserved for uncertain situations or if endovascular stenting is intended. Management consists either of primary repair or resection of the

injured area with subsequent grafting. However, in recent years, endovascular repair, also termed 'thor-acic aortic endografting for trauma' (TAET), has gained increasing importance in these patients, redu-cing not only events of spinal cord ischemia but also overall mortality compared to open approaches. Minor intimal tears or small pseudo-aneurysms may even be managed conservatively with close follow-up.

In these often polytrauma patients, bridging to surgery or intervention, in order to allow treatment of imminently threatening injuries, is occasionally necessary. In this phase, besides cardiopulmonary stabilization, the administration of short-acting beta-blocking agents to control the heart rate and to decrease the mean arterial pressure to approximately 60 mmHg is crucial.

Hilar vessels

Injuries to the hilar vessels may initially be controlled by direct occlusion with a finger or hilar placement of a soft vascular clamp proximal to the injury (on occasion an intrapericardial access to the hilum must be chosen). Optimal treatment consists of direct repair since pneumonectomy is associated with poor outcome in these patients. Peripheral pulmonary artery lesions may be repaired or the affected lobe or segment may be resected.

Major thoracic veins

Major thoracic venous injuries are very uncommon. Caval lesions may result in hemothorax or pericardial tamponade, which is associated with intrapericardial injuries. If repair proves to be difficult or impossible, injured subclavian or azygous veins can be ligated. Injuries of the thoracic inferior or superior vena cava and innominate vein may require shunt placement to facilitate repair.

Systemic air embolism

Systemic air embolism is usually described following central penetrating lung injury or severe central lung laceration due to blunt trauma, followed by positive-pressure ventilation, which then results in air being forced into the low-pressure pulmonary venules or even the great vessels (depending on the injury). With the air gaining access to the aorta and the coronary arteries, manifestations range from seizures and arrhythmias to cardiac arrest. Resuscitation requires thoracotomy, immediate clamping of the pulmonary hilum and aspiration of the air from the left ventricle and ascending aorta. Experience with hyperbaric oxygen therapy has generally been good in patients with air embolism from other causes and may be considered after successful closure of the 'fistula'.

Missile embolization

Embolization to the pulmonary arteries is usually treated with surgical removal or interventional techniques. A chest radiograph taken immediately preceding incision or intraoperative fluoroscopy is mandatory to detect more distal embolization that may occur during positioning. Asymptomatic patients with small distal fragments may be treated expectantly. Occasionally, missile emboli may migrate through a patent foramen ovale or from central parenchymal or vascular injury to gain access to the left side of the heart and subsequently to the systemic circulation.

Cardiac injuries

Blunt cardiac injuries are mostly seen in traffic accidents, while other causes are falls, assaults or sporting injuries. Injuries are highly variable and range from mild contusions, which occasionally also may trigger dysrhythmia, to severe tissue injuries such as valvular or cardiac chamber rupture. Therefore, patients may be asymptomatic, may show signs of pericardial tamponade or possibly die in the field because of exsanguinating injuries. In penetrating cardiac injuries, mortality is about 70 to 80% depending on the location and severity of injury. Due to the size and degree of exposure, ventricular injuries mostly involve the right (43%) or left ventricle (34%). Right (16%) or left atrial injuries (7%) are less common. Patients who reach the hospital before suffering from cardiac arrest have a high probability of survival. Valvular injuries or injuries of the coronary arteries usually lead to impaired cardiac function in long-term follow-up.

Cardiac contusion

Cardiac contusions typically occur in forceful blunt trauma of the anterior chest wall, with a prevalence of around 20%. Electrocardiography is the diagnostic tool of choice to detect any rhythm or conduction disorders, which occur in around 1.5% of blunt chest trauma victims. The role of serum troponin and myocardial creatine kinase levels is still unclear, since these parameters may express some sort of myocardial injury, but they cannot predict cardiac complications.

Commotio cordis

Commotio cordis, also called 'sudden cardiac death', occurs during sporting or recreational activities in usually otherwise healthy individuals and results from a blow to the heart, presumably arriving just into the ascending part of the T-wave (vulnerable period) and thus leading to ventricular arrhythmia. Prompt resuscitation and defibrillation are crucial; nevertheless, survival rates are generally relatively poor and in the range of 15%.

Pericardial tamponade

Cardiac tamponade is more common due to penetrating rather than blunt thoracic trauma. Since the pericardial sac is made of rather inelastic fibrotic tissue, already small amounts of blood (100–400 ml) can severely impair cardiac function. The typical clinical signs of tamponade include arterial hypotension, elevated venous pressure (resulting in distended neck veins) and muffled heart tones. But these signs, also referred to as 'Beck's triad', are only clearly present in about 10–30% of patients. It is not unusual that associated injuries lead to hypovolemia and hypotension; consequently neck veins are inconspicuous, and blood pressure is low anyway. Low QRS voltage on electrocardiogram may be another hint to pericardial tamponade. Since pericardial ultrasonography has become an integral part of FAST, which is routinely performed in most emergency departments, ultrasonographic diagnosis is made with an accuracy of about 90% (in the hands of an experienced operator). Subsequently, performed subxiphoid pericardiocentesis may then definitively confirm diagnosis and temporarily stabilize the patient's hemodynamic situation, until operative exploration through left thoracotomy (alternatively median sternotomy) in the operating theatre is possible. In patients who do not respond to the usual measures of resuscitation for haemorrhagic shock and in whom cardiac tamponade is strongly suspected, direct pericardiocentesis may be justified. Be aware that clotted pericardial blood may result in negative (i.e. 'dry') pericardiocentesis.

Myocardial laceration

Small wounds are controlled with direct finger pressure, while larger ones may be controlled by insertion of a balloon catheter (Foley). But care has to be taken not to obstruct blood in- or outflow and not to apply too much traction, resulting in extension of the laceration. Atrial injuries may be controlled by placing a Satinsky clamp across the wound. Injuries to the atria and left ventricle can usually be directly sutured using 0 (ventricle) or 3/0 (atrium) non-absorbable monofilament suture material. When suturing right ventricular injuries, Teflon pledgets (or a piece of pericardium) are advisable to prevent cut-through of the stitches. Small coronary arteries (diameter < 1 mm) may be ligated, while larger vessels should be re-anastomosed. Tears near a coronary can be repaired by mattress suture technique.

In penetrating cardiac injuries, luxation of the heart is mandatory in order not to miss posterior cardiac wounds; however, this manoeuvre has to be carried out carefully and only for a short time, since it leads to a decreased venous return, bradycardia and eventually ventricular fibrillation.

Valvular lesions

Injuries of the cardiac valves are rather uncommon findings in thoracic trauma patients. Depending on the nature of the injury (papillary muscle or leaflet disruption) and location, victims either die shortly after the event or reach the emergency department in a state of cardiogenic shock. If applicable, reconstruction can be delayed until the patient has sufficiently recovered.

Resuscitative thoracotomy

Emergency department thoracotomy may be life-saving in selected patients only.

In **blunt trauma** victims, signs of life must be present on admission to the emergency department; otherwise immediate thoracotomy is of extremely limited benefit.

Signs of life include detectable blood pressure, respiratory motor effort, cardiac electrical activity or pupillary response.

In contrast to penetrating thoracic trauma, blunt trauma victims who present with pulseless electrical activity (PEA) on arrival are not candidates for emergency thoracotomy.

In **penetrating injury**, outcomes are generally better when the aforementioned criteria are respected; furthermore, indications may be extended to patients with PEA. A relative indication for resuscitative thoracotomy is given in patients who show signs of life in the field, sustaining witnessed cardiac arrest within ≤15 minutes of pre-hospital CPR.

The following manoeuvres can be accomplished with emergency thoracotomy:

- Evacuation of pericardial tamponade and treatment of underlying injury
- Control of exsanguinating intrathoracic hemorrhage (i.e. initial blood loss 1,500 ml and/or 300 ml/h and hemodynamically unstable patient)
- Open cardiac massage (closed heart massage is ineffective in hypovolemic patients with cardiac arrest)
- Cross-clamping of descending aorta in order to reduce infra-diaphragmatic blood loss and redistribute blood to vital organs (i.e. brain, heart and lungs).

Technique

Resuscitative thoracotomy is a left antero-lateral thoracotomy through the fifth intercostal space with the patient in a supine position. Consider right antero-lateral thoracotomy only in patients without cardiac arrest who suffer from hypotension due to right-sided injuries. Depending on the injuries which have to be addressed, the approach can be extended either laterally (injuries of the descending aorta or intended supradiaphragmal cross-clamping), upwards through the sternum (hemiclamshell approach), to reach the vascular structures of the superior mediastinum or to the contralateral side (clamshell approach) for full exposure of the heart and the right hilum.

Literature

1   Bernardin B, Troquet JM. Initial management and resuscitation of severe chest trauma. *Emerg Med Clin North Am* 2012 May; 30(2):377–400. Review.

2   Peytel E, Menegaux F, Cluzel P, et al. Initial imaging assessment of severe blunt trauma. *Intensive Care Med.* Nov 2001; 27(11):1756–61.

3   Onat S, Ulku R, Avci A, et al. Urgent thoracotomy for

penetrating chest trauma: analysis of 158 patients of a single center. *Injury* 2011 Sep; 42(9): 900–4.

4   Carretta A, Melloni G, Bandiera A et al. Conservative and surgical treatment of acute posttraumatic tracheobronchial injuries. *World J Surg* 2011 Nov; 35(11):2568–74.

5   Moore FO, Goslar PW, Coimbra R, et al. Blunt traumatic occult pneumothorax: is observation safe? Results of a prospective AAST multicenter study. *J Trauma* May 2011; 70(5):1019–25.

6   Cothren C, Moore EE, Biffl WL. Lung-sparing techniques are associated with improved outcome compared with anatomic resection for severe lung injuries. *J Trauma* 2002; 53:483–7.

7   Cohn SM, Dubose JJ. Pulmonary contusion: an update on recent advances in clinical management. *World J Surg* 2010 Aug; 34(8): 1959–70. Review.

8   Pettiford BL, Luketich JD, Landreneau RJ. The management of flail chest. *Thorac Surg Clin* 2007 Feb; 17(1):25–33. Review.

9   Tanaka H, Yukioka T, Yamaguti Y et al. Surgical stabilization or internal pneumatic stabilization?

A prospective randomized study of management of severe flail chest patients. *J Trauma* 2002; 52:727.

10 Harston A, Roberts C. Fixation of sternal fractures: a systematic review. *J Trauma* 2011 Dec; 71(6):1875–9. Review.

11 Richards EC, Wallis ND. Asphyxiation: a review. *Trauma* 2005; 7:37–45. Review.

12 Asensio JA, Chahwan S, Forno W, et al. Penetrating esophageal injuries: multicenter study of the American Association for the Surgery of Trauma. *J Trauma* 2001; 50(2):289.

13 Hanna WC, Ferri LE, Fata P, et al. The current status of traumatic diaphragmatic injury: lessons learned from 105 patients over 13 years. *Ann Thorac Surg* 2008 Mar; 85(3):1044–8.

14 McGrath EE, Blades Z, Anderson PB. Chylothorax: aetiology, diagnosis and therapeutic options. *Respir Med.* 2010 Jan; 104(1):1–8. Epub 2009 Sep 18. Review.

15 Boffa DJ, Sands MJ, Rice TW, et al. A critical evaluation of a percutaneous diagnostic and treatment strategy for chylothorax after thoracic surgery. *Eur*

J Cardiothorac Surg. 2008 Mar; 33(3):435–9.

16 Scaglione M, Pinto A, Pinto F, et al. Role of contrast-enhanced helical CT in the evaluation of acute thoracic aortic injuries after blunt chest trauma. *Eur Radiol* 2001; 11:2444–8.

17 Xenos ES, Minion DJ, Davenport DL, et al. Endovascular versus open repair for descending thoracic aortic rupture: institutional experience and meta-analysis. *Eur J Cardiothorac Surg* 2009 Feb; 35(2):282–6.

18 Miller KR, Benns MV, Sciarretta JD, et al. The evolving management of venous bullet emboli: a case series and literature review. *Injury* 2011 May; 42(5): 441–6.

19 Sybrandy KC, Cramer MJM, Burgersdijk C. Diagnosing cardiac contusion: old wisdom and new insights. *Heart* 2003 May; 89(5):485–9. Review.

20 Working Group, Ad Hoc Subcommittee on Outcomes, American College of Surgeons–Committee on Trauma. Practice management guidelines for emergency department thoracotomy. *J Am Coll Surg* 2001; 193:303–9.

Epidemiology and etiology

Despite patients' reluctance to seek out medical attention, hyperhidrosis is not as rare a disorder as would be perceived and has historic roots in the medical literature. The condition is divided into primary and secondary hyperhidrosis. Secondary hyperhidrosis is a generalized sweating typically affecting the entire body and is consequent to underlying metabolic, neoplastic, infectious or endocrine conditions[1]. Some examples of these conditions include diabetes mellitus, hyperthyroidism, carcinoid syndrome, malignancies such as lymphoma, tuberculosis, systemic shock, heart failure, Parkinson's disease and spinal cord injuries[2]. In contrast, primary (idiopathic) hyperhidrosis is typically focal and is defined as the production of sweat by eccrine glands that is beyond the body's physiological parameters for thermo-regulation[3]. Usually this is an exaggerated response to a physiological stress or emotional/psychological stimulus[4]. Moreover, primary hyperhidrosis is subcategorized based on location (palmar, plantar, axillary or craniofacial). For the purposes of this chapter, the term 'hyperhidrosis' will be used to refer more specifically to primary hyperhidrosis.

The incidence of hyperhidrosis varies in the literature. An earlier Israeli study reported incidence rates of 0.6–1.0%[5]. More recent evidence suggests that the prevalence of hyperhidrosis is higher, ranging from 2.8% in the United States to 4.6% in specific parts of China[6,7]. An estimate suggests that the condition affects roughly 7.8 million individuals in the United States[6]. The variability in epidemiologic data reflects two principles characteristic of hyperhidrosis. First, the definition of hyperhidrosis is unclear, largely leading to subjective reliance for diagnosis, as well as the potential for over- or under-reporting. Second,

individuals suffering the condition often do not seek medical care, either due to social discomfort or to a lack of knowledge of possible treatment options[1,8].

Commonly, individuals are diagnosed early in adulthood, considering the role of pubertal heightening of the disorder. Gender distribution is equal, with the greatest prevalence existing among working-age adults. Moreover, a genetic predilection appears to exist, with 25–50% of cases demonstrating an autosomal dominant pattern of inheritance of variable penetrance[1,10,11]. This familiar pattern of inheritance appears to be more strongly correlated with individuals presenting prior to the age of 20. Focally, the most common site for *severe* disease appears to be palmoplantar hyperhidrosis of the palms and soles[9]. Other common sites for severe disease include the combination of the palms and axillae (15–20%), the axillae alone (5–10%) and craniofacial region (5%)[3].

Pathophysiology

The human body contains an uneven distribution of up to 4 million sweat glands throughout the body. Palmar density (700 glands/cm^2) is greater than other less populated parts of the body (the back with 64 glands/cm^2, the forehead with 180 glands/cm^2). Interestingly, different body parts perspire secondary to different stimuli and with different purposes. Sweating from the forehead, back and torso primarily serves a thermoregulatory function.[12] Palmoplantar sweating, in contrast, appears to be triggered by cortical function, responding to various emotional signals/stresses. Furthermore, there exist three types of sweat glands: eccrine, apocrine and apoeccrine–with the latter being only recently described in the axilla and sharing morphological and functional similarities to the other two.[1] Eccrine

Core Topics in Thoracic Surgery, ed. Marco Scarci, Aman Coonar, Tom Routledge and Francis Wells. Published by
Cambridge University Press. © Cambridge University Press 2016

glands are more abundant (approximately 3 million) – preferentially located in the palms, axillae and soles of the feet – with only 5% being functional at any point in time. These glands respond to sympathetic activation via the cholinergic neurotransmitter acetylcholine.[13] In comparison, apocrine glands are less numerous, located strictly in the axillae and urogenital area, and are activated during puberty via adrenergic nerve fibres, secreting a more odorous and viscid sweat directly into hair follicles.[14]

The exact pathophysiology of hyperhidrosis remains largely unclear but does appear to be primarily induced by autonomic (via the sympathetic chain) over-stimulation of the eccrine glands. Sweating appears to be a disproportionate response to emotional stress but is often spontaneous and episodic.[15] The sympathetic chain and eccrine glands are both histologically and functionally normal, suggesting that this is a central disease process, primarily affecting the portion of the hypothalamic sweat center controlling the palms and soles.[16] This cortical involvement of the disease is supported by the notion that patients typically do not experience emotional sweating in states of sleeping or sedation.[17]

Thoracolumbar sympathetic nerve fibres arise from the anterior column of the grey matter and travel with the anterior nerve roots to the sympathetic chain located vertically, parallel and adjacent to the vertebral column on either side. Pre-ganglionic fibres travel through the *white rami communicantes* to the corresponding ganglia. The thoracic sympathetic trunk contains 12 ganglia, which are located in front of the heads of the ribs posteriorly, covered by a thin layer of parietal pleura. Each ganglion is attached to the other via nervous cords measuring 1–2 mm in width – creating the sympathetic trunk. Aberrant anatomy composed of collateral nerves, double chains and Kuntz fibres (communicating sympathetic rami) may exist and require careful attention in the operative setting.[1] This apparatus serves as the means by which cortical thermoregulatory control is achieved via the hypothalamic preoptic sweat center.

The most probable explanation for focal hyper hidrosis is neurogenic over-activity of the reflex circuits innervating the eccrine glands. The exact nature and specifics linking this hyper-excitability to primary hyperhidrosis is unclear.[2] Recent evidence suggests generalized autonomic dysfunction (affecting both the sympathetic and parasympathetic nervous systems) as the key determinant in the

pathophysiology of hyperhidrosis[18]. Nonetheless, it is clear that the thoracic sympathetic ganglia (particularly at the levels of T2 and T3) is a centre-point in the mechanism of primary hyperhidrosis – serving as the passage way between the hypothalamus and the end organ, that is the eccrine glands[19].

Clinical presentation

Hyperhidrosis affects men and women equally, with the peak incidence being highest among younger working-age adults and the disorder being rare prior to the age of 12[20]. It is important to note that the incidence does not correspond with the onset of symptoms. Of note, women are more likely to seek medical attention (47.5 vs 28.6%).[21] No standardized definitions or quantitative measures exist for diagnostic purposes. Nonetheless, normal quantities of sweat have been determined to be <1 ml/m^2/min in one study. Hyperhidrotic patients can produce sweat in the excess of 40 ml/m^2/min[22]. Those quantitative thresholds obviously differ between individuals, with smaller individuals and women producing less sweat overall. As such, the parameters provided are reserved for research purposes and are difficult to apply in the clinical setting. Accordingly, diagnosis of hyperhidrosis is most commonly based on subjective patient reporting[2].

The majority of patients present due to the social implications and associated limitations of the disorder, which are most pronounced in the upper limb, particularly palmar hyperhidrosis[23,24]. Consequent to their condition, up to 35% of patients report decreased amounts of time spent pursuing leisure activities, and 22% report occupational consequences with decreased time spent at work[20]. In terms of morbidity, hyperhidrosis does not have a physiological bearing but nonetheless is significantly debilitating to patients. The Hyperhidrosis Disease Severity Scale is a simple four-point scale created to distinguish the extent of the psychosocial morbidity experienced by patients. A summary of the scale, as proposed by Strutton et al., is provided in Table 27.1[20].

Patient evaluation and indications for treatment

As mentioned previously, hyperhidrosis is relatively more common than patient presentation would indicate, a fact best supported by patient reluctance to

Table 27.1 Hyperhidrosis Disease Severity Scale

Points	Severity
1	Never noticeable, never interfering
2	Tolerable, sometimes interfering
3	Barely tolerable, frequently interfering
4	Intolerable and always interfering

Table 27.2 Diagnostic criteria for primary hyperhidrosis

Major criteria	Focal, visible, excessive sweating ≥6 months in the absence of secondary causes
Minor criteria (at least two)	Bilateral and symmetrical involvement At least one episode per week Impairment of daily activities Onset at age ≤25 Positive family history Cessation of sweating during sleep

seek care secondary to a lack of knowledge of the available treatment options[1]. Delineating the nature and specific presentation of hyperhidrosis is essential in providing patients with the most appropriate treatment. Disease onset, pattern (volume, areas involved, duration and nocturnal symptoms) and severity are important initial determinants used to identify the role for surgical intervention. Moreover, diligence must be taken in order to rule out secondary systemic causes of sweating[2].

Hornberger et al. suggested a set of diagnostic criteria to be employed in the diagnosis of primary hyperhidrosis. These include (1) focal, visible, excessive sweating for at least 6 months in the absence of secondary causes and (2) at least two of the following – bilateral symmetrical sweating, frequency of at least one episode per week, impairment of daily activities, age at onset <25 years, positive family history and cessation of sweating during sleep[25]. Essential to establishing the diagnosis and stratifying patients to optimal treatment options (surgical vs non-operative) is the careful delineation of the burden of disease on quality of life. Patients with more severe and debilitating disease (usually those with palmoplantar conditions) typically tend to be more satisfied with surgical intervention and are more likely to tolerate the associated side effects and possible complications that can occur[26]. Four characteristics have been associated with higher rates of satisfaction following thoracic sympathectomy. These include profound palmar sweating (with dripping), quantitatively elevated level of palmar sweating, bimodal onset (infancy or puberty) with symptoms worsening at the time of puberty and increasing stimulation of sweating with ordinary hand lotion or other tactile stimuli (Table 27.2)[27]. The Society of Thoracic Surgeons expert consensus panel outlined in 2011 the 'ideal candidate' for sympathectomy to be relatively young (<25), with early onset of disease, a BMI < 28, a resting heart rate > 55 bpm and no evidence of sweating during sleep[28].

The initial assessment of the patient should entail a detailed history and physical examination aimed at specifying risk factors, delineating the burden of disease on the patient quality of life and ruling out causes of secondary hyperhidrosis. The diagnosis is typically based on the presence of sweating that leads to functional impairment. Investigations are typically limited to ruling out secondary infections, metabolic or endocrine causes of hyperhidrosis. Diagnostic tests specific to idiopathic hyperhidrosis are not commonly used, but the most pertinent ones include gravimetric testing, the Minor starch-iodine test and the ninhydrin test. These are typically non-invasive and assess the presence and severity of sweating production at skin level. Essentially, once a patient's condition is deemed existent, and the extent clearly outlined, treatment is sought out – with different therapeutic options being offered based on the level of severity[2,3,26].

Surgical vs non-surgical treatment options

Treatment of hyperhidrosis is not solely surgical. In fact, a variety of non-operative therapeutic options exist, which are typically reserved for mild to moderate forms of the condition. The majority of these consist of topical agents that are applied directly to the affected area. These include: aluminum chloride hexahydrate ($AlCl_3 \cdot 6H_2O$), which blocks the lumen of eccrine glands, and anticholinergic agents, which function to decrease the local cholinergic impulse at the end organ of the eccrine gland[3]. Typically, topical agents are used as first-line treatment due to their ease of application and relative economic viability. The main side effect is skin irritation[11]. Oral agents in the form of anticholinergic muscarinic receptor competitive blockers are not as commonly used due to significant degree of side effects[3].

Iontophoresis (the passage of a galvanic current through skin that is submerged in water) has been used as first-line therapy for more severe cases. The principal function of iontophoresis is that the passage of current tends to disrupt and block the eccrine ducts. Contraindications to treatment include pacemakers, pregnancy and implanted metal devices[16,29]. Botulinum toxin intradermal injections can also be used in the treatment of hyperhidrosis. The toxin works to inhibit the release of the cholinergic neuro transmitter acetylcholine at the synaptic junction. Botulinum toxin therapy (similar to iontophoresis) can be used in the setting of failed topical therapy and is considered by many to be first-line treatment in the setting of craniofacial hyperhidrosis. Improved clinical outcomes occur within 2 weeks of treatment and will last on average 6–8 months[3]. Contraindications to treatment include hypersensitivity to albumin and history of peripheral neuropathies or neuromuscular junction disorders[15,30]. The main limiting factor for the usage of botulinum toxin injections is the fact that the effect is temporary, and the cost of treatment is substantial.

The Canadian Hyperhidrosis Advisory Committee recently used an evidence-based approach to outline a treatment of hyperhidrosis primarily based on the location and severity of the disorder. Essentially, for palmorplantar and axillary mild forms of the disease, first-line therapy should consist of topical aluminum chloride, with botulinum toxin and iontophoresis therapy as second-line options in refractory cases. The latter two options are reserved as first-line treatment options for severe cases, as well as craniofacial hyperhidrosis. According to the expert consensus panel, surgical intervention should be reserved for refractory cases that do not respond to any of the aforementioned treatment modalities[11]. It is important to note, however, that surgery is the only therapeutic option that offers permanent benefit, which is likely why it is becoming more actively sought out as compared to botulinum toxin intradermal injections[31].

Surgery in the treatment of hyperhidrosis is not a new phenomenon. However, with the emergence of minimally invasive thoracoscopy, surgery has emerged as a viable option in the treatment of particularly palmar and plantar hyperhidrosis. Thoracic sympathectomy has evolved with time from an invasive and technically demanding procedure to a simple minimally invasive, bilateral same-day operation[1,26,27]. With this progression and increased accessibility, the role of surgery in the treatment of hyperhidrosis has significantly developed. Initially, sympathectomy was performed via an open posterior approach (using paramedian incision around the vertebrae followed by resection of the proximal 3 cm of rib), as well as a supraclavicular approach (via dissection of the scalene muscle insertion without breaching of the pleura). More refined and potentially less morbid techniques were later developed, including the anterior transthoracic approach using a thoracotomy incision and the transaxillary approach entering the second intercostal space for more direct visualization of the sympathetic trunk in the superior sulcus. The latter approach has generated widespread acceptance, and is likely the next most feasible option in the case of failed thoracoscopic sympathectomy[26].

Surgical principles of thoracic sympathectomy

The first minimally invasive thoracic sympathectomy was performed in the 1950s by Kux, who described an endoscopic technique for the procedure[32]. Thoracoscopic sympathectomy for palmar hyperhidrosis emerged as the most definitive treatment in the early 1990s, and since then, several facets of the procedure have been under contention[33]. The procedure is performed with single or double-lumen endotracheal ventilation, with the patient in the supine position and in deep reverse Trendelenburg. This allows the non-ventilated lung to fall away from the superior sulcus. Bilateral sympathectomies can be performed during the same procedure, and patients may not require a chest tube following lung re-expansion. Insufflation of the hemithorax with carbon dioxide (not exceeding 10 mmHg in order to avoid tension pneumothorax) may be performed in order to increase the working space and improve visualization. Disruption of the sympathetic chain takes place on the anterior surface of the corresponding dorsal rib, with the level of thoracic chain disruption (T2, T3, T4, etc.) corresponding to the rib[26]. An important technical principle to consider is the presence of a communicating sympathetic ramus that crosses the second rib (Kuntz nerve). It may be prudent to attempt to locate this communicating nerve, if present, since incomplete disruption may lead to failure of the procedure with persistent transmission of sympathetic stimuli down the thoracic sympathetic chain[1,26]. However, it is unclear at the moment if there is any definitive benefit in disrupting the nerve of Kuntz, and some authors even doubt the existence of the nerve as an anatomical entity.

Variation exists with regards to the method of disruption as well as the level of disruption. The latter two principles comprise the majority of the controversy regarding thoracic sympathectomy in the treatment of hyperhidrosis[1,26,28,34].

It is important to establish definition in the case of such controversies. 'Sympathectomy' is defined as the removal/excision of the entire ganglion (ganglionectomy). This contrasts with 'sympathotomy', which is a mere disruption of the chain at the level of above the ganglion[26]. The majority of sympathetic input to the palms is derived at the level of T2. Transection of the stellate ganglion (T1) is associated with higher rates of Horner's syndrome. Moreover, it appears as though the higher the level of disruption, the greater is the risk of post-operative compensatory sweating (the most pertinent complication of thoracic sympathectomy)[35]. Several studies have attempted to identify the appropriate level and extent of disruption that would lead to the optimal results while minimizing compensatory sweating. Chang et al. compared disruption at T2 vs T3 vs T4 and reported comparable rates of improvement of palmar hyperhidrosis but greater incidence of compensatory sweating in the higher levels (93, 92 and 80%, respectively). The severity of the compensatory sweating was significantly less in the T4 group, but gustatory sweating was greater in that group (11.4% in T4, 23.1% in T3 and 5.8% in T2).[36] Moreover, it appears as though the extent of disruption (single vs multiple levels) may be a factor in compensatory sweating, with single-level disruption being associated with decreased rates of post-operative complications[37,38].

Several methods of sympathetic chain disruption exist, each with varying benefits and risks. Resection of the sympathetic ganglion (ganglionectomy) more accurately defines a true sympathectomy[26]. While more complete, this technique may potentiate increased rates of post-operative compensatory sweating[35]. Transection of the chain is usually performed superior to the rib and is typically performed using thermo-ablative methods via cautery. The advantage to this approach is that it necessitates less dissection and is relatively simple to perform[26]. Clipping over

the sympathetic trunk can be performed over the level of the rib or both above and below the ganglion (corresponding to a functional ganglionectomy). Although it requires more pleural dissection in order to clearly delineate the sympathetic chain, the main advantage of clipping is its reversibility, particularly in the case of severe compensatory sweating. Reversal (which entails simple removal of the clips) is not perfect, with higher failure rates outside a 2-week post-operative time window secondary to permanent perineural damage[39]. However, a few reports have shown acceptable results of up to 50% clinical reversibility when reversal is performed less than 6 months after the original sympathectomy[40].

The Society of Thoracic Surgeons Expert Consensus for the Surgical Treatment of Hyperhidrosis established the importance of a standardized nomenclature with regard to details of the operative approach used to perform the sympathectomy. This nomenclature is to include both the level and method of interruption of the sympathetic trunk. With regards to the anatomical level of interruption, it was felt that a rib-oriented approach is perhaps more appropriate than using the thoracic spine as the point of reference. Accordingly, a disruption at a specific level refers to interruption of the sympathetic chain above the corresponding rib. This allows for more clarity and transferability from patient to patient and takes into consideration the probability of anatomical variation that can cloud the accuracy of reporting based on the thoracic spine[28].

The panel also further outlined specific surgical guidelines based on disease site. For palmar hyperhidrosis, although having higher rates of compensatory sweating, the recommendation was to perform either a multi-level R3–R4 or single-level R4 interruptions. The latter is associated with lower rates of compensatory sweating, with the unfortunate potential for moister hands. In the case of palmoplantar hyperhidrosis, an R4–R5 disruption is recommended. The same holds true for patients who demonstrate axillary form of hyperhidrosis (even if combined with other sites of disease). In as much, craniofacial hyperhidrosis is to be treated with an R3 interruption, which has the dual effect of treating the condition, without the extra risk of Horner's syndrome and compensatory sweating that are associated with the R2 disruption. With regards to the method of interruption, there appears to be no specific recommendation made – implying that all forms are adequate in ensuring that there is enough separation between the ends of the chain to prevent regrowth.[28]

Complications and side effects

At the time of surgery, certain considerations must be taken in order to avoid potentially dangerous and life-threatening complications. The greatest complication of thoracic sympathectomy is failure of the procedure. Overall, failure rates are low, ranging from 0.2–3.7% in the literature[41]. Technical aspects are often the culprit, leading to failed thoracic sympathectomies. These include anatomical variations (Kuntz nerve, pleural adhesions and aberrant anatomy), nerve regeneration and incomplete disruption of the chain[41]. The latter is likely the greatest cause of failed sympathectomies[42]. Intraoperative pulse oxymetry can be used to monitor adequate disruption during clipping and transection. The instantaneous physiological response to sympathetic disruption is peripheral vasodilation, which can be depicted via change in the amplitude reading suggestive of increased peripheral circulation[43]. Moreover, left-sided sympathetic chain stimulation (particularly the stellate ganglion) can trigger ventricular tachycardia, and in some cases disruption of the sympathetic chain can lead to significant bradycardia. The latter cardiac complication can be a long-term side effect requiring pacemaker insertion – essentially sympathectomy leads to a beta-blockade effect, decreasing sympathetic tone to the heart and, in turn, decreasing heart rate and blood pressure. In fact, thoracic sympathectomy can uncommonly be used in the treatment of prolonged QT syndrome that is refractory to medical treatment[41,44].

The most significant and pertinent side effect pertaining to thoracic sympathectomy is the phenomenon of compensatory sweating, where the hyperhidrosis is essentially transferred from previously affected areas on the palms, feet and axillae to previously denervated areas[26,28,41]. Essentially, the body is separated into an anhidrotic segment above the nipple line and increased consequential sweating below the nipple line. Both mild (14–90%) and severe (1.2–31%) forms of compensatory sweating exist. The latter is characterized as split-body syndrome, where a part of the body previously suffering from excessive sweating becomes dead to sympathetic input, while the hidrotic segment of the body becomes hyperactive[41]. Conceptually, the number of functional eccrine sweat glands decreases by 40%, but the total amount of body sweating does not change – implying that residual sweat glands in previously unaffected parts compensate with increased sweat production. The exact mechanism by which this takes place is unclear but could potentially be the result of defective negative-feedback mechanisms that can no longer pass through the disrupted sympathetic chain. It is these severe forms of compensatory sweating that carry significant morbidity and functional detriment to patients, often leading to regret towards undergoing thoracic sympathectomy to treat their primary disorder[41,45].

As mentioned previously, the rates and severity of compensatory hyperhidrosis have been linked to two main technical concepts relating to thoracic sympathectomy: (1) the level of chain disruption and (2) the extent of disruption (single vs multi-level)[1,24,26,28]. A variety of evidence supports the notion that limiting the extent of resection decreases post-operative compensatory sweating. The level of selective disruption has also been associated with differential compensatory hyperhidrosis. T2 level disruption appears to have the highest rate of compensatory sweating, with lower levels having proportionately less. Accordingly, certain recommendations suggest sympathectomy at the T3–T4 level.[41] This is in relative contradiction to the notion that T2 level disruption typically leads to optimal outcomes in treating primary palmoplantar hyperhidrosis[28]. Treatment options for compensatory hyperhidrosis are limited, and the possibility of sympathectomy revision (mainly via removal of clips) exists, but to a limited extent[39]. Overall, the effect of compensatory sweating in consequence to idiopathic hyperhidrosis treatment is relative and subjective – based on patient values, tolerance and the initial morbidity associated with the primary disease[28].

Other less common side effects of thoracic sympathectomy include gustatory sweating, Horner's syndrome and phantom sweating. Gustatory sweating describes post-prandial facial sweating. The mechanism is unclear, but rates of gustatory sweating are lower than those of compensatory sweating (0–38%). Phantom sweating, on the other hand, is a sensation experienced by patients post-operatively, where sweat appears to be ready to secrete out of sweat glands, without its actual occurrence. Rates of phantom sweating vary in the literature from 0–59%. Finally, Horner's syndrome (with an incidence of 0.7–3%) is likely more of a concern in patients with craniofacial hyperhidrosis who may inadvertently receive an R2 interruption[28,41].

The aforementioned complications can occur relatively early post-operatively but typically employ a gradual and insidious course of onset, often developing over months. As such, expert consensus is that patient follow-up should occur at 1 month, 6 months, 1 year and yearly thereafter for at least 5 years[28]. Follow-up invokes on the surgeon a responsibility to adequately assess and address patient satisfaction and quality of life. As clearly outlined, more severe cases of hyperhidrosis tend to be more responsive and appreciative of surgical intervention[26,28,41]. Patients with facial blushing/sweating appear to have the least satisfaction, with those with palmoplantar hyperhidrosis having the most. Essentially, the post-operative complications of compensatory sweating (with its significant prevalence) is better tolerated by patients who had more severe primary disease. A study conducted in 2007 comparing patients receiving thoracic sympathectomy to counterparts who were refused coverage by insurance companies (although having the same indications) demonstrated that overall quality of life of the surgical arm (with regards to social, professional and cosmetic outcomes) was greater than in those not undergoing surgery. This is in the face of the potential adverse consequences of compensatory hyperhidrosis[46].

References

1   Shargall Y, Spratt E, Zeldin RA. Hyperhidrosis: what is it and why does it occur? *Thorac Surg Clin* 18 (2008): 125–32.

2   Solish N, Wang R, Murray CA. Evaluating the patient presenting with hyperhidrosis. *Thorac Surg Clin* 18 (2008): 133–40.

3   Gee S, Yamauchi PS. Nonsurgical management of hyperhidrosis. *Thorac Surg Clin* 18 (2008):141–55.

4   Glaser DA, Ladegaard L, Pilegaard HK. Primary focal hyperhidrosis: scope of the problem. *Cutis* 2007; 79(Suppl 5):5–17.

5   Adar R, Kurchi A, Zweig A et al. Palmar hyperhidrosis and its surgical treatment: surgical therapy hyperhidrosis. *Ann Surg* 1977; 186:37–41.

6   Strutton DR, Kowarlski JW, Glaser DA, et al. US prevalence of hyperhidrosis and impact on individual with axillary hyperhidrosis: results from a national survey. *J Am Acad Dermatol* 2004; 51:241–8.

7   Tu YR, Li X, Lin M, et al. Epidemiological survey of primary palmar hyperhidrosis in adolescent in Fuzhou of People's Republic of China. *Eur J Cardiothorac Surg* 2007; 31(4):737–9.

8   Solish N, Benohanian A, Kowalski JW. Prospective open-label study of botulinum toxin type A in patient with axillary hyperhidrosis: effects on functional impairment and quality of life. *Cuis* 2006; 77(Suppl 5): 17–27.

9   Lear W, Kessler E, Solish N, et al. An epidemiological study of hyperhidrosis. *Dermatol Surg* 2007; 33(1 Spec No.):S69–75.

10 Ro KM, Cantor RM, Lange KL, et al. Palmar hyperhidrosis: evidence of genetic transmission. *J Vasc Surg* 2002; 35(2):382–6.

11 Solish N, Bertucci V, Dansereau A, et al. A comprehensive approach to the recognition, diagnosis, and severity-based treatment of focal hyperhidrosis: recommendations for the Canadian Hyperhidrosis Advisory Committee. *Dermatol Surg* 2007; 33(8):908–23.

12 Hornberger J, Grimes K, Naumann M, et al. The multi-speciality working groupon the recognition diagnosis and treatment of primary focal hyperhidrosis: recognition, diagnosis and treatment of primary focal hyperhidrosis. *J Am Acad Dermatol* 2004; 51:274–86.

13 Kreyden OP, Scheidegger EP. Anatomy of the sweat glands, pharmacology of botulinum toxin, and distinctive syndromes associated with hyperhidrosis. *Clin Dermaol* 2004; 22:40–4.

14 Atkins JL, Butler PEM. Hyperhidrosis: a review of current management. *Plast Reconst Surg* 2002; 110(1):222–8.

15 Glaser DA, Hebert AA, Pariser DM, et al. Primary focal hyperhidrosis: scope of the problem. *Cutis* 2007; 79(Suppl 5):5–17.

16 Johnson RH, Spaulding, JM. Disorders of the autonomic nervous system. Chapter 10. Sweating. *Contemp Neurol Ser* 1974; 11:19–198.

17 Sato K, Kang WH, Saga K, et al. Biology of sweat glands and their disorders: normal sweat glands function. *J Am Acad Dermatol* 1989; 20:537–63.

18 Manca D, Valls-Sole J, Callejas MA. Excitability recovery curve of the sympathetic skin response in healthy volunteers and patients with palmar hyperhidrosis. *Clin Neurophysiol* 2000; 111(10):1767–70.

19 Kaya D, Karaca S, Barutcu I, et al. Heart rate variability in patients with essential hyperhidrosis: dynamic influence of sympathetic and

parasympathetic maneuvers. *Ann Noninvasive Electrocarciodol* 2005; 10(1):1–6.

20 Strutton DR, Kowalski JW, Glaser DA, et al. US prevalence of hyperhidrosis and impact on individuals with axillary hyperhidrosis: results from a national survey. *J Am Acad Dematol* 2004; 51(2):241–8.

21 Weksler B, Luketich JD, Shende M. Endoscopic Thoracic sympathectomy: at what level should you perform surgery? *Thorac Surg Clin* 18 (2008):183–91.

22 Sato K, Kang WH, Saga K, et al. Biology of sweat glands and their disorders. I. Normal sweat gland function. *J Am Acad Dermatology* 1989; 20(4):537–63.

23 Atkins JL, Butler PEM. Hyperhidrosis: a review of current management. *Plast Reconstr Surg* 2002; 110(1):222–8.

24 Amir M, Arish A, Weinstein Y, et al. Impairment in quality of life among patients in seeking surgery for hyperhidrosis (excessive sweating): preliminary results. *Isr J Psychiatry Relat Sci* 2000; 37(1):25–31.

25 Hornerger J, Grimes K, Naumann M, et al. Recognition, diagnosis and treatment of primary focal hyperhidrosis. *J Am Acad Dermatol.* 2004; 51(2):274–86.

26 Baumgartner FJ. Surgical approaches and techniques in the management of severe hyperhidrosis. *Thorac Surg Clin* 18 (2008):167–81.

27 Baumgartner FJ. Compensatory hyperhidrosis after thoracoscopic sympathectomy. *Ann Thorac Surg* 2005; 80:1161.

28 Cerfolio RJ, De Campos JR, Bryant AS, et al. The Society of Thoracic Surgeons Expert Consensus for the Surgical Treatment of Hyperhidrosis. *Ann Thorac Surg.* 2011 May; 91(5):1642–8.

29 Dolianitis C, Scarff CE, Kelly J, et al. Iontophoresis with glycopyrrolate for the treatment of palmoplantar hyperhidrosis. *Australas J Dermatol* 2004; 45(4):208–12.

30 Lowe NJ, Yamauchi PS, Lask GP, et al. Efficacy and safety of botulinum toxin type A in the treatment of palmar hypherhidrosis: a double-blind, randomized placebo-controlled study. *Dermatol Surg* 2002; 28(9):822–7.

31 Reisfeld R, Berliner KI. Evidence-based review of the nonsurgical management of hyperhidrosis. *Thorac Surg Clin* 18 (2008):157–66.

32 Kux E. Thoracic endoscopic sympathectomy in palmar and axillary hyperhidrosis. *Arch Surg* 1978; 113:264–6.

33 Lin C-C. A new method of thoracoscopic sympathectomy in hyperhidrosis palmaris. *Surg Endosc* 1990; 4:224–6.

34 Leseche G, Castier Y, Thabut G, et al. Endoscopic transthoracic sympathectomy for upper limb hyperhidrosis: limited sympathectomy does not reduce postoperative compensatory sweating, *J. Vasc Surg* 2003; 37:124–8.

35 Yazbek G, Nelson W, de Campos JRM, et al. Palmar hyperhidrosis–which is the best level of devervation using video-assisted thoracoscopic sympathectomy: T2 or T3 ganglion? *J Vasc Surg* 2005; 42:281–5.

36 Chang Y-T, Li H-P, Lee J-Y, et al. Treatment of palmar hyperhidrosis: T4 level compared with T3 and T2. *Ann Surg* 2007; 246:330–6.

37 Dewey TM, Hervert MA, Hill SL, et al. One-year follow-up after thoracoscopic sympathectomy for hyperhidrosis; outcomes and consequences. *Ann Thorac Surg* 2006; 81:1227–33.

38 Doolabh N, Horswell S, Williams M, et al. Thoracoscopic sympathectomy for hyperhidrosis: indications and results. *Ann Thorac Surg* 2004; 77:410–14.

39 Lin C-C, Mo L-R, Lee L-S, et al. Thoracoscopic T2-sympathetic block by clipping–a better and reversible operation for treatment of hyperhidrosis palmaris: experience with 326 cases. *Eur J Surg* 1998; 164(Suppl 580):13–16.

40 Sugimura H, Spratt EH, Compeau CG, et al. Thoracoscopic sympathetic clipping for hyperhidrosis: long-term results and reversibility. *J Thorac Cardiovasc Surg* 2009; 137(6):1370–6.

41 Dumont P. Side effects and complications of surgery for hyperhidrosis. *Thorac Surg Clin* 18 (2008):193–207.

42 De Campos JR, Kauffman P, Werebe E, et al. Quality of life, before and after thoracic sympathectomy: report on 378 operated patients. *Ann Thorac Surg* 2003; 76(3):886–91.

43 Klodell CT, Lobato EB, Willert JL, et al. Oximetry-derived perfusion index for intraoperative identification of successful thoracic sympathectomy. *Ann Thorac Surg* 2005; 80:467–70.

44 Hsu CP, Chen CY, Hsia JY, et al. Resympathectomy for palmar and axillary hyperhidrosis. *Br J Surg* 1998; 85:1504–5.

45 Shoenfield Y, Shapiro Y, Machtiger A, et al. Sweat studies in hyperhidrosis palmaris and plantaris: a survey of 60 patients before and after cervical sympathectomise. *Dermatologica* 1976; 152(5):257–62.

46 Boley T, Belangee K, Markwell S, et al. The effect of thoracoscopic sympathectomy on quality of life and symptom management of hyperhidrosis. *Ann Thorac Surg* 2003; 75:1075–9.

Index

AAH. *See* atypical adenomatous hyperplasia
AAT. *See* α-1 antitrypsin deficiency
abdominal closure, 245
ACCP, 9
achalasia, 229–31
  clinical presentation, 230
  diagnosis, 230
  etiology, 230
  indications for surgery, 231–2
  non-surgical management, 231
  operations, 232
  surgical results, 232
  testing, 231
  treatment, 230–1
acidic agents, 224
Actinomyces, 97
active drainage, 180–1
acute respiratory distress syndrome (ARDS), 194
adenocarcinoma
  clear cell, 130
  growth patterns, 130
  histological classification of, 131–2
  lung cancer, 130–1
  micropapillary, 130
  minimally invasive, 130–1
  risk-adjusted survival, 237
  signet ring, 130
adenocarcinoma in situ (AIS), 130–1
adenoid cystic carcinoma
  lung, 137
  trachea, 51–2
adenosquamous carcinoma
  histological classification of, 131–2
  lung, 131
adjuvant chemotherapy
  in elderly patients, 144
  lung cancer and, 140
  meta-analyses, 143
  molecular prognostic and predictive markers, 144–5
  optimal regimen, 143
  randomized phase III studies, 141
  stage I treatment, 143–4
Adjuvant Navelbine International Trial Association (ANITA) trial, 141–2
adjuvant radiotherapy, 145

AFB. *See* auto-fluorescence bronchoscopy
airway bypass tract stent placement, 82
airway obstruction, 254
alcohol, 86
ALK gene rearrangements, 134
alkali agents, 224
α-1 antitrypsin deficiency (AAT), 76
alveolar hemorrhage, 111
anastomosis, 53
Ancona, 182
ANITA trial. *See* Adjuvant Navelbine International Trial Association trial
anterior approach, VATS, 31–2
  advantages, 32
anterior mediastinal surgery, 161
anterior thoracotomies
  indications for, 31
  open approach in supine position, 30–1
  pitfalls, 31
antibiotics
  for bronchopleural fistula, 195–7
  for empyema, 88–9
  for lung abscess, 98
aorta, 263
APC. *See* argon plasma coagulation
ARDS. *See* acute respiratory distress syndrome
argon plasma coagulation (APC)
  complications, 42
  equipment, 42
  indications, 42
  results, 42
  therapeutic bronchoscopy, 41–2
aspergilloma, 96
aspergillosis
  cavernostomy for, 100–2
  complications, 97–101
  diagnosis, 99–100
  etiology, 99
  indications for surgery, 100
  invasive, 99
  management, 100
  microbiology, 99
  myoplasty for, 100
  operative approaches, 100–1
  pathophysiology, 99

  prognosis, 97–101
  thoracoplasty for, 100–1
  VATS for, 101
Aspergillus, 97
asthma, 48
atelectasis, 2, 19
atypical adenomatous hyperplasia (AAH), 129
auto-fluorescence bronchoscopy (AFB), 45
axillary thoracotomy
  indications and advantages, 28
  open approach in lateral decubitus, 28
  pitfalls, 28
azygos vein, 17
azygous venous system, 151–2

Bacteroides, 87
BAE. *See* bronchial artery embolization
balloon dilatation, 231
barium swallow, 228, 231
Barrett's esophagus, 242
benign tracheal tumors, 51–2
  squamous papilloma, 51
Beta-hemolytic streptococci, 87
bilateral thoracosternotomy
  clamshell incision, 30
  indications, 30
  open approach in supine position, 30
  pitfalls, 30
biologic lung reduction, 81–2
Blastomyces, 97
bleach, 224
blunt chest trauma, 253
BMI. *See* body-mass index
Bochdalek hernias, 216–17
body-mass index (BMI), 78–84
body plethysmography, 6–10
botulinum toxin, 230–1
Boyle's law, 6–10
brachytherapy (BT), 236
  complications, 44
  high dose rate, 43
  indications and results, 43–4
  low dose rate, 43
  medium dose rate, 43
  patient preparation, 43–4
  therapeutic bronchoscopy, 43–4

275

BRAF, 134
breast cancer, 174
bronchial artery embolization (BAE), 109–10
bronchial atresia, 59–60
bronchial lavage, 40
bronchial rupture, 255–6
bronchioalveolar carcinoma, 61, 130
bronchogenic cysts, 59
bronchopleural fistula, 45
  antibiotics for, 195–7
  bronchoscopy for, 196
  clinical presentation, 194
  definition, 193
  empyema and, 196
  etiology, 193
  imaging, 194–5
  large, 195–6
  post-operative factors, 193–4
  risk factors, 193–4
  surgical avoidance, 195
  treatment, 195–7
bronchopulmonary carcinoma, 64–5
bronchopulmonary neuroendocrine tumors, 135
bronchopulmonary sequestrations, 59–63
bronchoscopic laser
  classification, 42
  complications, 43
  indications for, 42–3
  methods for, 42–3
  results, 43
  therapeutic bronchoscopy, 41–2
bronchoscopic thermal vapor ablation (BTVA), 82
bronchoscopy, 48. *See also* therapeutic bronchoscopy
  for bronchopleural fistula, 196
  clearing of airway, 40
  diagnostic yield of, 118
  hemoptysis, 107, 109
  in lung abscess, 98
bronchospasm, 2
BT. *See* brachytherapy
BTS, 1–9
BTVA. *See* bronchoscopic thermal vapor ablation

calcium channel blockers, 230
CALGB9633 trial, 142–3
cancer specific methods (CSM), 43
Cantrell's pentalogy, 206
carbon monoxide, 4
carcinoid tumors, 131–2, 135–6
cardiac contusion, 264
cardiac injuries, 264
cardiac surgery, 203
cardiopulmonary bypass (CPBP), 153

cardiopulmonary exercise test (CPET), 1–8
caustic injuries, 242
caustics, ingestion of
  clinical presentation, 224
  common agents, 224
  initial management, 224–5
  long-term management, 225
  pathophysiology, 224
cavernostomy, 100–2
CCAM. *See* congenital cystic adenomatoid malformations
Centers for Medicare and Medicaid (CMS), 70
central diaphragm paralysis, 214
cervical mediastinoscopy, 124
cervical perforations, 245
cervical stimulation tests, 210–11
cervicothoracic CT scan, 210
cervicothoracic MRI, 210
chemotherapy. *See* adjuvant chemotherapy; neo-adjuvant chemotherapy
chest cavity access
  incision choice, 25
  minimally invasive approaches, 31–3
    hybrid approaches, 33–4
  open approach in lateral decubitus
    axillary thoracotomy, 28
    muscle-sparing antero-lateral thoracotomy, 27–8
  open approach in supine position
    bilateral thoracosternotomy, 30
    median sternotomy, 28–30
  open approaches in lateral decubitus, 25
    muscle-sparing postero-lateral thoracotomy, 26–7
    postero-lateral thoracotomy, 25–6
  patient positioning, 25
chest radiograph
  empyema, 92–3
  of eventration, 210–11
chest trauma
  airway obstruction in, 254
  aorta and, 263
  blunt, 253
  bronchial rupture and, 255–6
  cardiac contusion and, 264
  cardiac injuries and, 264
  chest wall in, 257
  commotio cordis, 264
  diaphragm in, 261–6
  esophageal injuries and, 261
  flail chest, 259
  hemothorax in, 256–7
  hilar vessels in, 263
  imaging studies, 254
  initial evaluation, 254

  intrathoracic trachea in, 255
  laryngotracheal injury and, 254–5
  lung contusion in, 257
  lung laceration in, 256–8
  missile embolization and, 264–6
  penetrating, 253–4
  pericardial tamponade and, 264
  pneumothorax in, 256
  from resuscitative thoracotomy, 265
  rib fractures in, 258–9
  sternoclavicular dislocation and, 255
  systemic air embolism, 263–4
  thoracic duct and, 262–6
  tracheal compression and, 255
  traumatic asphyxia, 260
chest tube drainage, 190–1
chest wall, 257
  defects, 260
chest X-ray, 64
  esophageal perforation, 243
chondroma, 51
chronic obstructive pulmonary disease (COPD), 69
  lung reduction in, 69–70
  NETT and, 77
cisplatin, 142–3
clavicle fractures, 260–1
clear cell adenocarcinoma, 130
clindamycin, 98
closing volume (CV), 2
CMS. *See* Centers for Medicare and Medicaid
CO_2 laser, 42
Cobb angle, 200
Coccidioides, 97
colorectal cancer, 173
commotio cordis, 264
compensatory sweating, 272
computed tomography (CT)
  cervicothoracic, 210
  for empyema, 87–8, 95–6
  esophageal perforation, 243
  in hemoptysis, 107
  in lung cancer staging, 123
congenital chest wall deformities, 199
  incidence of, 199
congenital cystic adenomatoid malformations (CCAM), 59–60
congenital diaphragmatic hernia, 216
congenital emphysema, 63–4
congenital pulmonary airway malformation (CPAM)
  with multiple cysts, 61
  prenatal exam, 59
contrast swallow, 243
COPD. *See* chronic obstructive pulmonary disease
CPAM. *See* congenital pulmonary airway malformation

CPBP. *See* cardiopulmonary bypass
CPET. *See* cardiopulmonary exercise test
CR, 86
C-reactive protein (CRP), 86
Cross trial, 237
CRP. *See* C-reactive protein
cryotherapy
  complications, 41
  indications for, 41
  instrumentation, 41
  results, 41
  therapeutic bronchoscopy, 41
Cryptococcus, 97
CSM. *See* cancer-specific methods
CT. *See* computed tomography
Cushing's syndrome, 135–6
CV. *See* closing volume
cystic fibrosis, 111
cystic lesions, 59–60
cystic lung malformations, 58
  post-natal diagnosis, 60–1

da Vinci, Leonardo, 199–200
da Vinci Surgical System, 158
DDR2, 135
diaphragm disorders, 209
  chest trauma and, 261–6
  ultrasound of, 210
diaphragmatic paralysis (DP), 209
  central, 214
  general considerations, 214
  reconditioning, 216
  results, 209–16
  surgical technique, 215
  technical aspects, 215
  unilateral, 209
diffuse esophageal spasm, 231
diffuse idiopathic neuroendocrine cell hyperplasia (DIPNECH), 129
diffusion constant, 4
Digivent, 182
DIPNECH. *See* diffuse idiopathic neuroendocrine cell hyperplasia
diverticuli, 227
  epiphrenic, 228
  indications for surgery, 228
  non-surgical management, 228
  operations, 228–9
  parabronchial, 229
  presentation, 227–8
  surgical complications, 229
  surgical results, 229
  thoracic, 228
  types, 227
double-lumen tube, 19
DP. *See* diaphragmatic paralysis
drug use, 86
Dumon stents, 45

dysphasia, 110
dyspnea, 1

EASE. *See* Exhale Airway Stents for emphysema trial
EBUS. *See* endobronchial ultrasound
EBV. *See* endobronchial one way valves; Epstein-Barr virus
EELV. *See* end-expiratory lung volume
EGFR. *See* epidermal growth factor
elderly patients, 144
electrocautery, 41
electrodiathermy, 41
electronic drainage systems, 181–2
electrophysiological study, 210–11
emphysema, congenital, 63–4
empyema
  alcohol and, 86
  antibiotics for, 88–9
  bacteriology of, 87
  bronchopleural fistula and, 196
  chest radiograph, 92–3
  in children, 92–7
  CT for, 87–8, 95–6
  diagnosis, 87
  drug use and, 86
  etiology, 86
  history of, 86
  imaging, 87–8
  indications for surgery, 89
  intrapleural fibrinolytics for, 89
  management, 88
  microbiology, 86–7
  open window thoracostomy for, 91
  operative approaches
    debridement, 90
    decortication, 90
    drainage, 89–90
  pathophysiology, 86–7
  pleural aspiration in, 88
  pleural fluid drainage for, 88
  post-pneumonectomy, 91–6
  prognosis, 89
  stages of, 86–7
  thoracoplasty for, 90–1
  time scale, 86–7
  US for, 88
end-expiratory lung volume (EELV), 69–70
endobronchial one-way valves (EBV), 79–80
endobronchial ultrasound (EBUS), 11, 117
  combined EUS, 13
    patient selection, 13–14
  complications, 14–15
  linear probe, 11–12
    in isolated mediastinal lymphadenopathy diagnosis, 14

lung cancer staging, 124
  mediastinoscopy and, 18–19
  radial probe, 11
  training, 15
Endobronchial Valve for Emphysema Palliation Trial (VENT), 79–80
endoscopic ultrasound (EUS), 12, 235–6
  combined EBUS, 13
    patient selection, 13–14
endoscopy
  esophageal perforation, 243, 245–7
  tracheal masses, 52
  tracheal stenosis, 52
EphA2, 134
epidermal growth factor (EGFR), 133
epinephrine, 109
epiphrenic diverticuli, 228
Epstein-Barr virus (EBV), 127–8
ERCC1. *See* excision repair cross-complementation group 1
erlotinib, 133
ERS, 9
ERV. *See* expiratory reserve volume
esophageal cancer
  clinical presentation, 234–5
  epidemiology, 234
  etiology, 234
  investigations, 235
  staging, 235–6
  surgical anatomy, 234
  surgical outcomes, 239
  surgical treatment, 236
  systemic, 236–7
  treatment, 236–9
esophageal injury, 261
esophageal perforation, 240
  abdominal closure, 245
  caustic injuries, 242
  cervical perforations, 245
  chest X-ray, 243
  clinical features, 242–3
  contrast swallow, 243
  CT, 243
  endoscopy, 243, 245–7
  esophagectomy, 245
  etiology, 240–1
  extra-luminal causes, 242
  foreign-body injury, 241–2
  iatrogenic injuries, 240–1
  infections and, 242
  initial management, 244–5
  intraluminal causes, 240–1
  intrathoracic closure, 245
  malignancy and, 242
  non-operative management, 245
  operative injuries, 242
  pathophysiology, 240
  results, 247–8

esophageal perforation (cont.)
symptoms and signs of, 242–3
thoracoscopy for, 245
traumatic, 242
treatment, 244
esophagectomy
for esophageal perforation, 245
minimally invasive, 238
robotic, 163
ESTS, 9
EUS. *See* endoscopic ultrasound
eventration, 209
chest radiograph of, 210–11
contraindications for surgery,
210–11
electrophysiologic study of, 210–11
full-night polysomnography, 210
indication for surgery, 210–11
open thoracic approach, 211
plication, 211
pulmonary function tests, 210
surgical objectives, 211
surgical results, 211
excision repair cross-complementation
group 1 (ERCC1), 144–5
exercise, 77–8
exercise testing
complex, 1–8
intermediate, 8
lung function assessment, 7–8
shuttle walk test, 8
simple, 8
six-minute walk test, 8
stair climbing, 8
Exhale Airway Stents for Emphysema
(EASE) trial, 82
expiratory airflow, 2
expiratory reserve volume (ERV), 1–2
external thoracic venous system, 152
extra-thoracic metastases, 168–9

FEV1. *See* forced expiratory volume in
one second
FFB. *See* flexible fiberoptic
bronchoscope
FGF. *See* fibroblast growth factor
FGFR1, 134
fibroblast growth factor (FGF), 58
Fick's law, 4
58 Fr bougie, 229
fine-needle aspiration (FNA), 117
flail chest, 259
Fleischner Society, 117
flexible fiberoptic bronchoscope (FFB),
39
as diagnostic tool, 39
in therapeutic bronchoscopy, 39–40
floppy posterior fundoplication, 223
flow-volume loop, 2–6

FNA. *See* fine-needle aspiration
forced expiratory volume in one second
(FEV1), 2–4
ppo, 7
volume-time curve in, 3–6
forced vital capacity (FVC), 1–2
foreign bodies
injury, 241–2
retrieval, 40–1
FRC. *See* functional residual capacity
French Thoracic Cooperative Group,
145
full-night polysomnography, 210
functional residual capacity (FRC), 1–2
Fusobacterium, 87
FVC. *See* forced vital capacity

galactomannan antigen, 100
gas dilution, 4–6
gastroesophageal reflux disease
(GERD), 221
basic physiology, 221
indications for surgery, 221–2
operations, 222–3
Gastrografin, 53
gefitinib, 133, 142
GERD. *See* gastroesophageal reflux
disease
GGOs. *See* ground glass opacifications
Gianturco stents, 45
ground-glass opacifications (GGOs),
116
gustatory sweating, 272–3

Haemophilus influenzae, 87, 97
helium-neon aiming beam, 42
hemidiaphragm, 209
hemoptysis
bronchoscopy, 107, 109
causes, 105–6
CT in, 107
in cystic fibrosis, 111
definition, 105
epinephrine for, 109
examination, 106–10
investigations, 106–7
localizing, 109
management of, 107–8
massive, 105, 108–9
mortality rates, 105
Nd:YAG laser in, 109
patient history, 105–10
key aspects in, 107
stable patients, 109
surgery, 110–11
vasculitis and, 111
hemostasia, 26, 30
hemothorax, 256–7
heparin, 153

HER2 status, 235
hernia sac removal, 226–7
hiatal hernias, 225
clinical presentation, 225–6
complications, 227
indication for surgery, 226
surgical results, 227
type I, 225
type II, 225
type III, 225
type IV, 225
hilar vessels, 263
Histoplasma, 97
Horner's syndrome, 272–3
HOXb-5, 58
human papilloma virus (HPV), 127–8
hydrops, 59–60
hypercalcemia, 128
hyperechogenic lesions, 59–60
prenatal treatment of, 60
hyperhidrosis
clinical presentation, 268–9
complications, 272–3
diagnostic criteria, 269
disease severity scale, 269
epidemiology, 267
etiology, 267
non-surgical treatment, 269–70
pathophysiology, 267–8
patient evaluation, 268–9
surgical side effects, 272–3
surgical treatment, 269–70
thoracic sympathectomy, 270–2
hypertensive lower esophageal
sphincter, 231
hypoxemia, 14–15

IALT. *See* International Adjuvant Lung
Cancer Trial
iatrogenic injuries, 240–1
iatrogenic tracheoesophageal fistula, 53
immunohistochemical (IHC) analysis,
144–5
induction chemotherapy, 146–7
infectious tracheoesophageal fistula, 53
inframammary skin, 30
infrastomal lesions, 49
inhalation injury, 50
innominate artery, 17
innominate vein, 30–3
intercostal spaces, 30
internal mammary artery injury, 203
internal thoracic venous system, 152
International Adjuvant Lung Cancer
Trial (IALT), 142
International Registry of Lung
Metastases, 167–8
intracystic mucinous cell clusters, 61
intraluminal obstruction, 50

intrapleural fibrinolytics, 89
intrapleural pressure, 2
  airflow, 183
  tube thoracostomy, 181–5
intrathoracic closure, 245
intrathoracic trachea, 255
isolated mediastinal lymphadenopathy,
    14

Jarcho-Levin syndrome, 207
JBR10 trial, 140–1
Jeune's disease, 206–7

Kaplan-Meier estimates, 74–5
Kirsten rat sarcoma viral oncogene
    homolog (KRAS), 133–4
Klebsiella pneumoniae, 87, 97
KRAS. *See* Kirsten rat sarcoma viral
    oncogene homolog
K-ras mutations, 61

laparoscopic partial fundoplication,
    229
laparoscopy
  history, 214
  results, 214
  technical aspects, 214
large cell carcinoma
  histological classification of, 131–2
  lung, 131
  neuroendocrine, 136
laryngeal stenosis, 49
laryngotracheal injury, 254–5
lateral decubitus, open approaches in,
    25
  muscle-sparing antero-lateral
    thoracotomy, 27–8
  muscle-sparing postero-lateral
    thoracotomy, 26–7
  postero-lateral thoracotomy, 25–6
lateral suture, 212
lateral thoracotomy, 171
left anterior mediastinoscopy, 124
left carotid artery, 17
left recurrent nerve, 17
lepidic predominant adenocarcinoma,
    130
LES. *See* lower esophageal sphincter
LigaSure, 19
linear probe EBUS, 11–12
  in isolated mediastinal
    lymphadenopathy diagnosis, 14
lobectomy, 7
  robotic surgical system, 161
  VATS, 160–1
    uniportal approach, 33
loculations, 19
lower esophageal sphincter (LES), 221
  hypertensive, 231

LU22, 145–6
lung
  biopsy, 31
  contusion, 257
  laceration, 256–8
  morphogenesis, 58
  small cell carcinoma, 136
lung abscess
  anaerobic bacteria in, 97
  antibiotics for, 98
  bronchoscopy in, 98
  clinical features, 97–8
  complications, 98–9
  diagnosis, 98
  etiology, 97
  indications for surgery, 98–9
  investigation, 98
  management, 98
  microbiology, 97
  pathophysiology, 97
  percutaneous drainage, 98
  prognosis, 99
  risk factors, 99
  segmental localization in, 97
lung cancer, 127
  adenocarcinoma, 130–1
  adenoid cystic carcinoma, 137
  adenosquamous carcinoma, 131
  adjuvant chemotherapy after surgical
    resection, 140
  ALK gene rearrangements in,
    134
  ANITA trial, 141–2
  atypical adenomatous hyperplasia,
    129
  BRAF in, 134
  CALGB9633 trial, 142
  carcinoid tumors, 135–6
  carcinoma in situ, 128–9
  clinical effects, 128
  DDR2 in, 135
  diagnosis, 12–13
  diffuse idiopathic neuroendocrine
    cell hyperplasia, 129
  EGFR in, 133
  EphA2 in, 134
  FGFR1 in, 134
  field effect, 129
  histological classification of, 131–2
  IALT, 142
  immunophenotypical characterization
    of, 131–2
  incidence, 127–8
  JBR10 trial, 140–1
  large cell carcinoma, 131
  mediastinoscopy and, 17–18
  meta-analyses, 142–3
  molecular prognostic and predictive
    markers, 144–5

mucoepidermoid carcinoma, 137
  non-small cell, 133
  p53 in, 134–5
  PIK3CA in, 134
  preinvasive lesions, 128
  primary pulmonary lymphoma,
    137–8
  prognosis, 128
  PTEN in, 134
  radical surgery for, 9
  risk factors, 127–8
  robotic surgical systems for, 160–1
  salivary gland tumors and, 136–7
  sarcomatoid carcinoma, 131–3
  squamous cell carcinoma, 129–30
  squamous dysplasia, 128–9
  staging, 12–13
    cervical mediastinoscopy, 124
    clinical presentation, 121
    CT in, 123
    EBUS, 124
    groups, 121–2
    invasive staging, 124
    investigations, 123
    left anterior mediastinoscopy,
      124
    migration, 124–5
    MRI in, 123
    multi-disciplinary team, 122–3
    PET in, 123
    radionuclide bone scans, 123–4
    scalene biopsy, 124
    supraclavicular node biopsy, 124
    systems, 121
    TNM, 17
    trans-thoracic needle biopsy,
      124
  targeted agents, 142
  UFT for, 142
  VATS for staging, 19–22
lung congenital malformations, 58
  post-natal treatment, 64–5
  pre-natal diagnosis, 59–60
  surgical procedures, 65
lung function assessment
  common measurements, 2–4
  examination, 1
  exercise testing, 7–8
  history, 1
  lung volume in, 1–2
  LVRS and, 77
  in pre-operative assessment, 8–9
  smoking history and, 1
  spirometry in, 2
  transfer factor in, 4
lung volume
  biologic reduction, 81–2
  BTVA for reduction of, 82
  in lung function assessment, 1–2

lung volume reduction surgery (LVRS), 69
  air leak following, 75–6
  α-1 antitrypsin deficiency in, 76
  BMI and, 78–84
  cardiopulmonary morbidity, 74–5
  in COPD, 69–70
  cost-effectiveness of, 78
  data analysis, 71–2
  effects of, 76
  exercise and, 77–8
  high risk for death subgroup, 73
  history of, 70
  lung function and, 77
  MS, 76
  non-surgical investigative
    approaches to, 79
  operative mortality, 74–5
  outcome prediction, 77
  outcome prediction in non-high-risk
    NETT patients, 73
  oxygenation and, 77
  patient selection, 76–7
  perfusion scintigraphy, 76–7
  pulmonary hemodynamics and, 77
  self-activating coils, 80–1
  surgical and anesthetic procedures, 71
  underperformance of, 78–9
  underutilization of, 78–9
  VATS, 76
    uniportal approach, 32
lung volumes, 4–6
LUNGART study, 145
LVRS. See lung volume reduction
    surgery
lymph nodes
  dissection, 238
  pulmonary metastasectomy and,
    168–72

M1a, 19
macro-cystic malformations, 60
MAGE-A3 antigen, 142
magnetic resonance imaging (MRI)
  cervicothoracic, 210
  in lung cancer staging, 123
major complication composite
  (MCC), 79–80
malignant tracheal tumors, 50–1
  adenoid cystic carcinoma, 51–2
  chondroma, 51
  squamous cell carcinoma, 51
malignant tracheoesophageal fistula, 53
MALT. See mucosa-associated
    lymphoid tissue
Mayo Clinic, 182
MCC. See major complication
    composite

median sternotomy
  advantages of, 29
  following thymectomy, 30–3
  LVRS, 76
  for mediastinal mass excision,
    30–3
  open approach in supine position,
    28–30
  pitfalls, 29
  SVC syndrome, 153
mediastinal mass, 30–3
mediastinal nodal disease, 19
mediastinal shift, 59–60
mediastinal staging, 13
  re-staging after neo-adjuvant
    chemotherapy, 14
mediastinoscopy, 13
  EBUS and, 18–19
  lung cancer and, 17–18
  surgical anatomy video of, 17
Medical Research Council, 212
  dyspnoea scale, 1
melanoma, 174
MIA. See minimally invasive
    adenocarcinoma
micropapillary adenocarcinoma,
    130
minimally invasive adenocarcinoma
    (MIA), 130–1
minimally invasive approaches, chest
    cavity access, 31–3
  hybrid approaches, 33–4
minimally invasive esophagectomy,
    238
minimally invasive repair (MIRPE)
  pectus carinatum, 205
  pectus excavatum, 201
minimally invasive thoracic surgery,
    158
MIRPE. See minimally invasive repair
missile embolization, 264–6
MIST2. See Multi-Centre Intrapleural
    Sepsis Trial 2
Montgomery type stents, 45
Morgagni-Larrey hernias, 217
  VATS of, 216–17
motility disorders, 229
MRI. See magnetic resonance imaging
mucoepidermoid carcinoma, 137
mucosa-associated lymphoid tissue
    (MALT), 137–8
Multi-Centre Intrapleural Sepsis Trial 2
    (MIST2), 89
multicystic malformation, 60
multistation N2 disease, 19
multistation N3 disease, 19
muscle-sparing antero-lateral
    thoracotomy
  indications, 28

open approach in lateral decubitus,
    27–8
  pitfalls, 28
muscle-sparing postero-lateral
    thoracotomy
  indications and advantages, 27
  open approaches in lateral decubitus,
    26–7
  operative view in, 26–7
  pitfalls, 27
myasthenia gravis, 161–2
myoplasty, 100
myotomy, 229
  robotic Heller, 163

National Cancer Institute of Canada
    (NCIC), 140–1
National Emphysema Treatment Trial
    (NETT), 70–1
  COPD and, 77
  cost-effectiveness in, 78
  exclusion criteria, 71–2
  inclusion criteria, 71
  long-term follow-up, 73–4
  LVRS outcomes in non-high-risk, 73
  primary outcomes, 72–3
NCIC. See National Cancer Institute of
    Canada
Nd:YAG laser, 42
  in hemoptysis, 109
needle aspiration, 190
neo-adjuvant chemotherapy
  mediastinal re-staging after, 14
  randomized phase III trials, 146
NETT. See National Emphysema
    Treatment Trial
neutrophil phagocytosis, 86–7
NICE guidelines, 107
nitrosaminoketone (NNK), 127–8
non-seminomatous testicular germcell
    tumor, 174
non-small cell lung cancer, 133
NOTCH-1c, 58
nutcracker esophagus, 231

open approach in lateral decubitus
  axillary thoracotomy, 28
  muscle-sparing antero-lateral
    thoracotomy, 27–8
open approach in supine position
  anterior thoracotomies, 30–1
  bilateral thoracosternotomy, 30
  median sternotomy, 28–30
open approaches in lateral decubitus,
    25
  muscle-sparing postero-lateral
    thoracotomy, 26–7
  postero-lateral thoracotomy, 25–6
open window thoracostomy, 91

operative injuries, 242
osteosarcoma, 173–4
oxygenation, 77

p53, 134–5
PAL. *See* prolonged air leak
parabronchial diverticuli, 229
paraneoplastic syndromes, 128
parietal pleura, 26
passive drainage, 180
PDT. *See* photodynamic therapy
pectus arcuatum, 204
pectus carinatum, 203–4
    minimally invasive repair, 205
    open repair, 204
    self-adjustable bracing for, 205
pectus excavatum, 199–201
    age of repair, 202–3
    cardiac surgery and, 203
    complications, 202
    development of, 200
    incision, 203
    internal mammary artery injury,
        203
    multi-disciplinary approach, 203
    prosthetic reconstruction, 201
    psychological impact of, 200
    resuscitation, 203
    symmetry of deformity, 203
    treatment, 200–1
penetrating chest trauma, 253–4
percutaneous drainage, 98
perfusion scintigraphy, 76–7
pericardial tamponade, 264
peripheral pulmonary nodule, 22
persistent mediastinal compressive
        effect, 59–60
PET. *See* positron emission
        tomography
PFS, 146–7
phantom sweating, 272–3
photodynamic therapy (PDT)
    in early-stage disease, 45
    in late-stage disease, 45
    phases of, 44
    results, 45
    therapeutic bronchoscopy, 44–5
    tissue destruction in, 44
PIK3CA, 134
platelet-derived growth factor-B, 58
pleural effusion, 19
pleural fluid drainage, 88
pleuropneumoblastoma, 61
plication
    eventration, 211
    history, 213
    results, 213–14
    technical aspects, 213
pneumatic dilation, 231

pneumothorax
    in chest trauma, 256
    chest tube drainage, 190–1
    clinical classification of, 188
    definition, 188–9
    epidemiology, 188–9
    follow-up, 191
    needle aspiration for, 190
    observation, 190
    pathogenesis, 189
    prevention, 191
    spontaneous, 188
        diagnostic approaches, 189–90
        primary, 188
        secondary, 188–9
    treatment, 190–1
Poland's syndrome, 205
    sternal cleft, 205–6
    sternal defects, 205
    thoracic ectopia cordis, 206
polypoid endobronchial growth, 135
polytetrafluoroethylene (PTFE), 150
PORT. *See* post-operative radiotherapy
positron emission tomography (PET),
        117
    in lung cancer staging, 123
posterior approach, VATS, 31
    advantages, 31
    pitfalls, 31
posterior crural closure, 223
posterolateral thoracotomy, 171
    indications and advantages, 26
    muscle-sparing, 26–7
    open approaches in lateral decubitus,
        25–6
    pitfalls, 26
    skin marks of, 26–33
postintubation stenosis
    infrastomal lesions, 49
    laryngeal stenosis, 49
    management, 49–50
    points of occurrence, 49
    stoma site obstruction, 49
    tracheal intramural lesions, 50–6
post-operative radiotherapy (PORT),
        145
post-pneumonectomy empyema, 91–6
post-therapeutic tracheal stenosis, 50
PPB. *See* pulmonary pleuroblastoma
predicted postoperative (ppo) lung
        function, 6–7
    confounding factors, 7–10
    FEV1, 7
    segment counting, 6–7
    transfer factor, 7
preinvasive lesions, 128
    histological classification of, 131–2
primary pulmonary lymphoma,
        137–8

primary spontaneous pneumothorax
        (PSP), 188
    epidemiology, 188–9
prolonged air leak (PAL)
    avoidance of, 179
    tube thoracostomy for, 179–80
proton pump inhibitors, 222
Pseudomonas aeruginosa, 87
PSP. *See* primary spontaneous
        pneumothorax
PTEN, 134
PTFE. *See* polytetrafluoroethylene
pulmonary angiography, 110
pulmonary blastoma, 132–3
pulmonary function tests, 210
pulmonary hemodynamics, 77
pulmonary metastasectomy, 167
    ablative techniques, 173
    breast cancer, 174
    colorectal cancer, 173
    for extra-thoracic metastases control,
        168–9
    five-year survival, 168
    for identification, 169
    indications for, 168
    lymph node involvement, 168–72
    melanoma, 174
    non-seminomatous testicular
        germcell tumor, 174
    osteosarcoma, 173–4
    pre-operative exam, 170
    primary tumor control, 168
    rationale for, 167–8
    for recurrent metastases, 168–73
    in soft tissue sarcoma, 173
    surgical approach, 170–2
    surgical resection, 169–70
    technique, 170
    VATS for, 171–2
pulmonary pleuroblastoma (PPB),
        64–5

radial probe EBUS, 11
radiation therapy
    tracheal masses, 52
    tracheal stenosis, 52
radiofrequency ablation (RFA), 41–2
radionuclide bone scans, 123–4
Ravitch technique, 201, 203
RB. *See* rigid bronchoscope
recurrent metastases, 168–73
reflux esophagitis, 242
renal cell carcinoma, 174
RESET trial, 81
residual volume (RV), 1–2, 69–70
resuscitative thoracotomy, 265
reverse Trendelenburg, 222
RFA. *See* radiofrequency ablation
rhabdomyosarcoma, 61

rib fractures, 258–9
right paratracheal nodal stations, 17
rigid bronchoscope (RB), 39
robotic surgical systems
    advantages, 159–60
    anterior mediastinal surgery, 161
    development of, 158
    disadvantages, 159–60
    esophagectomy, 163
    history of, 158
    lobectomies, 161
    for lung cancer, 160–1
    for myasthenia gravis, 161–2
    robotic Heller myotomy, 163
    thymomas, 162–3
RV. *See* residual volume

Salamanca group, 182
salivary gland carcinoma, 131–2
salivary gland tumors, 136–7
sarcomatoid carcinoma
    histological classification of, 131–2
    lung, 131–3
scalene biopsy, 124
scapular fractures, 261
scoliosis, 200
SCTS, 1–9
secondary spontaneous pneumothorax (SSP), 188
    causes of, 189
SEER. *See* Surveillance, Epidemiology, and End Results
segment counting, 6–7
self-activating coils for LVR, 80–1
self-adjustable bracing, 205
SGRQ. *See* St George's Respiratory Questionnaire
short gastric vessels, 223
short rib thoracic dysplasia (STRD), 206–7
shuttle walk test, 8
signet ring adenocarcinoma, 130
six-minute walk test, 8
small cell carcinoma
    histological classification of, 131–2, 136
    lung, 136
smoking history, 1
soft tissue sarcoma, 173
solid lung malformations, 61–3
solitary pulmonary nodule (SPN)
    definition, 115
    differential diagnosis, 115
    frequency of, 115
    further management of, 116
    high-risk nodules, 118
    initial evaluation, 115–16
    intermediate-risk, 117–18

low-risk nodules, 117
    risk stratification, 116
Southwest Oncology Group (SWOG), 146
SP. *See* spontaneous pneumothorax
spinal cord ischaemia, 110
spirometry
    in lung function assessment, 2
    morbidity and, 2–4
    rationale for, 2
SPN. *See* solitary pulmonary nodule
spondylocostal dysostosis, 207
spondylothoracic dysplasia, 207
spontaneous pneumothorax (SP), 188
    diagnostic approaches, 189–90
    primary, 188
        epidemiology, 188–9
    secondary, 188
        causes of, 189
squamous cell carcinoma
    histological classification of, 131–2
    lung cancer, 129–30
    risk-adjusted survival, 237
    trachea, 51
squamous dysplasia, 128–9
squamous papilloma, 51
SSP. *See* secondary spontaneous pneumothorax
St George's Respiratory Questionnaire (SGRQ), 71–2
stair climbing, 8
Stanford Research Institute, 158–9
Staphylococcus aureus, 87, 97
stay sutures, 229
stenosis, 50. *See also* tracheal stenosis
stents
    Dumon, 45
    Gianturco, 45
    indications for, 45
    instrumentation, 45
    methods, 45
    Montgomery type, 45
    therapeutic bronchoscopy, 45–6
    types of, 45–6
sternal cleft, 205–6
sternal defects, 205–6
sternal fractures, 259–60
sternal retractor, 29
sternoclavicular dislocation, 255
sternoclavicular joint, 261
sternocleidomastoid muscle, 30
sternum, 29
stoma site obstruction, 49
STRD. *See* short rib thoracic dysplasia
Streptococcus milleri, 87
Streptococcus pneumonia, 87, 97
subglottic stenosis, 53
superior vena cava, 17
    patch reconstruction of, 154

superior vena cava (SVC) syndrome
    anatomy, 151–2
    clinical presentation, 152
    definition, 150
    diagnosis, 152
    etiology, 150–1
    historical notes, 150
    median sternotomy for, 153
    pathophysiology, 152
    treatment, 153–5
supine position, open approach in
    anterior thoracotomies, 30–1
    bilateral thoracosternotomy, 30
    median sternotomy, 28–30
supraclavicular node biopsy, 124
Surveillance, Epidemiology, and End Results (SEER), 144
SVC syndrome. *See* superior vena cava syndrome
SWOG. *See* Southwest Oncology Group
systemic air embolism, 263–4

T2N0M0, 236
TBNA. *See* transbronchial needle aspiration
TEMLA. *See* transcervical extended mediastinal lymphadenectomy
therapeutic bronchoscopy, 39
    cancer-specific methods, 43
        brachytherapy, 43–4
        photodynamic therapy, 44–5
    classification of, 40
    FFB in, 39–40
    mechanical methods, 40–1
        bronchial lavage, 40
        bronchoscopic clearing of airway, 40
        foreign-body retrieval, 40–1
    methods, 40
    RB in, 39
    stents, 45–6
    thermal methods, 41–3
        argon plasma coagulation, 41–2
        bronchoscopic laser, 41–2
        cryotherapy, 41
        electrocautery, 41
        electrodiathermy, 41
        radiofrequency ablation, 41–2
thoracic diverticuli, 228
thoracic duct, 262–6
thoracic ectopia cordis, 206
thoracic great vessels, 263
thoracic sympathectomy, 270–2
thoracic trauma. *See* chest trauma
thoracoabdominal ectopia cordis, 206
thoracolumbar sympathetic nerve, 268

thoracoplasty
  for aspergillosis, 100–1
  for empyema, 90–1
thoracoscopy, 245
thoracotomy, 2. *See also specific types*
thymectomy, 162
  median sternotomy following, 30–3
thymomas, 162–3
tidal volume (TV), 1–2
tissue plasminogen activator (t-PA), 89
titanium implants, 201
TLC. *See* total lung capacity
TNF-α. *See* tumor necrosis alpha
TNM staging, 121
  groups, 122
  lung cancer, 17, 121–2
  multi-disciplinary team, 122–3
  seventh edition, 122
total lung capacity (TLC), 1–2, 69–70
t-PA. *See* tissue plasminogen activator
trachea
  compression, 255
  intramural lesions, 48–56
    post-intubation stenosis, 50–6
  obstructive lesions of, 48
tracheal masses
  endoscopy, 52
  operative treatment of, 52–3
  radiation therapy, 52
tracheal resection, 52
tracheal stenosis
  endoscopic treatment, 52
  idiopathic, 50
  infection due to, 50
  operative treatment of, 52–3
  post-therapeutic, 50
  radiation therapy, 52
tracheoesophageal fistula, 53
  anastomotic complication, 54
  closure, 55
  esophageal origin, 53–4
  etiologies of, 53
  extrinsic, 54
  iatrogenic, 53–4
  infectious, 53
  malignant, 53–5
  operative treatment of, 54–5
  post-intubation, 54–6
  resection, 55

  stent-related, 54
  tracheal origin, 53–4
  traumatic, 54, 56
tracheomalacia, 48
transabdominal laparoscopic Nissen
    fundoplication operation,
    222–3
  complications, 223
  results, 223
transbronchial needle aspiration
    (TBNA), 11–12
transcervical extended mediastinal
    lymphadenectomy (TEMLA),
    14, 18
transfer factor, 4
  ppo, 7
trans-thoracic needle biopsy, 124
traumatic asphyxia, 260
traumatic esophageal perforation, 242
traumatic tracheal stenosis, 50
tube thoracostomy
  active drainage in, 180–1
  double, 185
  electronic drainage systems, 181–2
  intrapleural pressure, 181–5
  non-suction, 180
  passive drainage in, 180
  for prolonged air leak, 179–80
  randomized trials, 180, 185
  single, 185
  standardization of terminology,
    180–1
  suction, 180
tuberculosis, 99
tumor necrosis alpha (TNF-α), 87
TV. *See* tidal volume

UDP. *See* unilateral diaphragmatic
    paralysis
UFT. *See* uracil/tegafur
Ultracision, 19
ultrasound (US). *See also*
    endobronchial ultrasound;
    endoscopic ultrasound
  diaphragm, 210
  for empyema, 88
unilateral diaphragmatic paralysis
    (UDP), 209
  clinical presentation, 210

uniportal approach, VATS, 32
  advantages, 33
  lobectomy, 33
  lung volume reduction surgery, 32
  pitfalls, 33
uracil/tegafur (UFT), 142
US. *See* ultrasound

vagal nerves, 222
VAMLA. *See* video-assisted
    mediastinal lymphadenectomy
vasculitis, 111
VATS. *See* video-assisted thoracoscopic
    surgery
VENT. *See* Endobronchial Valve for
    Emphysema Palliation Trial
vertebral venous system, 152
video-assisted mediastinal
    lymphadenectomy (VAMLA),
    18
  pericardial biopsy and window,
    19–22
video-assisted thoracoscopic surgery
    (VATS), 31–3
  anterior approach, 31–2
    advantages, 32
  for aspergillosis, 101
  camera position, 31
  debridement, 90
  decortication, 90
  diagnostic procedures with, 31
  history of, 158
  lobectomy, 160–1
  for lung cancer staging, 19–22
  LVRS, 76
  of Morgagni-Larrey hernias, 216–17
  posterior approach, 31
    advantages, 31
    pitfalls, 31
  for pulmonary metastasectomy,
    171–2
  uniportal approach, 32
    advantages, 33
    lobectomy, 32
    LVRS, 32
    pitfalls, 33

wedge resection, 22
whole lung lavage. *See* bronchial lavage

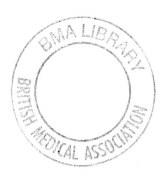